Equine Nutrition

Editors

PATRICIA HARRIS
MEGAN SHEPHERD

VETERINARY CLINICS OF NORTH AMERICA: EQUINE PRACTICE

www.vetequine.theclinics.com

Consulting Editor
THOMAS J. DIVERS

April 2021 • Volume 37 • Number 1

ELSEVIER

1600 John F. Kennedy Boulevard • Suite 1800 • Philadelphia, Pennsylvania, 19103-2899

http://www.vetequine.theclinics.com

VETERINARY CLINICS OF NORTH AMERICA: EQUINE PRACTICE Volume 37, Number 1
April 2021 ISSN 0749-0739, ISBN-13: 978-0-323-76171-0

Editor: Katerina Heidhausen
Developmental Editor: Ann Gielou Posedio

Veterinary Clinics of North America: Equine Practice (ISSN 0749-0739) is published in April, August, and December by Elsevier Inc., 360 Park Avenue South, New York, NY 10010-1710. Business and Editorial Offices: 1600 John F. Kennedy Blvd., Suite 1800, Philadelphia, PA 19103-2899. Subscription prices are $293.00 per year (domestic individuals), $766.00 per year (domestic institutions), $100.00 per year (domestic students/residents), $334.00 per year (Canadian individuals), $820.00 per year (Canadian institutions), $365.00 per year (international individuals), $820.00 per year (international institutions), $100.00 per year (Canadian students/residents), and $180.00 per year (international students/residents). To receive student/resident rate, orders must be accompanied by name of affiliated institution, date of term, and the signature of program/residency coordinator on institution letterhead. Orders will be billed at individual rate until proof of status is received. Foreign air speed delivery is included in all *Clinics* subscription prices. All prices are subject to change without notice. **POSTMASTER:** Send address changes to *Veterinary Clinics of North America: Equine Practice*, 3251 Riverport Lane, Maryland Heights, MO 63043. Customer Service (orders, claims, online, change of address): Elsevier Health Sciences Division, Subscription **Customer Service, 3251 Riverport Lane, Maryland Heights, MO 63043. Tel: 1-800-654-2452 (U.S. and Canada); 314-447-8871 (outside U.S. and Canada). Fax: 314-447-8029. E-mail: journalscustomerservice-usa@elsevier.com (for print support);** E-mail: **journalsonlinesupport-usa@elsevier.com (for online support).**

Reprints. For copies of 100 or more of articles in this publication, please contact the Commercial Reprints Department, Elsevier Inc., 360 Park Avenue South, New York, NY 10010-1710. Tel.: 212-633-3874; Fax: 212-633-3820; E-mail: reprints@elsevier.com.

Veterinary Clinics of North America: Equine Practice is covered in *MEDLINE/PubMed (Index Medicus), Excerpta Medica, Current Contents/Agriculture, Biology and Environmental Sciences,* and *ISI.*

Contributors

CONSULTING EDITOR

THOMAS J. DIVERS, DVM
Diplomate, American College of Veterinary Internal Medicine; Diplomate, American College of Veterinary Emergency and Critical Care; Steffen Professor of Veterinary Medicine, Department of Clinical Sciences, Section of Large Animal Medicine, College of Veterinary Medicine, Cornell University, Ithaca, New York, USA

EDITORS

PATRICIA HARRIS, MA, PhD, VetMB, MRCVS
Diplomate, European College of Veterinary and Comparative Nutrition; RCVS specialist Veterinary Clinical Nutrition (equine); Head of Equine Studies Group, WALTHAM Petcare Science Institute, WALTHAM-on-the-Wolds, Melton Mowbray, United Kingdom

MEGAN SHEPHERD, DVM, PhD
Diplomate, American College of Veterinary Nutrition; Clinical Assistant Professor, Nutrition, Department of Large Animal Clinical Sciences, Virginia-Maryland College of Veterinary Medicine, Blacksburg, Virginia, USA

AUTHORS

RUTH BISHOP, BSc (Hons)
Diploma in Equine Science; Equine Nutritionist, Premier Nutrition Ltd, Rugeley, United Kingdom

PASCALE CHAVATTE-PALMER, DVM, PhD, HDR
Université Paris-Saclay, UVSQ, INRAE, BREED, Jouy-en-Josas, France; Ecole Nationale Vétérinaire d'Alfort, BREED, Maisons-Alfort, France

MARCIO COSTA, DVM, PhD
Assistant Professor, Department of Veterinary Biomedical Sciences, University of Montreal, Saint-Hyacinthe, Canada

DAVID A. DZANIS, DVM, PhD
Diplomate, American College of Veterinary Nutrition; Chief Executive Officer, Regulatory Discretion, Inc, Santa Clarita, California, USA

CARRIE J. FINNO, DVM, PhD
Diplomate, American College of Veterinary Internal Medicine; Associate Professor, Population Health and Reproduction, University of California, Davis School of Veterinary Medicine, Davis, California, USA

CAROLYN HAMMER, DVM, PhD
Department of Animal Sciences, North Dakota State University, Fargo, North Dakota, USA

PATRICIA HARRIS, MA, PhD, VetMB, MRCVS
Diplomate, European College of Veterinary and Comparative Nutrition; RCVS specialist Veterinary Clinical Nutrition (equine); Head of Equine Studies Group, WALTHAM Petcare Science Institute, WALTHAM-on-the-Wolds, Melton Mowbray, United Kingdom

MYRIAM HESTA, DVM, PhD
Diplomate, European College of Veterinary and Comparative Nutrition; Associate Professor, Nutrition, ECAN Equine and Companion Animal Nutrition, Department of Veterinary Medical Imaging and Small Animal Orthopaedics, Faculty of Veterinary Medicine, Ghent University, Merelbeke, Belgium

NICOLA JARVIS, BVetMed, Cert AVP (Equine Medicine), CertAVP (Equine Surgery Soft Tissue), MRCVS
Senior Veterinary Surgeon, Redwings Horse Sanctuary, Hapton, Norfolk, United Kingdom

KRISHONA L. MARTINSON, PhD
Professor and Equine Extension Specialist, Department of Animal Science, University of Minnesota, St Paul, Minnesota, USA

ERICA C. McKENZIE, BSc, BVMS, PhD
Professor, Department of Clinical Sciences, Carlson College of Veterinary Medicine, Oregon State University, Corvallis, Oregon, USA

HAROLD C. MCKENZIE III, DVM, MS, MSc (VetEd)
Diplomate, American College of Veterinary Internal Medicine (Large Animal Internal Medicine); Professor, Large Animal Medicine, Department of Large Animal Clinical Sciences, Virginia Maryland College of Veterinary Medicine, Virginia Tech, Blacksburg, Virginia, USA

BRIAN D. NIELSEN, PhD, PAS
Diplomate, American College of Animal Nutrition; Professor, Equine Exercise Physiology, Department of Animal Science, Michigan State University, East Lansing, Michigan, USA

NERIDA RICHARDS, PhD, RAnNutr
Equilize Horse Nutrition Pty Ltd, Tamworth, New South Wales, Australia

MORGANE ROBLES, PhD
Institut National de la Recherche Scientifique (INRS), Centre Armand Frappier Santé-Biotechnologies, Laval, Quebec, Canada; Université Paris-Saclay, UVSQ, INRAE, BREED, Jouy-en-Josas, France; Ecole Nationale Vétérinaire d'Alfort, BREED, Maisons-Alfort, France

MEGAN SHEPHERD, DVM, PhD
Diplomate, American College of Veterinary Nutrition; Clinical Assistant Professor, Nutrition, Department of Large Animal Clinical Sciences, Virginia-Maryland College of Veterinary Medicine, Blacksburg, Virginia, USA

BURT STANIAR, PhD
Penn State University, University Park, Pennsylvania, USA

MERI STRATTON-PHELPS, DVM
Diplomate, American College of Veterinary Internal Medicine (Large Animal Internal Medicine); Diplomate, American College of Veterinary Nutrition; President, All Creatures Veterinary Nutrition Consulting

KRISTINE L. URSCHEL, BSc, PhD
Associate Professor, Department of Animal and Food Sciences, University of Kentucky, Lexington, Kentucky, USA

INGRID VERVUERT, DVM
Professor, Institute of Animal Nutrition, Nutrition Diseases and Dietetics, Faculty of Veterinary Medicine, Leipzig University, Leipzig, Germany

Contents

> Nutrition and management have enabling and supporting roles to play in the health, welfare, and performance of equines. Poor or inappropriate nutrition may therefore impose limits on an animal's ability to perform and adversely affect health and welfare. Understanding the gastrointestinal tract from a nutrition perspective can help to reduce the risk of certain clinical problems. This article outlines key factors with respect to the equine digestive tract and discusses relevant aspects of ration formation. Forage is highlighted, because inappropriate forage provision is one of the key limitations in many horse diets.

> Inappropriate nutrition is a priority welfare challenge. Nutritional mistakes are common and can lead to adverse events, such as poor growth and performance, colic, laminitis, and obesity. A detailed nutritional assessment involving evaluating the equine patient, current diet/ration, and management is essential in creating an effective nutritional plan. Goal(s) should be established and used to inform the plan. Management or resource barriers should be considered. Effective communication and a team-based approach versus an authoritarian one are likely to enhance the success of the nutritional plan. Developing a plan should be an interactive process, adjusting as needed after intentional monitoring.

> Forage is the most important feed component of a horse's diet and often determines overall long-term health. With differences between available forage types, suitable forages must be carefully selected based on a horse's nutrient and physiologic requirements. The selection of inappropriate forage can have dire consequences. Forages can be broadly divided into cool and warm season grasses and legumes. Each type of forage has its own nutritional and non-nutritional aspects that must be considered when selecting forages. And almost all forages are low in some critical minerals and vitamins, requiring a majority of horses receive targeted supplementation for optimum health.

polysaccharide storage myopathy and recurrent exertional rhabdomyolysis, can be managed in part by restricting dietary nonstructural carbohydrate intake.

VETERINARY CLINICS OF NORTH AMERICA: EQUINE PRACTICE

RELATED SERIES

Veterinary Clinics of North America: Food Animal Practice
https://www.vetfood.theclinics.com/

Preface

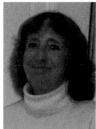

Patricia Harris, MA,PhD, VetMB, MRCVS,   Megan Shepherd, DVM, PhD, DipACVN
DipECVCN

Editors

In this digital age, looking for the definition of Nutrition on the Internet comes up with the following: "Nutrition is the science that interprets the nutrients and other substances in food in relation to maintenance, growth, reproduction, health and disease of an organism. It includes food intake, absorption, assimilation, biosynthesis, catabolism and excretion." Wikipedia February 2020 or the Cambridge Dictionary states: "the substances that you take into your body as food and the way that they influence your health" and "the process of taking in and using food, or the scientific study of this." Both of these perfectly adequate definitions of nutrition fail to consider the art of nutrition, which is essential when dealing with an animal, such as the horse, that cannot be reasoned with or shown the scientific evidence and may have an independent approach to the feed provided! This issue on equine nutrition therefore tries to provide information with respect to both the Science and the Art of Nutrition. Each article has multiple authors, often from different regions of the world, united in their interest, knowledge, and passion for the topic being discussed. This issue is not meant to serve as an all-inclusive textbook; rather, the aim is to provide a solid framework to give readers the foundation from which to work with the equines in their care and/or to act as an aide-memoire on those areas to consider when dealing with specific cases.

This book starts with an overview by Harris and Shepherd of the key concepts to consider when feeding equines and a review on conducting a nutrition assessment by Hesta and Shepherd. In the next article by Richards and colleagues a review of the nutrient content of different forages is provided. The next 5 articles by Hesta and Costa, Jarvis and McKenzie, Shepherd and colleagues, Urschel & McKenzie focus on the nutritional management of gastrointestinal issues, weight management, muscle health and the broodmare. The next chapter by Vervuert and Stratton-Phelps gives some nutritional insights into certain nutraceuticals and in the final chapter Bishop and Dzanis provide important guidance on feed and supplement regulation in both the U.S. and Europe.

Finally, as passionate believers in the power of nutrition to positively or negatively influence the health, welfare, behavior, and performance of the horse, we as the editors

Vet Clin Equine 37 (2021) xi–xii
https://doi.org/10.1016/j.cveq.2021.01.003
0749-0739/21/© 2021 Published by Elsevier Inc.

hope that this issue will inspire current and future veterinarians to embrace the 'area' of nutrition and harness its power when advising on and managing equines.

We would like to express our appreciation to all the authors for collaborating to create quality content in each article.

Patricia Harris, MA, PhD, VetMB, MRCVS, DipECVCN
Equine Studies Group
Waltham Petcare Science Institute
Waltham-on-the-Wolds
Melton Mowbray, UK

Megan Shepherd, DVM, PhD, DipACVN
Department of Large Animal
Clinical Sciences
Virginia-Maryland College of
Veterinary Medicinev
Blacksburg, VA, USA

E-mail addresses:
Pat.harris@effem.com (P. Harris)
meshephe@vt.edu (M. Shepherd)

What Would Be Good for All Veterinarians to Know About Equine Nutrition

Patricia Harris, MA, PhD, VetMB, MRCVS, DipECVCN[a],*,
Megan Shepherd, DVM, PhD, DACVN[b]

KEYWORDS

- Microbial fermentation • Forage • Digestion • Ration formulation

KEY POINTS

- Horses (taken to mean all equines) are fundamentally non-ruminant herbivores. This means that they are suited to eating high-fiber diets because of continual microbial fermentation, mainly within the caecum and colon.
- Good hygienic quality, long-stem forage should ideally be the foundation of most equine diets. Horses at a healthy weight (ie, not overweight or underweight) should ideally be fed forage ad libitum (to minimize time between meals) and at least 1.5% of their bodyweight (BW) in dry matter (DM) per day.
- If additional energy provision is required, consider alternative forages, more digestible fiber sources, and/or gradually introduced vegetable oil/fat. If cereals/grains or cereal/grain-based feeds, are fed, the following precautions should be implemented because of the associated risk with gastric ulceration and the limited capacity to digest starch in the small intestine:
  - Restrict the starch and sugar content per meal (<1 g/kg BW/meal).
  - Feed small, and if needed more frequent meals (ie, <2 kg/500 kg horse/meal).
  - Ensure grains (other than oats) have been appropriately processed/cooked.

INTRODUCTION

Veterinarians/veterinary surgeons are often considered by horse owners, and sometimes themselves, to be a (or even the) major source of good quality, unbiased, knowledge with respect to equine nutrition.[1–3] This is perhaps not surprising given that nutrition (taken here to include the diet and nutritional management) influences equine

[a] Head of Equine Studies Group, WALTHAM Petcare Science Institute, Waltham-on-the-Wolds, Melton Mowbray, Leics LE14 4RT, UK; [b] Department of Large Animal Clinical Sciences, Virginia-Maryland College of Veterinary Medicine, Phase II Duck Pond Drive, Virginia Tech Mail Code 0442, Blacksburg, VA 24061, USA
* Corresponding author.
E-mail address: Pat.harris@effem.com

Vet Clin Equine 37 (2021) 1–20
https://doi.org/10.1016/j.cveq.2020.11.001
0749-0739/21/© 2020 Elsevier Inc. All rights reserved.

health, behavior, performance, and welfare. However, various surveys have suggested, in the United Kingdom and the United States, that veterinarians often have low confidence when talking about nutrition, especially complex nutrition situations.[2–5] Low confidence might be caused by lack of recent continuing professional development. Roberts and Murray[4] found that most responding veterinarians had not recently attended any equine nutrition continuing professional development. Furthermore, Nichols[2] reported that 75% of veterinarians had not received any nutrition continuing professional development in the past year, mainly because they had chosen to spend their time on other topics (41%) but also because no suitable courses had been offered at the symposium/conference they had attended (~21%). In addition, many equine veterinarians do not seem to be satisfied with the level of equine nutrition education they received at university/veterinary school.[2] A survey of 14 veterinary schools in Europe and the Middle East[6] suggested that whereas the university deans and faculty members all recognized that nutrition (all species) was important (averaged four out of five in importance), 41% of those surveyed said they were not satisfied with the nutritional skills and performance of their graduates. This article addresses the previously mentioned issue and provides a base for all those veterinarians working with horses, and serves as a background resource to the other more specific articles in this issue.

Nutrition in its broadest sense promotes and supports health, welfare, performance, and behavior. Conversely, when inappropriately addressed, nutrition has the potential to cause adverse welfare, reduce performance, cause unwanted behaviors, and directly or indirectly increase the risk of certain clinical conditions. These aspects are discussed in more detail in the subsequent articles, whereas this article concentrates on some of the basic underlying principles, such as considering the gastrointestinal tract (GIT)/digestive tract from a nutritional perspective and the importance of forage. Details of nutrient requirements are not covered in this article and readers are advised to look at reference books[7–9] for more details.

BASIC OVERVIEW OF THE EQUINE GASTROINTESTINAL TRACT

Horses are herd-living, non-ruminant, hindgut fermenting, primarily grazing herbivores that have evolved with a specialized GIT capable of using a wide range of plant species. These feed materials are hydrolyzed and/or fermented by the microbiota found throughout the GIT, to yield energy and nutrients. Naturally the horse is a trickle feeder that forages for up to 15 hours per 24-hour period and rarely spends more than a 3-hour period without foraging.[10] The following provides a brief overview of the GIT and its physiology; further information is found in the references provided.[8]

Mouth

- Mobile equine lips enable selective grazing, with the potential to avoid eating small particles in feed, such as vitamin and mineral pellets.
- Saliva (>99% water): up to 35 to 40 L/d in an adult 500- to 600-kg horse; pH of 8.6 to 9.1
  - Only produced during chewing.
  - Contains virtually no digestive enzymes (eg, amylase 0.44 μ/mL vs 98 μ/mL in pigs[11]).
  - Primarily acts as a lubricant.
  - Contains bicarbonate, a key gastric buffer.
- Dry matter (DM) content of any swallowed bolus depends mainly on
  - The physical nature and composition of the feed.

- o The time taken for mastication[12,13] which is
  - ■ Influenced by the density and how easily the feed is broken down.[14,15]
  - ■ The size of the head/jaws.[16]
- o Forage (in particular long-stem) takes longer to chew than cereal-based or pelleted feed, resulting in more saliva being produced and subsequently a lower DM of the swallowed bolus (~11%–15% vs ~35% DM).[12]
- o The addition of appropriate amounts (~15%–20% of the meal) of chopped/short fiber that is chaff (eg, chopped soft alfalfa, dried grass, and/or straw) to cereal or complementary feeds may be beneficial in slowing down the rate of eating[15–17] and stimulate saliva production.
- The chewing cycle is complex[14] and
  - o Reduces particle sizes, thereby supporting optimal digestion.
  - o Releases soluble nutrient components that can then be digested prececally.[18]
  - o Long-stem forage promotes a fuller range of dental excursions to promote more even dental wear; whereas restricted movement with easily commutable feeds, such as cereals/pellets, increases the risk of abnormal dentition including hooks.[14]

Stomach

- Capacity of 8 to 15 L: adult 500-kg horse.
- Naturally, because of the trickle feeding pattern of ingestion, the stomach is never empty.
- Feed is retained for approximately 85 to 300 minutes postprandially depending on type and size of meal.[18]
- Hydrochloric acid is secreted at a variable rate even when the stomach is empty,[19] which increases the risk of gastric ulceration, especially if not provided with forage regularly.[20]
  - o Controversy over potential risks of therapeutically reducing gastric acid output over the long-term with respect to possibly
    - ■ Reducing barrier function against bacterial colonization.[21]
    - ■ Influencing calcium balance (and fracture risk).[22,23]
- Size and composition of a meal influences the
  - o pH gradient within the stomach[18] through the
    - ■ Amount of saliva produced and gastric acid secreted.
    - ■ Nature and stratification of the feed material within the stomach.
  - o Rate of gastric emptying varies, but in general[24–26]
    - ■ Liquids empty more rapidly than solids.
    - ■ Water can bypass the stomach contents (ie, no reason not to provide water constantly because post-prandial drinking does not flush out the stomach contents).
    - ■ Larger meals have a greater rate of emptying than smaller meals, one reason for reducing the size of meals.
    - ■ Starch and oil slows gastric emptying, regardless of meal size.
- Contains a diverse bacterial community even when fasted,[27,28] mainly influenced by, and influencing, the following:
  - o Starch digestion: the high proportion of amylolytic bacteria can rapidly digest starch and produce primarily lactic acid then acetate as main end-products.[18,28]
  - o The DM content of the ingesta and gastric lumen pH influence the intensity and effectiveness of intragastric fermentation.
- Secretes pepsin and lipase,[18] which are potentially important to protein and fatty acid digestion. However, the exact role in equine digestion is unknown.

- Fructans in grass are potentially hydrolyzed to some extent by gastric acid[29] or microbial fermented in the stomach.

Small Intestine

- Comparatively short
  - Ingesta rate of passage is therefore
    - Relative quick.
    - Depends on the amount of food entering.
    - When large meals are fed, because of shortened transit time, even nutrients that otherwise may have been digested in the small intestine (SI) reach the hindgut where they may be rapidly fermented.[18]
- No gallbladder, therefore
  - Bile is continually produced.
  - Bile salt excretion, important for fat digestion, depends on an intact enterohepatic circulation.
- Pancreatic secretion
  - Up to 25 L/d in an average-sized horse.[30]
  - ~ pH 8 caused by high bicarbonate content.
  - Apparently continuous.
- Basic digestive processes are similar to those of other monogastric animals
  - Dietary nonstructural carbohydrates (NSC) and proteins are hydrolyzed by the pancreatic and intestinal brush border enzymes.[18,31–34]
  - Concentrations of amylase and trypsinogen within the pancreatic juice are low, compared with other species.[35]
- Starch digestion is limited, and digestion depends in particular on[12,13,36–39]
  - The feedstuff, including availability to the digestive enzymes (eg, the extent to which any outer husk or hull has been broken down).
  - The ratio of amylose to amylopectin within the starch granule (more amylopectin typically more glucose availability) and the nature of the starch granule (especially important for corn).
  - The effect of any processing
    - Thermal treatment of certain grains (eg, corn and barley) required to swell and gelatinize the starch, to improve SI starch digestibility.
- Transport mechanisms for glucose and fructose is believed to be similar to those in other species. There is limited capacity to transport glucose compared with an omnivorous mammal, such as the pig,[40,41] which adds to the reduced ability to digest starch and sugar in the SI.
- Less is known about protein and fat assimilation,[42] although equine pancreatic tissue contains high concentrations of lipase,[43] which means the horse can digest large intakes of oil when adapted.
- Complex microbiota is reviewed in Myriam Hesta and Marcio Costa's article, "How Can Nutrition Help with Gastrointestinal Tract-Based Issues," elsewhere in this issue.
  - Varies by region, especially foregut (stomach and SI) versus hindgut (cecum, colon), thus feces has limitations in representing the full GIT.[44–46] Furthermore, the microbiota of the gastrointestinal (GI) lumen versus mucosa vary.[45]
  - Likely plays a role in SI digestion (and in the health of the GIT and the whole animal including its immune system).[18]
    - Insoluble fibers are not hydrolyzed in the SI (the β-glycosidic bond is not degraded by mammalian SI enzymes[10,47]), but microbial fermentation does occur.[48,49]

Hind Gut

- No mucosal enzymes.
- No significant active transport mechanisms for hexose sugars.
- Digestion and absorption of residual carbohydrates relies on microbial fermentation undertaken by a complex microbiome (mainly bacteria but also fungi and to a lesser extent protozoa[50–52]) and absorption of
  - End-products of fermentation in particular from the intense fibrolytic activity: short-chain or volatile fatty acids (VFA) predominantly acetate, then propionate, and then butyrate.[48]
    - Butyrate is key in supporting intestinal cell energy supply and health.
    - Acetate and propionate are primary energy precursors for the horse[53] and at least 50% of absorbed energy in forage-fed horses is derived from VFAs from microbial fermentation.[53,54]
    - Acetate is aerobically oxidized to ATP/energy[55] or stored as triglyceride in adipose and skeletal tissue.[56]
    - Propionate is predominantly converted into glucose by the liver and supports blood glucose.[57]
  - Water passively follows VFA[58,59] and sodium absorption.
  - Microbial fermentation influences the pH of the gut lumen with slowly fermented carbohydrates, such as cellulose, the most abundant carbohydrate in most forages, promoting a near neutral pH.[48]
- Fermentation processes[29,48,54,60–65] depend on
  - The amount and the temporal influx of fermentable material arriving from the SI.
    - Increasing proportions of NSC (starch and water-soluble sugars) favour the production of lactate and propionate at the expense of acetate.
  - Yielding less net energy than if absorbed as glucose.
  - Resulting in decreased cecal and/or colonic pH, with an increased risk of clinical conditions including colic, diarrhea, and laminitis.
- Water balance and plasma volume through the transmucosal movement of water[48,60,61] depends on
  - The ileocecal flow of DM and its composition.
  - The rate of production and absorption of VFAs
    - Fiber in the hindgut can act as fluid reservoir (which is particularly relevant for horses undergoing endurance-type exercise).
- Contribution of hindgut protein to the amino acid pool is controversial.[48,66]
  - Prececal protein availability is currently considered to be key.
- Dietary composition, obesity, and age can influence the composition of the GI microbiota significantly[48,51,67–69] but, at the moment, consistent specific microbiome signatures for age and obesity and other specific clinical conditions have not been found, perhaps because of different organisms being able to support the same function. However, in general forage-based diets result in more diverse populations of microbes than starch-based diets.
  - The small core microbiome in the horse is thought to increase the risk of digestive upsets with dietary change.[51]
  - The influence of the individual animal on the microbiome response to a dietary challenge seems to be important.[69]
- Most macrominerals and trace elements given to horses are absorbed in the SI, as are most of the dietary vitamins.[7,70,71] Phosphorus, however, is absorbed mainly in the hind gut and high phosphorus intakes, especially in the form of

plant phytates, may interfere with calcium absorption in the SI. Most of the water-soluble B vitamins are synthesized in the large intestine of a healthy horse, provided with an adequate forage diet, through the action of resident microbiota.[71]

Water

Horses should have clean drinking water available at all times.[72] Water intake and requirements are influenced by total DM consumed,[7] DM content of feed (higher with hay vs pasture),[73] protein intake,[74] sweat production,[75] water salinity,[76] water temperature,[7,77] ambient temperature, and interhorse variability. In general[7,72]

- Require ∼3 to 5 L water/kg feed for horses on an all-hay diet versus ∼2 to 4 L/kg on a hay-grain diet.
- With a sweat loss of 5 L and 10-kg DM intake (7.5 kg forage and 2.5 kg complementary feed) a 500-kg horse at an ambient temperature of 20°C needs ∼25 to 45 L of water.
  - In warmer climates (>25°C–30°C daytime temperature), intakes may be increased by 15% to 30%.
  - Lack of water, even with short periods of turnout, may increase gastric ulceration[20] and colon impaction risk.[73]

Forage

The terms "forage" and "roughage" are typically used interchangeably to refer to the high-fiber feed component of the horses' diet. Forage includes grasses and legumes and may be fed fresh (ie, pasture) or preserved (eg, long-stem hay, chopped hay, haylage). Roughage typically refers to high-fiber by-product feeds (eg, straw, cereal hulls, beet pulp). "Foraging" is taken to refer to all feed intake activities, regardless of feed type or management practices. Ideally horses should be fed sufficient fresh or preserved forage to prevent prolonged periods (ie, >5 hours, especially during daylight hours) without the opportunity to forage.[10]

Forage Types

Types of forage include cool-season grasses (eg, Orchard Grass, Timothy), warm-season grasses (eg, Bermuda grass), cool-season legumes (eg, alfalfa, clover), and warm-season legumes (eg, kudzu). Cool-season grasses store energy (oversupply of sugars produced during photosynthesis) primarily in the form of fructan. Warm-season grasses store energy primarily in the form of starch; and unlike fructan, starch storage is self-limiting.[47] Therefore, cool-season grasses have the potential to be high in NSC, specifically water-soluble carbohydrate (WSC), particularly in cooler climates. See Myriam Hesta and Megan Shepherd's article, "How to Perform a Nutritional Assessment in a First Line/General Practice," in this issue regarding forage assessment, Nerida Richards and colleagues' article, "Nutritional and Non-Nutritional Aspects of Forage," in this issue for more information regarding potential risks and toxicities associated with different forages and Megan Shepherd and colleagues' article, "Nutritional Considerations When Dealing with an Obese Adult Equine," in this issue regarding use of forage types for managing the obese horse.

Good pasture management is key for preventing weed development and to support grazing[78] and forage production. Knowledge of common local toxic plants is helpful. Furthermore, veterinarians can consult with extension agents (United States) regarding ways to improve a farm's pastures.

Forage Nutrient Content

Forage nutrient content is influenced by maturity, leaf/stem ratio, plant species and morphology, soil quality, water and nutrient availability, sunlight, and harvesting and storage methods.[10] As a plant matures, the cell wall (structural fibers) increases and cell contents (eg, crude protein) decrease, resulting in a reduction of the leaf/stem ratio. Furthermore, energy density and total tract digestibility (and often palatability) tend to decrease with increasing maturity.[15] Legumes are typically higher in protein and calcium than grasses. The ability of a forage to meet a horse's protein and amino acid requirements, when fed to meet the energy need, varies by region. For example, grasses in the mid-Atlantic region of the United States generally meet protein needs. However, hays in the United Kingdom are unlikely to meet protein needs, often even for horses at maintenance, and certainly not the essential amino acid requirements for performance horses (reviewed in Kristine L. Urschel and Erica C. McKenzie's article, "Nutritional Influences on Skeletal Muscle and Muscular Disease," in this issue). Most forage does not provide all adequate essential vitamins and minerals, even for maintenance. An appropriate balancer is therefore needed. Furthermore, the balancer chosen should be dependent on whether legume or grass-based forages are provided. Forage-based deficiencies are reviewed in Nerida Richards and colleagues' article, "Nutritional and Non-Nutritional Aspects of Forage," in this issue.

Forage Preservation

When fresh forage (ie, pasture) is not available or appropriate, preserved forage is needed.[10] Forage may be preserved by drying (ie, hay) or primarily through exclusion of air (ie, haylage) or via microbial fermentation coupled with exclusion of air (ie, silage). Feeding preserved forage often changes the dynamics of feeding management typically from a more ad libitum regimen to meal-feeding, although efforts to reduce the time between forage meals or extend the time foraging is required. Digestibility and palatability tend to reflect primarily maturity at harvesting and the forage type and species.

Hay

Forage may be preserved through drying in the field or by combining field and barn drying to a final DM content, ideally greater than 85%. Bales with too high a moisture content have a higher risk of fungal spores/bacteria and mycotoxin development. Hay moisture may be positively influenced by unsuitable weather conditions at cutting time and especially during wilting, insufficient turning and drying before baling, and improper storage. Feed and forage of a poor hygienic quality increase the risk of respiratory disease and GIT disorders (reviewed in Myriam Hesta and Marcio Costa's article, "How Can Nutrition Help with Gastrointestinal Tract-Based Issues," in this issue). Overtly dusty and moldy hay should not be fed (identified by plumes of dust when hay is moved or presence of black mold spots/plaques on the hay and/or the smell of mold). However, there may be no obvious signs that hay is of poor hygienic quality. If there are any concerns, the hay may be tested for mold spores. Additionally, hay may be steamed, which may help under certain circumstances. Be vigilant for contamination by way of plants or foreign bodies. Proper storage (eg, storing hay in a dry environment) is essential for maximizing feed hygiene.

Silage

Silage is made by harvesting plant material with a high water content (>50% and more typically 63%–68% moisture), often chopping, then packing in an airtight environment (silos or bales sealed with stretch film). The WSCs in the forage are fermented by anaerobic lactic acid bacteria; when the pH is sufficiently low, undesirable microbial growth should be inhibited. Silage pH can therefore be used as an indicator of the quality of the ensiling. Silage is less commonly fed to horses than haylage, at least in United Kingdom and United States.

Haylage

Haylage is produced by semi-drying (harvested typically at 30%–45% moisture) then storing air-tight in an anaerobic environment by wrapped in a stretch film, usually polyethylene. Final moisture content, however, is variable (from 20%–50%) making it difficult to feed on a DM basis without analysis. Fermentation is restricted so haylage generally contains lower concentrations of fermentation products (eg, lactic acid) than silage and pH cannot be used as a quality indicator. Furthermore, the WSC content of haylage may not be significantly lower than the fresh forage it was made from, because of the restricted fermentation. Therefore, haylage cannot be assumed in general to be lower in WSC than pasture or hay.[10] It is essential that haylage bales are stored appropriately to minimize the risk of damage from mammals and birds. This may necessitate storage away from hedgerows, the use of protective netting over the bales, and even surrounding them with a low electric fence (eg, strands 1–3 feet from the ground).

- Once the airtight seal is breached, microorganisms and fungi can rapidly grow.
- Seal integrity (tightness) is crucial to reduce fungal growth and is better when more layers of stretch film are used (recommended at least eight), especially with higher DM haylage.[10,79]
- When visible fungi are seen on the surface the risk is that the whole bale is affected.[79–81]
- The WSC content of haylage may be reduced slightly or not at all from the fresh forage from which it was harvested.
- Recently, concerns have been raised that haylage may contain high levels of unknown/unrecognized metabolites, which may not be desirable.[81]
- It is not uncommon for owners to underfeed haylage (and therefore structural fiber) especially when feeding on an as-fed weight basis as for hay, and not accounting for the higher moisture. Underfeeding also typically occurs when feeders wish to feed haylage but they have concerns with potential weight gain or behavioral issues because of its typically higher (because often cut when less mature) feed (energetic) value and potential increased palatability compared with hay.[15]

Forage Hygiene

The hygienic[10,82,83] and nutritional quality of forage and the quantity fed and the suitability of its nutritional make-up are key areas to be considered during any nutritional evaluation (reviewed in Myriam Hesta and Megan Shepherd's article, "How to Perform a Nutritional Assessment in a First Line/General Practice"; Nerida Richards and colleagues' article, "Nutritional and Non-Nutritional Aspects of Forage," in this issue). This is particularly important where there is a generalized failure to perform or thrive and/or if digestive disturbances are present (eg, recurrent colic, gastric ulcers, abnormal droppings/manure). A guide to the types and acceptable levels of bacteria, molds, and yeasts in different types of forages have been determined.[83] Mycotoxins are chemically robust and thermally resistant, thus difficult to eliminate. Steaming hay may not destroy mycotoxins, although specific washing of grains may reduce the contamination.[84] Soaking hay increases the bacterial count, although the importance of this on subsequent health is currently unknown.[85,86]

Consider limiting the length of time of soaking, especially in hot weather, to between 1 and 3 hours (the soaking fluid should be treated as effluent and appropriately disposed of). It is also important to realize that hay can contain mold spores in absence of mycotoxins; conversely, haylage can contain mycotoxins in absence of mold spores.[81] More information is required with respects to the role mycotoxins, fermentation metabolites, and certain bacteria (present either pre- or post- soaking) play in horse health.

INTRODUCING NEW FEED, INCLUDING FORAGE

Poor feed choice/poor ration management and rapid changes in feed, including rapid change in forage, can lead to GI microbiota changes and a decrease in pH, which increases the risk of clinical complications, such as diarrhea, colic,[87–89] and laminitis. Small changes should be made gradually over 3 to 5 days. Furthermore a 2-week, and possibly more than 3-week, adaptation period may be required, especially if the nutrient composition (energy source, protein level, WSC) is unknown or known to differ considerably.[10] Moving from pasture to a stabled environment also influences gut motility potentially increasing the risk of GI disturbances.[73] Finally, contamination of feed and forage with noxious agents, poisonous plants, and substances against the rules of competition/racing is important to consider (reviewed in Ruth Bishop and David A. Dzanis' article, "Staying on the Right Side of the Regulatory Authorities"; Nerida Richards and colleagues' article, "Nutritional and Non-Nutritional Aspects of Forage," in this issue).

HOW MUCH CAN HORSES EAT?

Voluntary DM intake varies (1.5%–5.5% body weight [BW][7,10,15,90]) depending on the individual, feed type availability, season, pasture management (eg, if there are lawns and troughs then intakes depend on whether individuals graze the rough areas) and so forth. But some key practical factors to consider are

- Feed plus forage (fresh or preserved) intake of ponies can approach 5% of BW as DM when they have 24-hour access.[90,91]
- Ponies can consume ~1% of their BW as pasture DM within 3 hours.[92]
- Feed/forage intake by horses is typically lower at ~2% to 2.5% BW/d on a DM basis.
- Horses are selective grazers and NSC content may positively influence selection.[93]
- The contribution of pasture to the daily DM intake is roughly estimated by[9]
  - Subtracting the amount of supplemental feeds/forage provided from an estimated daily DM intake level (eg, 3%–4% of BW for ponies out at grass for >16–18 h/d; 2%–3% BW for horses).
  - Time at pasture
    - For horses, 0.4% BW as DM per 3 hour of turnout; up to a maximum of 1% BW when turned out during the day and stabled at night.
    - For ponies, the rates and maximum values may be double that for horses.
  - Depending on pasture type and yield/biomass, as a starting point aim to provide healthy animals with the following[9,94] in addition to any pasture:
    - 24 hours stable, 100% daily forage allowance.
    - 4 to 8 hours pasture, 50% to 75% daily forage allowance.
    - 8 to 12 hours pasture, 25% to 50% daily forage allowance.
    - 24 hours pasture, 0% to 25% daily forage allowance.

However, BW and Body Condition Score (BCS) needs to be monitored; forage access should be altered as needed to maintain target BCS.

- An adequate intake of forage/complementary feed is difficult to achieve for some equines in intensive work, especially when under certain additional stress (eg, overtraining). In this situation it may help to stop adding any chaff to the complementary feed and offer separately or offering small amounts of multiple forms of forage may be beneficial to voluntary intake.[95]
- In general, it is recommended not to feed cereals/grains or feeds that result in raised blood insulin levels within 2 to 3 hours of most types of competition or hard exercise. Feeding small amounts (1–2 kg) of forage, via methods to extend intake time (eg, use of double but not treble haynets, or small-holed haylage nets) if required, is recommended (especially to reduce the risk of gastric ulceration) within these 2 to 3 hours of competition.[96]

HOW MUCH FORAGE SHOULD BE FED?

Horses at a healthy weight (ie, not overweight) should ideally be fed forage ad libitum and at least 1.5% of their BW in DM per day.[9,10,96] For example, a 500-kg horse should be offered a minimum of 7.5-kg DM forage/per day, which equates to 8.5 kg of a 90% DM hay, or 11 kg of a 70% DM haylage. Even horses in high-intensity work should be fed at least 1.25% of BW (eg, 6.25 kg DM for a 500-kg horse) in DM as forage. This means in practice

- When limit-feeding forage (eg, overweight horse), consider ways to extend intake time (reviewed in Megan Shepherd and colleagues' article, "Nutritional Considerations When Dealing with an Obese Adult Equine," in this issue).
- Higher intakes may be fed or consumed by horses, as long as healthy/target BCS is maintained.
- If BCS rises above target, even when feeding the minimum recommended intake, forage/feeds with lower energy content should be fed rather than reducing the DM forage intake (reviewed in Megan Shepherd and colleagues' article, "Nutritional Considerations When Dealing with an Obese Adult Equine," in this issue).

MAKING UP A RATION

The ration should reflect the individual equine's nutrient needs (including enhancements/restrictions for managing disease), available feeds, and palatability. Ideally long-stem forage should be the foundation of any diet, because it supports psychological and physiologic health and well-being.[9,10] However, adjustments may be needed under certain clinical circumstances. For example, animals with severe chewing difficulties may need to be fed high-fiber/forage pellets soaked into a mash form (reviewed in Nicola Jarvis and Harold C. McKenzie's article, "Nutritional Considerations When Dealing with an Underweight Adult or Senior Horse"; Megan Shepherd and colleagues' article, "Nutritional Considerations When Dealing with an Obese Adult Equine," in this issue). Details of nutrient requirements and recommendations are found in textbooks[7–9] and are not described in detail here.

Some individual animals, depending on life stage, workload, or a clinical reason, require more energy than ad libitum forage can provide. This has resulted in the inclusion of cereals/grains, by-product feeds (eg, brans), and/or oil in many diets. When additional energy is required, things to consider include

- Feeding less mature forage, which provides more energy.
- Adding more digestible fiber sources (eg, soya hulls, beet pulp) or a commercially prepared, nutritionally balanced complementary feed with a high fiber content and low or restricted levels of starch.
- Supplementing with nonrancid, feed-grade vegetable oil,[7,9,97,98] which
  - Has a high energy density with no sugar or starch.
  - Needs to be fed consistently for several weeks to gain any possible additional metabolic benefits.[98,99]
  - Should be introduced gradually, over several days or weeks, depending on the volume being added, to help avoid digestive disturbances (loose and oily manure).
  - Can typically be fed at up to 1 mL of oil/kg BW/d, divided among the meals.
    - One standard measuring cup contains 250 mL (8 fluid ounces) of vegetable oil ($\sim$225 g) and provides approximately 1.8 Mcal (7.6 MJ) of digestible energy (DE; equivalent to the energy provided in $\sim$0.6 kg oats or $\sim$0.5 kg corn). For a 500-kg horse in moderate work (daily DE needs of 26 Mcal) adding 500 mL oil/d provides about 14% of the DE requirement.
  - The authors recommend the additional provision (on top of normal requirements) of at least 1 to 1.5 IU vitamin E per milliliter of supplemental oil.
  - Check the overall nutritional balance of the diet. Oil only provides calories and no additional vitamins (vitamin E content variable) or minerals.
- With respect to the addition of cereals/grains (eg, oats)
  - These are not nutritionally balanced: imbalanced Ca/P ratio; low content of quality amino acids (eg, the first limiting amino acid lysine) and typically little trace minerals.
  - Contain different amounts of starch:
    - Oats contain around 40%, barley around 50% to 55%, and corn around 60%.
    - Prececal starch digestibility varies with the amount and type of grain and the nature of any mechanical or thermal processing. For example, oat starch (up to 2 g/kg BW) can have a prececal digestibility of greater than 80%, compared with $\sim$35% for corn starch.
    - Heat treatments, such as micronization, extrusion, and steam flaking, significantly improve the prececal starch digestibility of barley and corn.[39] Grains (other than oats) in compound or complementary feeds should always be cooked.[26,36,39,100]
  - Currently recommend a safe upper limit for starch and sugar intake of $\leq$1 g/kg BW per meal (and wherever possible <2 g/kg BW/d) from the nonforage feed portion (reviewed in Myriam Hesta and Marcio Costa's article, "How Can Nutrition Help with Gastrointestinal Tract-Based Issues," in this issue).[20,96]
  - Where necessary, increase the number of, rather than the size of, meals, offering no more than 0.4 kg of feed/100 kg of BW at a time that is up to 2 kg/meal for a 500-kg horse.
  - Always feed by weight not volume. This applies to all feeds because the relationship between weight and volume varies. For example, oats weigh less for a given volume than corn (resulting in an $\sim$45% relative value to corn if measure by volume vs $\sim$85% by weight) so replacing the same number of cups/scoops of corn by oats effectively means feeding less in weight of oats and much less energy.
  - Although custom-adding single ingredients, such as cereals, to the ration potentially offers a certain amount of ration flexibility, their use is problematic without sufficient knowledge or experience.[101]

- Coarse mixes/sweet feeds/textured/hard feeds are complementary feeds or concentrates formulated to be fed alongside forage and contain a mixture of several ingredients: typically based on grains, fiber sources, vegetable oil/fat, protein sources, vitamins, and minerals. Complete feeds are fiber-enhanced (eg, from beet pulp, alfalfa meal, soybean hulls) and are often formulated such that they may be fed without forage. Sugar and starch levels depend on which ingredients are being used and at what inclusion level.
  - These products can provide as much energy as pure cereals but can have restricted (defined here as <25%) or low starch (defined here as <10%, if they are based primarily on highly digestible fiber sources plus oil with almost no grain) content. Note, there are currently no regulatory maximum definitions for feeds labeled as restricted or low starch.
  - Labels should provide an indication of the provided level of certain (but usually not all) nutrients but, depending on the country and the legislative requirements, the values given may represent maximums or minimums or the actual analytical value may fall within set limits of the declared value (reviewed in Ruth Bishop and David A. Dzanis' article, "Staying on the Right Side of the Regulatory Authorities," in this issue).
  - Label information, and any additional information on the manufacturer's Web site, may give an indication of the suitability of a diet for its intended purpose but additional or confirmatory analysis may be required especially in complex cases.

Beyond Energy

Horse rations should be based on forage and then, if required, alternative sources of energy may be added to the diet to meet the individual's energy needs. Depending on which sources are added,[101] the ration may then require balancing for protein, including the essential amino acids, and then vitamins and minerals/trace elements using other feedstuffs.

- The dietary protein requirement is a function of amino acid needs, the amino acid composition of the dietary protein, and the digestibility of the protein (reviewed in Kristine L. Urschel and Erica C. McKenzie's article, "Nutritional Influences on Skeletal Muscle and Muscular Disease," in this issue). Practically, the horse's essential amino acid requirements must be met from protein sources that are digested in the SI.
- Additional protein over maintenance (1.5 g crude protein/kg BW) may be needed with exercise and training because of the accompanying muscular development, the need for muscle repair, and to replenish the nitrogen lost in sweat (~20–25 g/kg sweat loss) (reviewed in Kristine L. Urschel and Erica C. McKenzie's article, "Nutritional Influences on Skeletal Muscle and Muscular Disease," in this issue).
- Quality and nature of the protein fed is important especially in growing horses and those in hard or repetitive work. The amount of additional lysine needed depends on the hay and pasture being fed. For example, alfalfa and other legumes are higher in lysine than many meadow hays and grasses (reviewed in Kristine L. Urschel and Erica C. McKenzie's article, "Nutritional Influences on Skeletal Muscle and Muscular Disease"; Morgane Robles and colleagues' article, "Nutrition of Broodmares," in this issue).
- Peas, beans, linseed, soyabeans, and alfalfa meal are typically used as feed ingredients[7,101] to provide additional good-quality protein
  - Peas typically contain ~15 to 18 g lysine/kg DM and 8 to 10 g threonine/kg DM.

- Full-fat soya beans are ~40% protein (as fed) with high levels of essential amino acids (lysine ~24 g/kg DM or ~36 g lysine/kg DM of defatted soyabean meal).
- Need to consider other factors when using these ingredients. For example, the potential presence of antinutritive factors (eg, as in uncooked soyabean), palatability, and the need to account for the energy they provide.

Once the ration has been balanced with respect to the protein and amino acid intake, an assessment as to how closely the ration matches mineral and vitamin requirements needs to be made.[7,70,71,96] Obvious deficiencies are addressed through using specific supplements or more generic commercial balancers.

- Balancers are nutrient-dense complementary feeds, typically providing high-quality protein, delivering essential amino acids, such as lysine, and vitamins and minerals.
  - Are usually formulated to be fed at a much lower intake than conventional complementary feeds.
  - Are not provided as a significant source of energy, although they contribute some calories to the ration depending on their formulation.
  - Many horses and ponies especially in light to moderate work can be fed appropriately through just forage (grass fresh or preserved) and a balancer.
  - Are essential to provide if feeding soaked forage (because of leaching of essential water-soluble nutrients) or to animals on a weight loss regimen (to ensure adequate nutrient intake during energy restriction) and for many areas if on a forage-based diet or forage-straight cereal-based ration (discussed previously).
- It has been suggested, for example, that traditional rations may not offer all of the optimal nutritional components, especially where high performance horses are concerned, and that feed 'supplements' may be of benefit under some circumstances.[102,103] Supplements are discussed further in Ruth Bishop and David A Dzanis' article Staying on the right side of the regulatory authorities and Ingrid Ververt and Meri Stratton-Phelps' article, "The Safety and Efficacy in Horses of Certain Nutraceuticals that Claim to Have Health Benefits," in this issue.

Dry Matter Versus As-Fed

DM basis refers to the feed or forage after the moisture has been removed by a drying oven, whereas the term "as-fed" refers to a feed as it would be fed to a horse. Only the DM contains nutrients, so more feed needs to be fed on an as-fed basis to match requirements if two feeds with the same nutrient content on a DM basis are fed but one contains more water. Most complementary feeds, such as cereals, cubes, pellets, and so forth, contain around 10% moisture with a DM content of 88% to 92%. Fresh grass is highly variable depending on species, environment, and so forth but as a guide approximately 20% DM (cool season grass). Hay should have more than 85% DM and as an easy guide an average figure of 90% DM is used for calculations. The amount of forage in the ration should be calculated on a DM basis rather than an as-fed basis because of the low fiber/DM content of some immature hays, especially alfalfa, and haylages/silages. Requirements are given in a variety of ways. It is important to check which units are being used. Two of the most common are

1. Per kilogram DM feed intake: animals must therefore be fed appropriate amounts of feed for their age, reproductive status, workload, and so forth. This is therefore not

suitable to apply to animals on a weight-loss diet which are being fed restricted amounts.

2. Amounts per day on an as-fed basis either on an absolute BW basis or (under some systems) a metabolic BW basis.

REQUIREMENTS OR RECOMMENDATIONS

Maintenance requirement is defined as the daily intake that maintains constant BW and body composition and the health of a healthy adult horse with zero retention at a defined level of low activity in comfortable surroundings. For some nutrients, additional amounts are needed with exercise to cover, for example, the nutrient losses in sweat and to aid in the repair processes. Growth and reproductive status also impose their own additional demands (reviewed in Morgane Robles and colleagues' article, "Nutrition of Broodmares," in this issue).

The amount of any nutrient that should be provided in the ration can be given as a 'requirement' and therefore should be considered (practically) as a minimal level to sustain life or as a 'recommendation', which implies that either a safety margin has been built-in or it allows for the absence of complete requirement data. 'Optimal' intakes are of value especially when a particular system (eg, the immune system) may benefit from increased intakes (eg, horses in stressful circumstances, such as intense physical activity or travel for athletic competition). Although currently most optimal recommendations are based on personal experiences or beliefs and may have little or no scientific basis, they are helpful in designing rations. Many nutrition texts and feeding standard publications[7] present recommendations or a mixture of requirements and recommendations. However, in using any such reference publication it is always important to note that horses are individuals and vary in their metabolic efficiency (eg, some horses are good doers/easy keepers), temperament, health status (including level of parasitic burden), appetite, likes and dislikes, and other variables. Therefore, recommendations can only provide general guidance.

DIFFERENT SYSTEMS

Different ways of expressing requirements/recommendations are used around the world. For example, with respect to energy, DE is the most commonly used system in the United Kingdom and United States, with the Metabolizable or Net Energy systems gaining popularity in parts of mainland Europe.[104,105] All have advantages and disadvantages, but the main practical take home message is that the various systems and units should not be mixed: just use one system for identifying the requirements and how feeds can supply such requirements. For this issue DE and absolute (rather than metabolic) BW are used mainly. Reference is still made, where appropriate, to the two units of energy commonly used in the horse industry: the joule predominantly in Europe, and the calorie in the United States (4.184 J = ~1 calorie).

DISCLOSURE

The authors have no commercial or financial conflicts of interest to declare.

REFERENCES

1. Murray J-AMD, Bloxham C, Kulifay J, et al. Equine nutrition: a survey of perceptions and practices of horse owners undertaking a massive open online course in equine nutrition. J Equine Vet Sci 2015;35(6):510–7.

2. Nichols JL. Identifying equine veterinarians continuing educational needs in equine nutrition. Doctor of Philosophy degree thesis Oklahoma State University; 2018.
3. Parker A, Mastellar S, Bott-Knutson R, et al. Upper Midwest veterinarian perceptions and confidence levels regarding equine nutrition topics. J Equine Vet Sci 2018;69:108–14.
4. Roberts JL, Murray J-A. Survey of equine nutrition: perceptions and practices of veterinarians in Georgia, USA. J Equine Vet Sci 2013;33(6):454–9.
5. Roberts JL, Murray J-A. Equine nutrition in the United States: a review of perceptions and practices of horse owners and veterinarians. J Equine Vet Sci 2014;34(7):854–9.
6. Becvarova I, Prochazka D, Chandler M, et al. Nutrition education in European veterinary schools: competencies of European veterinary graduates in nutrition. In proceedings of the 15th annual AAVN clinical nutrition and research symposium proceedings 2015 Indianapolis June 3rd :14- 15. J Vet Med Educ 2016; 43(4):349–58.
7. NRC (National Research Council). Nutrient requirements of horses, 6th revision. Washington, DC: National Academy Press; 2007.
8. Geor RJ, Harris PA, Coenen M, editors. Equine applied and clinical nutrition. London (United Kingdom): Elsevier; 2013.
9. Harris PA, Geor RJ. Nutrition for the equine athlete: nutrient requirements and key principles in ration design. In: Hinchcliff KW, Kaneps AJ, Geor RJ, editors. Equine sports medicine & Surgery. 2nd Edition. New York (NY): Elsevier; 2014. p. 797–818.
10. Harris PA, Ellis AD, Fradinho M, et al. Review of feeding conserved forage to horses: recent advances and recommendations. Animal 2017;11(6):958–67.
11. Varloud M. Activité amylolytique des secretions salivaires. In: implication des micro-organismes de l'estomac dans la digestion de l'amidon par le cheval. Thesis presented to the National Agricultural Institute of Paris-Grignon; 2006. p. 62–8.
12. Meyer H, Coenen M, Gurer C. Investigations of saliva production and chewing in horses fed various feeds. East Lansing (MI): Proceedings of the Equine Nutrition and Physiology Society; 1985. p. 38–41.
13. Meyer H, Coenen M, Prost D. Digestive physiology of the horse. Feed insalivation and passage in the equine upper intestinal tract. J Anim Physiol Anim Nutr 1986;56:171–83.
14. Bonin SJ, Clayton HM, Lanovaz JL, et al. Comparison of mandibular motion in horses chewing hay and pellets. Equine Vet J 2007;39:258–62.
15. Cuddeford D. Factors affecting feed intake. In: Geor RJ, Harris PA, Coenen M, editors. Equine clinical and applied nutrition. London (United Kingdom): Elsevier; 2013. p. 64–89.
16. Campbell T, Doughty H, Harris P, et al. Factors affecting the rate and measurement of feed intake for a cereal based meal in horses. J Equine Vet Sci 2020;84: 102869.
17. Ellis AD, Thomas S, Arkell K, et al. Adding chopped straw to concentrate feed: the effect of inclusion rate and particle length on intake behaviour of horses. Pferdeheilkunde 2005;21:35–6.
18. Merritt AM, Julliand V. Gastrointestinal physiology. In: Geor RJ, Harris PA, Coenen M, editors. Equine clinical and applied nutrition. London (United Kingdom): Elsevier; 2013. p. p3–32.

19. Merritt AM, Sanchez L, Burrow JA, et al. Effect of GastroGard™ and three compounded oral omeprazole preparations on 24 h intragastric pH in gastrically cannulated mature horses. Equine Vet J 2003;35:691–5.

20. Luthersson N, Nielsen KH, Harris PA, et al. Risk factors associated with equine gastric ulceration syndrome in 201 horses in Denmark. Equine Vet J 2009;4(7): 625–30.

21. Javsicas LH, Sanchez LC. The effect of omeprazole paste on intragastric pH in clinically ill neonatal foals. Equine Vet J 2009;40(1):41–4.

22. Caston SS, Fredericks DC, Kersh KD, et al. Short-term omeprazole use does not affect serum calcium concentrations and bone density in horses. J Equine Vet Sci 2015;35:714–23.

23. Pagan JD, Petroski L, Mann A. Hauss A. Omeprazole reduces calcium digestibility in Thoroughbred horses. J Equine Vet Sci 2020;86:102851.

24. Geor RJ, Harris PA, Hoekstra KE, et al. Effect of corn oil on solid phase gastric emptying in horses. In Proceedings of the American College Veterinary Internal Medicine 2001;67:288.

25. Sutton DG, Bahr A, Preston T, et al. Validation of the 13C-octanoic acid breath test for measurement of equine gastric emptying rate of solids using radioscintigraphy. Equine Vet J 2003;35(1):27–33.

26. Meyer H, Radicke A, Kienzle E, et al. Investigations of preileal digestion of oats, corn and barley starch in relation to grain processing. In: proceedings of the 13th Equine Nutrition Physiology Symposium, Gainesville, FL. 1993:92.

27. Al Jassim RA, Scott PT, Trebbin AL, et al. The genetic diversity of lactic acid producing bacteria in the equine gastrointestinal tract. FEMS Microbiol Lett 2005; 248(1):75–81.

28. Varloud M, Fonty G, Roussel A, et al. Postprandial kinetics of some biotic and abiotic characteristics of the gastric ecosystem of horses fed a pelleted concentrate meal. J Anim Sci 2007;85:2508–16.

29. Ince JC, Longland AC, Moore-Colyer MJS, et al. In vitro degradation of grass fructan by equid gastrointestinal digesta. Grass Forage Sci 2014;69(3):514–23.

30. Kitchen DL, Burrow JA, Heartless CS, et al. Effect of pyloric blockade and infusion of histamine or pentagastrin on gastric secretion in horses. Am J Vet Res 2000;61(9):1133–9.

31. Kienzle E, Radicke S. Effect of diet on maltase, sucrase and lactase in the small intestinal mucosa of the horse. J Anim Physiol a Anim Nutr 1993;70:97–103.

32. Dyer J, Merediz EF, Salmon KS, et al. Molecular characterisation of carbohydrate digestion and absorption in equine small intestine. Equine Vet J 2002; 34(4):349–58.

33. Richards N, Choct M, Hinch GN, et al. Examination of the use of exogenous a-amylase and amyloglucosidase to enhance starch digestion in the small intestine of the horse. Anim Feed Sci Technol 2004;114:295–330.5.

34. Dyer J, Al-Rammahi M, Waterfall L, et al. Adaptative response of equine intestinal NA+/glucose co-transporter (SGLT1) to an increase in dietary soluble carbohydrate. Pflugers Arch 2009;458:419–30.

35. Kienzle E, Radicke S, Landes E, et al. Activity of amylase in the gastrointestinal tract of the horse. J Anim Physiol a Anim Nutr 1994;72:234–41.

36. Kienzle E. Small intestinal digestion of starch in the horse. Revue de Medecine Veterinaire (France) 1994;145:199–204.

37. Meyer H, Radicke S, Kienzle E, et al. Investigations on preileal digestion of starch grain, potato and manioc in horses. Zentralbl Veterinarmed A 1995;42: 371–81.

38. Kienzle E, Pohlenz J, Radicke S. Microscopy of starch digestion in the horse. J Anim Physiol a Anim Nutr 1998;80:213–6.
39. Julliand V, De Fombelle A, Varloud M. Starch digestion in horses: the impact of feed processing. Livest Sci 2006;100(1):44–52.
40. Fernandez Castano Meredi E, Dyer J, SalmonKSH, Shirazi-Beechey SP. Molecular characterisation of fructose transport in equine small intestine. Equine Vet J 2004;36:532–8.
41. Woodward AD, Fan MZ, Geor RJ, et al. Characterization of d-glucose transport across equine jejunal brush border membrane using the pig as an efficient model of jejunal glucose uptake. J Equine Vet Sci 2013;33(6):460–7.
42. Cehak A, Schröder B, Feige K, et al. In vitro studies on intestinal peptide transport in horses. J Anim Sci 2013;91(11):5220–8.
43. Lorenzo-Figueras M, Mrisset SM, Morisset J, et al. Digestive enzyme concentrations and activities in healthy pancreatic tissue of horses. Am J Vet Res 2007;68:1070–2.
44. Dougal K, Harris PA, Edwards A, et al. A comparison of the microbiome and the metabolome of different regions of the equine hindgut. FEMS Microbiol Ecol 2012;82:642–52.
45. Ericsson AC, Johnson PJ, Lopes MA, et al. A microbiological map of the healthy equine gastrointestinal tract. PLoS One 2016;11(11):e0166523.
46. Su S, Zhao Y, Liu Z, et al. Characterization and comparison of the bacterial microbiota in different gastrointestinal tract compartments of Mongolian horses. Microbiologyopen 2020;9:e1020.
47. Longland A, Byrd B. Pasture nonstructural carbohydrates and equine laminitis. J Nutr 2006;136:2099S–102S.
48. Argenzio RA, Southworth M, Stevens CE. Sites of organic acid production and absorption in the equine gastrointestinal tract. Am J Physiol 1974;226:1043–50.
49. Moore-Colyer MJS, Lumbis K, Longland A, et al. The effect of five different wetting treatments on the nutrient content and microbial concentration in hay for horses. PLoS One 2014;9(11):e114079.
50. Daly K, Shirazi-Beechey SP. Design and evaluation of group-specific oligonucleotide probes for quantitative analysis of intestinal ecosystems: their application to assessment of equine colonic microflora. FEMS Microbiol Ecol 2003;44:243–52.
51. Dougal K, de la Fuente G, Harris PA, et al. Characterisation of the faecal bacterial community in adult and elderly horses fed a high fibre, high oil or high starch diet using 454 pyrosequencing. PloS One 2014;9(2):e87424.
52. Edwards JE, Schennink A, Burden F, et al. Domesticated equine species and their derived hybrids differ in their fecal microbiota. Anim Microbiome 2020;2:8.
53. Geor RJ. Endocrine and metabolic physiology. In: Geor RJ, Harris PA, Coenen M, editors. Equine clinical and applied nutrition. London: Elsevier; 2013. p. 33–63.
54. Glinsky MJ, Smith RM, Spires HR, et al. Measurement of volatile fatty acid production rates in the cecum of the pony. J Anim Sci 1976;42:1465–70.
55. Pethick DW, Rose RJ, Bryden WL. Gooden JM. Nutrient utilisation by the hindlimb of thoroughbred horses at rest. Equine Vet J 1993;25(1):41–4.
56. Suagee JK, Corl BA, Crisman MV, et al. De novo fatty acid synthesis and NADPH generation in equine adipose and liver tissue. Comp Biochem Physiol B Biochem Mol Biol 2010;155(3):322–6.
57. Simmons HA, Ford EJ, Su S, et al. Gluconeogenesis from propionate produced in the colon of the horse. Br Vet J 1991;147(4):340–5.

58. Shirazy-Beechey SP. Molecular insights into dietary induced colic in the horse. Equine Vet J 2008;40:414–21.

59. Nedjadi T, Moran AW, Al-Rammahi MA, et al. Characterization of butyrate transport across the luminal membranes of equine large intestine. Exp Physiol 2014; 99(10):1335–47.

60. Clarke LL, Argenzio RA, Roberts MC. Effect of meal feeding on plasma volume and urinary electrolyte clearance in ponies. Am J Vet Res 1990;51:571–6.

61. Clarke LL, Roberts MC, Argenzio RA. Feeding and digestive problems in horses: physiologic responses to a concentrated meal. Vet Clin North Am Equine Pract 1990;6:433–50.

62. Hintz HF, Argenzio RA, Schryver HF. Digestion coefficients, blood glucose levels, and molar percentage of volatile fatty acids in intestinal fluid of ponies fed varying forage-grain ratios. J Anim Sci 1971;33:992–5.

63. Willard JG, Willard JC, Wolfram SA, et al. Effect of diet on cecal pH and feeding behaviour of horses. J Anim Sci 1977;45:87–93.

64. Radicke S, Kienzle E, Meyer H. Preileal apparent digestibility of oats and corn starch and consequences for cecal metabolism. In: proceedings of the 12th Equine Nutrition Physiology Symposium. Calgary (Canada): Canada; 1991. p. 43.

65. Daly K, Proudman CJ, Duncan SH, et al. Alterations in microbiota and fermentation products in equine large intestine in response to dietary variation and intestinal disease. Br J Nutr 2012;107(7):989–95.

66. Woodward AD, Holcombe SJ, Steibel JP, et al. Cationic and neutral amino acid transporter transcript abundances are differentially expressed in the equine intestinal tract. J Anim Sci 2010;88(3):1028–33.

67. Willing B, Vörös A, Roos S, et al. Changes in faecal bacteria associated with concentrate and forage-only diets fed to horses in training. Equine Vet J 2009;41(9):908–14.

68. Morrison PK, Newbold CJ, Jones E, et al. The equine gastrointestinal microbiome: impacts of age and obesity. Front Microbiol 2018. https://doi.org/10.3389/fmicb.2018.03017.

69. Morrison PK, Newbold CJ, Jones E, et al. Effect of age and the individual on the gastrointestinal bacteriome of ponies fed a high-starch diet. PLoS One 2020; 15(5):e0232689.

70. Coenen M. Macro and trace elements in equine nutrition. In: Geor RJ, Harris PA, Coenen M, editors. Equine clinical and applied nutrition. London (United Kingdom): Elsevier; 2013. p. 190–230.

71. Zeyner A, Harris PA. Vitamins. In: Geor RJ, Harris PA, Coenen M, editors. Equine clinical and applied nutrition. London (United Kingdom): Elsevier; 2013. p. 168–89.

72. Cymbaluk NF. Water. In: Geor RJ, Harris PA, Coenen M, editors. Equine clinical and applied nutrition. London (United Kingdom): Elsevier; 2013. p. 80–95.

73. Williams S, Horner J, Orton E, et al. Water intake, faecal output and intestinal motility in horses moved from pasture to a stabled management regime with controlled exercise. Equine Vet J 2015;47:96–100.

74. Oliveira C aA, Azevedo JF, Martins JA, et al. The impact of dietary protein levels on nutrient digestibility and water and nitrogen balances in eventing horses. J Anim Sci 2015;93:229–37.

75. Harris PA, Schott11 HC. Nutritional management of elite endurance horses. In: Geor RJ, Harris PA, Coenen M, editors. Equine clinical and applied nutrition. London (United Kingdom): Elsevier; 2013. p. 272–88.

76. Butudom P, Schott HC, Davis MW, et al. Drinking salt water enhances rehydration in horses dehydrated by frusemide administration and endurance exercise. Equine Vet J 2002;34(S34):513–8.
77. Butudom P, Barnes DJ, Davis MW, et al. Rehydration fluid temperature affects voluntary drinking in horses dehydrated by furosemide administration and endurance exercise. Vet J 2004;167(1):72–80.
78. Longland AC. Pastures and pasture management. In: Geor RJ, Harris PA, Coenen M, editors. Equine clinical and applied nutrition. London (United Kingdom): Elsevier; 2013. p. 332–50.
79. Schenck J. Filamentous fungi in wrapped forages. Doctoral thesis. Swedish University of Agricultural sciences; 2019.
80. O'Brien M, O'Kiely P, Forristal PD, et al. Visible fungal growth on baled grass silage during the winter feeding season in Ireland and silage characteristics associated with the occurrence of fungi. Anim Feed Sci Technol 2017;139: 234–56.
81. Andersen B, Phippen C, Frisvad J, et al. Fungal and chemical diversity in hay and wrapped haylage for equine feed. Mycotoxin Res 2020;36(2):159–72.
82. Wichert B, Nater S, Wittenbrink MM, et al. Judgement of hygienic quality of roughage in horse stables in Switzerland. J Anim Physiol Anim Nutr (Berl) 2008;92:432–7.
83. Kamphues J. Feed hygiene and related disorders in horses. In: Geor RJ, Harris PA, Coenen M, editors. Equine clinical and applied nutrition. London (United Kingdom): Elsevier; 2013. p. 367–80.
84. Trenholm HL, Charmley LL, Prelusky DB, et al. Washing procedures using water or sodium carbonate solutions for the decontamination of three cereals contaminated with deoxynivalenol and zearalenone. J Agric Food Chem 1992;40(11): 2147–51.
85. Moore-Colyer MJ, Hyslop JJ, Longland AC, et al. The mobile bag technique as a method for determining the degradation of four botanically diverse fibrous feedstuffs in the small intestine and total digestive tract of ponies. Br J Nutr 2002;88: 729–40.
86. Moore-Colyer M, Longland A, Harris P, et al. Mapping the bacterial ecology on the phyllosphere of dry and post soaked grass hay for horses. PLOS One 2020; 15(1):e0227151.
87. Cohen ND, Gibbs PG. Woods AM. Dietary and other management factors associated with colic in horses. J Am Vet Med Assoc 1999;215(1):53–60.
88. Durham A. Intestinal disease. In: Geor RJ, Harris PA, Coenen M, editors. Equine clinical and applied nutrition. London (United Kingdom): Elsevier; 2013. p. 568–81.
89. Curtis L, Burford JH, England GCW. Freeman SL. Risk factors for acute abdominal pain (colic) in the adult horse: a scoping review of risk factors, and a systematic review of the effect of management-related changes. PLoS One 2019; 14(7):e0219307.
90. Dugdale A, CurtisGC, Cripps P, et al. Effects of season and body condition on appetite, body mass and body composition in ad libitum fed pony mares. Vet J 2011;190:329–37.
91. Longland AC, Ince J, Harris PA. Estimation of pasture intake by ponies from liveweight change during six weeks at pasture. J Equine Vet Sci 2011;31:275–6.
92. Longland A, Barfoot C, Harris P. Effects of grazing muzzles on intakes of dry matter and water-soluble carbohydrates by ponies grazing spring, summer

and autumn swards, as well as autumn swards of different heights. J Equine Vet Sci 2016;40:26–33.

93. Allen E, Sheaffer C, Martinson K. Forage nutritive value and preference of cool-season grasses under horse Grazin. Crop Economics, Production & Management Agronomy 2013;105(3):679–84.

94. Harris P, Dunnett C. Nutritional tips for veterinarians. Equine Vet Educ 2018; 30(9):486–96.

95. Goodwin D, Davidson HPB, Harris PA. Responses of horses offered a choice between stables containing single or multiple forages. Vet Rec 2007;160(16): 548–51.

96. Harris PA, Coenen M, Geor RJ. Controversial areas in equine nutrition and feeding management: the editors' views. In: Geor RJ, Harris PA, Coenen M, editors. Equine clinical and applied nutrition. London (United Kingdom): Elsevier; 2013. p. 455–68.

97. Kronfeld DS, Holland JL, Rich V, et al. Fat digestibility in *Equus caballus* follows increasing first order kinetics. J Anim Sci 2004;82:1773–80.

98. Warren LK, Vineyard KR. Fat and fatty acids. In: Geor RJ, Harris PA, Coenen M, editors. Equine clinical and applied nutrition. London (United Kingdom): Elsevier; 2013. p. 136–55.

99. Pagan JD, Geor R, Harris PA, et al. Effects of fat adaptation on glucose kinetics and substrate oxidation during low intensity exercise. Equine Vet J 2002;(Suppl34):33–8.

100. McLean BML, Hyslop JJ, Longland AC, et al. Physical processing of barley and its effects on intra-caecal fermentation parameters in ponies. Anim Feed Sci Technol 2000;85(1):79–87.

101. Lindberg JE. Feedstuffs for horses. In: Geor RJ, Harris PA, Coenen M, editors. Equine clinical and applied nutrition. London (United Kingdom): Elsevier; 2013. p. 319–21.

102. Harris PA, Harris RC. Ergogenic potential of nutritional strategies and substances in the horse. Livest Prod Sci 2005;92:14–165.

103. Williams CA. Specialized dietary supplements. In: Geor RJ, Harris PA, Coenen M, editors. Equine clinical and applied nutrition. London (United Kingdom): Elsevier; 2013. p. 351–66.

104. Harris PA. Energy requirements of the exercising horse. Annu Rev Nutr 1997;17: 185–210.

105. Ellis A. Energy systems and requirements. In: Geor RJ, Harris PA, Coenen M, editors. Equine clinical and applied nutrition. London (United Kingdom): Elsevier; 2013. p. 96–112.

How to Perform a Nutritional Assessment in a First-Line/General Practice

Myriam Hesta, DVM, PhD[a],*, Megan Shepherd, DVM, PhD, DipACVN[b]

KEYWORDS

- Horse • Equine • Body condition score (BCS) • Forage • Nutrition • Ration • Diet
- Communication

KEY POINTS

- A nutrition assessment is a vital aspect of equine patient evaluation.
- A patient's physiologic status (eg, healthy adult, pregnant mare, or athlete) and presence of disease (eg, obesity, gastric ulcers, or myopathy) should inform nutritional goals.
- The current diet, feeding management, owner resources, and facilities should inform recommendations/suggestions.
- Effective communication influences the thoroughness of a diet history and owner compliance.

INTRODUCTION

Nutrition recommendations often are sought out to enhance athletic[1–3] or reproductive performance[4] and help manage specific diseases/conditions (eg, gastrointestinal disease, weight management, myopathy, and developmental orthopedic disease)[4]; see the chapters. Proper nutrition, however, is important for health maintenance and disease prevention and avoidance of toxic plants.[5] Therefore, in addition to a traditional physical examination (eg, assessing temperature and cardiac, respiratory, and intestinal auscultation), a nutrition assessment[6] should be a vital aspect of equine patient assessment. Early correction of common nutritional mistakes is fundamental for prevention of nutrition-related diseases.[4]

Evaluating the equine patient itself as well as its current (and sometime previous) diet/ration and management is essential in creating the most effective nutritional

[a] ECAN Equine and Companion Animal Nutrition, Department of Veterinary Medical Imaging and Small Animal Orthopaedics, Faculty of Veterinary Medicine, Ghent University, Salisburylaan 133, Merelbeke 9820, Belgium; [b] Department of Large Animal Clinical Sciences, Virginia-Maryland College of Veterinary Medicine, Phase II Duck Pond Drive, Virginia Tech Mail Code 0442, Blacksburg, VA 24061, USA
* Corresponding author.
E-mail address: Myriam.hesta@ugent.be

Vet Clin Equine 37 (2021) 21–41
https://doi.org/10.1016/j.cveq.2020.12.001
0749-0739/21/© 2020 Elsevier Inc. All rights reserved.

plan (**Table 1**). Energy and nutrient requirements may be estimated after assessing the equine itself. After a diet/ration evaluation, the need for change or adjustment may be determined and, if needed, in turn has to be monitored and readjusted as required. Optimal communication is crucial not only for a detailed and correct nutrition anamnesis/history but also to increase compliance and assure nutritional advice is applied correctly by the owner.

Formal global guidelines for conducting a nutrition assessment for small animals exists.[6] Guidelines for conducting a nutrition assessment for equines, however, are limited.[7–9] This article is meant to guide the general practitioner through conducting a nutrition assessment and to provide practical tips that can be used in the field. Appreciating that there are different approaches to conducting a nutrition assessment, the authors share their perspectives from practice and personal experiences. This article does not provide an exhaustive review; for more details on specific nutritional recommendations for healthy and diseased equines, see other chapters.

ASSESS THE EQUINE
Consider the Signalment (Age, Sex, Breed, Life Stage, and Performance)

- Foals need a nutritional plan based on their age (neonatal, before/after weaning, yearling, and so forth) and that differs from that of adults.[10]
- Pregnant or lactating mares and breeding stallions in the season have specific nutritional needs.[10] See Robles and colleagues' article, "Nutrition of Broodmares," in this issue.
- Healthy senior horses with a decreased body condition may benefit from a highly digestible diet with higher protein content.[11] Geriatric equines with severe dental disease, osteoarthritis, or pituitary pars intermedius dysfunction have specific needs.[11–15] Senior horses may become more insulin dysregulated with age and this may influence their nutritional management.[11] See Robles and colleagues' article, "Nutrition of Broodmares," in this issue.
- Some breeds appear to be predisposed to nutritionally sensitive conditions (obesity, equine metabolic syndrome, polysaccharide storage myopathy, and so forth).[16,17] See Shepherd and colleagues' article, "Nutritional Considerations

Table 1
Nutrition assessment outline: key considerations when evaluating 3 categories (horse, diet/ration, and management)

Assess the Horse	Assess the Diet/Ration	Assess the Management
• Age	• Water quality	• Who cares for the horse
• Gender	• Forage type	(owner, caregiver, trainer, etc.)
• Life stage	(fresh or processed;	• Environment
• Activity	grass or legume)	• Water accessibility
• BW	• Forage quality and	• Forage accessibility
• BCS	hygiene	• Use of slow feeders
• Cresty neck score	• Forage quantity	• Pasture management
• Muscle condition	• Complementary feed	• Complementary feed accessibility
• Appetite	nutrient profile	• Feeding frequency
• Oral health	• Complementary feed	• Number of hours between meals
• Fecal quality	manufacturer quality	
• Clinical abnormalities	control	
	• Complementary feed	
	quantity	

When Dealing with an Obese Adult Equine," and Urschel and McKenzie's article, "Nutritional Influences on Skeletal Muscle and Muscular Disease," in this issue

- Donkeys[18,19] and ponies have unique needs compared with horses. The digestive capacity of donkeys is higher compared with horses, and the diet should be high in fiber and low in nonstructural carbohydrates. A typical ration for adult donkeys should consist of 70% to 75% straw and 25% to 30% grass hay, grazing, or green fodder for most of the time of the year.[19] Many ponies appear to be metabolically efficient and often regarded as easy keepers.[20] See Shepherd and colleagues' article, "Nutritional Considerations When Dealing with an Obese Adult Equine," in this issue.
- Appropriate ration and nutritional management, which go further than meeting basic nutrient requirements for maintenance, allow the athlete to train, compete, and perform according to its athletic potential.[3]

Measure/Estimate Body Weight

- Properly calibrated scales are most precise but rarely practical/available. Therefore, on the farm, an equine's weight may be estimated using (1) a weight tape calibrated for equines or (2) plugging morphometric measurements into an equation (discussed later).[21] To be able to compare data over time, the same methodology, positioning, and timing are crucial. Different equations exist for different groups of equines (eg, foals and ponies) because 1 general equation may not be appropriate for all equines. See Shepherd and colleagues' article, "Nutritional Considerations When Dealing with an Obese Adult Equine," in this issue.
  - Adult body weight (BW) (kg) = girth (cm) 1.486 × length (cm) 0.554 × height (cm) 0.599 × neck (cm) 0.173]/Y[22]
    - Girth measured just behind elbow
    - Y = 3596 for Arabians, 3606 for ponies, and 3441 for stock horses
  - Foal BW (kg) = girth $(m)^3 \times 90$[23]
    - Rough guide, not as accurate as Staniar's below
    - Girth = caudal to the olecranon tuber, 2.54 cm caudal to the highest point of the withers and at the end of exhalation
    - For example, if girth circumference was 120 cm or 1.2 m, then calculated BW is 156 kg.
  - Thoroughbred foal BW (kg)[24]
    - First, calculate Vt + I (Volume of trunk and legs)= $([(G^2 \times B) + 4(C^2 \times F)])/4\pi$, then
    - If Vt + I < 0.27 m^3, weight (kg) is estimated as Vt + I × 1093
    - If Vt + I ≥ 0.27 m^3, weight (kg) is estimated as Vt + I × 984 + 24
    - G = girth circumference; C = carpus circumference; B = length of body; F = length of forelimb
- Calculate growth rate for the suckling foal/weanling/yearling. Growth rate is influenced by breed[25] and season.[26] Foals' weight can be estimated based on the expected mature weights; they are approximately 10%, 46%, 56%, 64%, and 76% of the mature weights at birth and 6 months, 9 months, 12 months, and 18 months of age, respectively.[27,28]
- Compare current weight with the previous weight in the medical record to determine if there is unintended weight change:
  - If unintended weight loss, see Jarvis and McKenzie's article, "Nutritional Considerations When Dealing with an Underweight Adult or Senior Horse," in this issue

○ If unintended weight gain, see Shepherd and colleagues' article, "Nutritional Considerations When Dealing with an Obese Adult Equine," in this issue

Assign a Body Condition Score

- Although there are multiple body condition score (BCS) systems, the authors recommend using a 9-point scale (**Table 2**).[29–32]
- Although a BCS of 4/9 to 6/9 generally is considered ideal, the authors consider a 4/9 to 5/9 a healthier target for a majority of situations.
  ○ For athletic equines, a 4/9 to 5/9 helps maximize power-to-weight ratio.
  ○ For equines with joint disease, a 4/9 to 5/9 likely is superior to a 6/9.
  ○ A score of 6/9 may be appropriate in certain situations, such as older horses prone to weight loss during winter and breeding mares around parturition with a history of high milk production.

Energy consumed, and more specifically utilized, is less than energy expenditure. Consider the following factors:

- General nutrition factors
  ○ Inadequate forage quality or quantity? Based on BW, forage intake should exceed 1.5% on dry matter (DM) basis.[33] Furthermore, forage does not meet the energy requirements if quality does not match needs (ie, high-quality forage for performing equines).[34,35]
  ○ If forage does not meet the energy needs, a high-energy complementary feed may be included. Some high-energy feeds, however, also are high in starch, and starch can negatively alter hindgut microbes and decrease total tract feed digestibility.[36] Furthermore, feed processing influences starch availability and thus impact.[37]
  ○ Too much starch and sugar (>1 g starch/kg BW/meal)[4,10] in combination with too low forage intake increases the risk of gastrointestinal disease.
  ○ Social competition and group feeding may influence feed access.
- Nutrition factors in performing equines
  ○ Mismatch between ration provided and nutrient needs, for example
    ■ High-intensity and/or long duration of training in combination with inadequate energy and nutrient intake. Amounts provided theoretically meet energy requirements but they exceed the maximum DM intake for that individual.
  ○ Inappropriate concentrates/complementary feeds
- Disease factors
  ○ Suboptimal appetite
    ■ Secondary to pain
      • Oral disease
      • Gastrointestinal disease (gastric ulcers or colic)
      • Orthopedic problems (including neck, limbs, and jaw) and inappropriate way of feeding that limits access (eg, feeding on the ground if neck pain)[38]
      • Other causes of pain
    ■ Secondary to other disease factors
      • In particular, liver disease, gastric ulcers, colitis, hyperlipidemia, dental disease; see Jarvis and McKenzie's article, "Nutritional Considerations When Dealing with an Underweight Adult or Senior Horse," in this issue
  ○ Loss of nutrients (eg, protein losing enteropathy, proteinuria) or inadequate nutrient digestion, absorption, and utilization

Table 2
Body condition score descriptors by region

Body Condition Score	Description	Sites	A Crest of Neck	B Withers	C Behind the Shoulder	D Over the Ribs	E Along the Back	F Tailhead Region
1	Poor (extremely emaciated, no fatty tissue felt)		Bone structures prominent	Bone structure prominent	Bone structure prominent	Bones project prominently	Bones project prominently	Bone prominent
2	Very thin (emaciated)		Structures discernible	Structures discernible	Structures discernible	Bones prominent	Slight fat covering over vertebrae; bones prominent	Bone prominent
3	Thin		Structures faintly discernible	Structures faintly discernible	Structures faintly discernible	Slight fat layer felt but easily seen	Fat built up about halfway on vertebrae	Bone prominent
4	Moderately thin		Not obviously thin	Not obviously thin	Not obviously thin	Faint outline	Slight ridge	Fat felt
5	Moderate		Blends smoothly into body	Rounded	Rounded	Easily felt not seen	Level	Fat beginning to feel spongy
6	Moderately fleshy		Fat beginning to be deposited	Fat beginning to be deposited	Fat beginning to be deposited	Fat feels spongy	May have slight crease	Fat feels soft
7	Fleshy		Noticeable fat deposited	Noticeable fat deposited	Noticeable fat deposited	Felt but noticeable fat deposition	May have crease	Fat is soft
8	Fat		Prominent crest of neck	Filled with fat	Filled with fat	Difficult to feel	Crease	Fat prominent
9	Extremely fat		Bulging fat	Budging fat	Budging fat	Patches of fat	Obvious crease	Budging

Adapted from Henneke DR, Potter GD, Kreider JL, et al. Relationship between Condition Score, Physical Measurements and Body-Fat Percentage in Mares. *Equine Vet J* 1983;15:371–372 with permission.

- ■ Proper mastication is the first step in the digestive process, which can be upset by dental disease. Quids and corn dollies may indicate dental disease but they also can be consumed by other horses when group fed so their presence missed. Increased fecal fiber length also may be a sign of dental disease, although it not always is present.[39]
- ■ Inadequate access to food or water (eg, joint disease/mobility limitations; inability to move to or access the resources)
- See also Jarvis and McKenzie's article, "Nutritional Considerations When Dealing with an Underweight Adult or Senior Horse," in this issue.

Energy consumed is in excess of energy expenditure due to overfeeding, reduced mobility, being metabolically efficient.
- See also Shepherd and colleagues' article, "Nutritional Considerations When Dealing with an Obese Adult Equine," in this issue regarding diagnosing obesity.
- Owners tend to underscore overweight and obese equines.[40,41]
- Although a 9/9 is the upper limit of the 9-point BCS system, a BCS above the 9-point scale limits may be given.
- Not all equines with a BCS of 6/9 need a weight loss program prescribed. The authors, however, consider 6/9 overweight; therefore, further weight gain should be prevented and owners should be informed.
- General nutrition factors
  - ○ Overestimation of BW and/or energy requirements
    - ■ See Shepherd and colleagues' article, "Nutritional Considerations When Dealing with an Obese Adult Equine," in this issue regarding estimating BW.
  - ○ Underestimation of feed quality, especially forage
  - ○ Ad libitum feeding, unlimited/uncontrolled pasture access. Ponies can consume up to 5% of their BW on DM basis over 24 hours[42,43] or up to 1% in a 3-hour period.[44,45] The latter also highlights that just limiting duration of pasture turn out may not be enough to prevent overeating.
  - ○ Feeding a diet/ration that is too energy dense, relative to the equine's voluntary DM intake. Feeding a high-quality forage and/or concentrates/complementary feeds to an equine with relatively low energy requirements (eg, inactive horse, easy keeper, or donkey)
  - ○ Feeding by volume (eg, flakes) instead of weight with underestimation of the quantity and quality of forage and/or concentrates
  - ○ Fed extras by people other than care taker (neighbors, parents, or children)
- Nutrition factors in the competing equine
  - ○ Overestimation of level of work, which includes consideration for both intensity and duration of activity
- See Shepherd and colleagues' article, "Nutritional Considerations When Dealing with an Obese Adult Equine," in this issue regarding estimating target BW.

Cresty Neck Score

- Cresty neck score (0 [no visual or palpable crest] to 5 [large droopy crest]) is an indicator of regional adiposity.
- A cresty neck score greater than 2 can be associated with insulin dysregulation and in some studies was more predictive than BCS.[46,47]

Assess Muscle Condition

- A formal muscle condition scoring for universal use in all equines does not exist, unlike for canine and feline patients.[48] An equine's topline, or muscle along the

dorsal spinous processes, however, is a common site for assessing muscle mass, with dorsal spinous process definition signaling suboptimal muscle mass.
- Suboptimal muscle condition, that is, poor topline
  - Secondary to inadequate dietary energy and/or protein intake and/or quality
  - Secondary to disuse
    - Poor fitness
    - Undertraining or overtraining or inappropriate training
    - Joint disease
    - Back pain
    - Neurologic disease
- Continuing the Assessment for the Healthy Equine (eg, Health Maintenance/Disease Prevention). Are natural feeding behavior principles (trickle feeders and multiple small meals) facilitated?[33]
  - Is forage given in an amount of at least 15 g DM per kg of BW (1.5% of BW) and ideally long-stem? (**Box 1**)[33]
  - Over how many meals are the daily feeds fed?
  - Is time between forage meals less than 5 hours, especially during day time?
  - How is forage offered? For example, if processed forage (eg, hay), is it limit/meal fed; if so, is it offered in a way to slow consumption rate and reduce time between meals (eg, slow feeder or hay net)? See Shepherd and colleagues' article, "Nutritional Considerations When Dealing with an Obese Adult Equine," in this issue regarding extending foraging time and using grazing muzzles.
  - See also Harris and Shepherd's article, "What Would Be Good for all Veterinarians to Know About Equine Nutrition," and Hesta and Costa's article, "How Can Nutrition Help with Gastrointestinal Tract-Based Issues," in this

---

Box 1
Example calculations

Quick calculations for nutritional screening: example for a 550-kg horse, 1 hour of moderate work per day

2 diet scenarios
1. 11.6 kg hay + micronutrient supplement
2. 10 kg hay + 1 kg of complementary feed (85% DM, 35% starch and sugar)

Minimum roughage intake: 1.5% BW on DM basis = greater than 8.25 kg DM or approximately 9.710 kg of hay (85% DM) but 13.750 kg of haylage (60% DM); 11.6 kg and 10 kg of hay, in situation 1 and situation 2, respectively, both are meeting the minimal requirements.

Maximum DM intake: 2.25% (light work): 12.375 kg DM. Situation 1: this horse eats 11.6 kg of hay = 9.9 kg DM (85% DM). The horse theoretically can eat this amount because it is less than the maximum DM intake. Situation 2: 10 kg hay, approximately 8.5 kg DM (85% DM) + concentrate: 1 kg, approximately 0.850 kg DM (85% DM), so 9.35 kg DM in total and less than the maximum DM intake; so, the horse can eat these amounts.

Maximum sugar and starch intake: situation 2: 1 kg of concentrates, approximately 350 g of starch and sugars in 1 day. 350/550/2 meals = 0.318 g of starch and sugar/kg BW/meal, so less than the limit of 1–2 g/kg BW/meal; so, this intake level is safe.

Conclusion from this example: both situation 1 (hay-only diet) and situation 2 (hay + small amount of complementary feed) are above the minimum roughage intake and below the maximum DM and maximum sugar and starch intake levels. Nutritional assessment can be continued by evaluating other nutrient intake and nutritional management.

issue regarding the importance of feeding to support healthy gastrointestinal tract function.

○ Evaluate feed storage to determine that feeds are kept dry and complementary feeds are sealed to be protected from rodents/vermin.

Continuing the Assessment for the Equine with a Nutritionally Sensitive/Responsive Condition/Disease

- If not healthy, how can the disease/condition(s) be managed nutritionally? Some example considerations:
  ○ If there is presence of gastrointestinal disease, then see Harris and Shepherd's article, "What Would Be Good for all Veterinarians to Know About Equine Nutrition," in this issue regarding the importance of feeding to support healthy gastrointestinal tract function and Hesta and Costa's article, "How Can Nutrition Help with Gastrointestinal Tract-Based Issues," in this issue regarding managing gastrointestinal tract issues.
  ○ If poor fecal quality (amount, consistency, and length of undigested fibers), then see Hesta and Costa's article, "How Can Nutrition Help with Gastrointestinal Tract-Based Issues," in this issue regarding managing gastro-intestinal tract issues.
  ○ If dental disease (eg, malocclusion, missing teeth, or evidence of quidding/dropping feed), then see Jarvis and McKenzie's article, "Nutritional Considerations When Dealing with an Underweight Adult or Senior Horse," in this issue (underweight senior) or Shepherd and colleagues' article, "Nutritional Considerations When Dealing with an Obese Adult Equine," in this issue (overweight) because not all equines with dental disease are thin. Consider fiber length and food form. In cases of insufficient chewing, forage with a reduced fiber length may be needed. In severe cases, the traditional forage may have to be replaced by a complete feed or soaked feed/mash or soup, ensuring that fiber requirements are still met by using other fiber sources (eg, beet pulp, alfalfa, or grass cubes).[49]
  ○ Observe the equine eating, is there evidence of quidding/dropping feed and discomfort?
  ○ If poor hair/hoof/skin quality, then consider fatty acid, micromineral, vitamin, and S-containing amino acid intake.
  ○ If abnormal behavior (eg, pica, coprophagia, or crib biting), consider ways to provide environmental enrichment, maximize forage in the diet, and minimize time between meals. See Shepherd and colleagues' article, "Nutritional Considerations When Dealing with an Obese Adult Equine," in this issue regarding making the hay last and grazing muzzles.
  ○ If myopathy, then see Richards and colleagues' article, "Nutritional and Non-Nutritional Aspects of Forage," in this issue regarding forage nutrient deficiencies and Urschel and McKenzie's article, "Nutritional Influences on Skeletal Muscle and Muscular Disease," in this issue regarding nutrition and muscle.
- Laboratory diagnostics[50] can help refine the assessment.

Establishing Energy and Nutrient Requirements for the Individual Equine

The National Research Council (NRC)[10] hosts a Web form that allows users to enter individual equine information under "Animal Specifications" and retrieve general daily energy and essential nutrient requirements (https://nrc88.nas.edu/nrh/). Many countries also have their specific energy systems and nutrient requirements (eg, CVB[51] in Belgium and the Netherlands Lelystad; INRA[52] in France Paris; and GEH[53] in Germany). For the veterinarian, it is important to not compare between systems, for example, a net energy with a digestible energy unit or digestible protein requirements with crude protein (CP) intakes. This makes it important for veterinarians to stay with 1 system with which they are familiar.

If There Are Multiple Equines on the Farm, Considerations for Managing the Herd

- Can individuals be grouped by life stage (weanlings, yearlings, or pregnant mares) or performance (athletes with similar training)?
- Consider grouping equines by BCS (eg, group that needs prescribed weight gain, group that needs to maintain current healthy weight, and group that needs prescribed weight loss). Caregivers should note, however, that overweight equines may be more dominant[54]; thus, social dynamics must be considered to create cohesive groups.
- Social dynamics within a herd may prohibit certain groupings.
- What is the social hierarchy; which equine(s) are likely to be pushed from food and shelter? Or the opposite, which equines are more likely to be overeating?

ASSESS THE DIET/RATION AND FEEDING MANAGEMENT

Being physically present, ideally during at least 1 feeding period, is preferred over a remote dietary assessment because it improves the accuracy of the gathered information.[55] It also gives the opportunity to weigh the concentrates, forage, and supplements; to check the quality of all feed by opening bins and bales; and to take representable subsamples for chemical analysis, if needed.

Consider the Environment/Housing

- The equine's environment influences feeds available.
  ○ What feeds are available in the region?
  ○ Is fresh pasture available? If so, consider actually physically evaluating it on the farm instead of relying on the owner's input. Also, consider how season influences pasture forage availability and quality.
- How many hours per day are spent in a stall? Can these be amended, if required (ie, potential negative effect of stall confinement in gastric ulcers); what is the ventilation in the stall (respirable particles from the feed/forage); and what is the bedding (ie, straw and ingestion with potential risk for colic/mycotoxins, and so forth)?
- How many hours per day are spent outside? In a dry lot (no fresh forage) or on pasture?
- When outside, is there shelter from sun/rain/wind?
- In cold climates/during cold seasons, are blankets/rugs available?
- How is drinking water offered and is it accessible (decreased water intake can lead to constipation and impaction) and potable?
  ○ Offered to the group or individually? Can an individual block the access?
  ○ What is the water offered in? Trough, bucket, automatic water dispenser, or stream? Are horses familiar with the automatic system? Could the system have failed?
  ○ Is the water accessible; can the equine(s) easily get to the water source? For example, equines with significant orthopedic discomfort may have a hard time getting to water in an unlevel area.
  ○ How often is the water trough/bucket cleaned and refreshed?

- In cold areas or during cold seasons, how is the water managed to prevent freezing? Some equines have water temperature preferences.
- Is algae present? Presence of algae suggests that the trough/bucket is past due for cleaning.
- What is the water quality? Although it is uncommon for water to be submitted for water quality testing (eg, total dissolved solids, coliform count, and hardness), this can be done and may be indicated in some circumstances (eg, enteroliths). If the water source is municipal/town, then a water quality should be tested regularly by the municipality, and analysis should be available to the farm owner. If the water source is a well/bore hole, then water quality testing is the responsibility of the farm owner.[56,57]
- Could water intake be quantified? This is rarely so but important to be aware of should water intake monitoring become essential to care (eg, postimpaction colic).
- Note, drinking water intake is lower with fresh pasture forage than with hay.

What Type of Forage Is Fed; What Is the Quality; How Much Is Fed; and How Is It Measured and How Is It Offered?

Forage type and format (see Harris and Shepherd's article, "What Would Be Good for all Veterinarians to Know About Equine Nutrition," and Richards and colleagues' article, "Nutritional and Non-Nutritional Aspects of Forage," in this issue)

- Different types of forage can have different nutrient contents. Legume type of forage, such as alfalfa, are higher in protein compared with grasses. Also, the type of grass may influence nutrient digestibility.
- Forage format (see Harris and Shepherd's article, "What Would Be Good for all Veterinarians to Know About Equine Nutrition," in this issue)
  - Pasture or preserved, for example, silage, haylage, hay, or straw
    - Differences in DM content between hay and haylage influence nutrient intake (less nutrient intake for haylage on an as-fed basis if has the same nutrient content on DM basis as hay).
    - Straw contains a low amount of protein, minerals, and vitamins compared with hay[10,51]; when large amounts are eaten, it may cause impaction in sensitive animals.[33]
  - Long-stem or chopped, cubed, or pelleted? Chewing time of pelleted hay is reduced by 75% compared with traditional hay.[58,59]
  - If pasture, how many hectares and with how many other equines and for how many hours per day?
    - If pasture, is there an even cover of grass, grass, and legume?
    - If pasture, what is the forage make-up, for example, even cover of grass, grass and legume, or weeds? Intake of poisonous plants like ragwort is more likely when grass availability is low.
  - See Harris and Shepherd's article, "What Would Be Good for all Veterinarians to Know About Equine Nutrition," in this issue for more information about forage format.

Forage quality (see Harris and Shepherd's article, "What Would Be Good for all Veterinarians to Know About Equine Nutrition," in this issue)

- Forage quality matters. For example, if an equine is fed 9.1 kg (20 lb) grass hay per day, calorie/energy provision is 14 Mcal (59 MJ) from a poor-quality grass hay

(1.54 Mcal [6.44 MJ] per kg, as fed) versus 18 Mcal (75 MJ) from a high-quality grass hay (1.98 Mcal [8.28 MJ] per kg, as fed); a difference of 4 Mcal (17 MJ) per day or 120 Mcal (502 MJ) per month!

- Forage quality may be assessed using visual/olfactory/tactile senses and nutrient analysis.[60]
  - Visual/olfactory/tactile assessment of forage includes evaluation of color, presence of foreign debris, aroma, presence of seed heads, and leaf-to-stem ratio. Ideally, hay should be low dust, free of debris (plastic, dead animals/insects), less than 5% debris (tree leaves and weeds), free of visual and olfactory evidence of mold, and not yellow in color.
  - Hay should feel dry outside and in; if moisture and warmth are felt between flakes, then the moisture content is too high.
  - As a guide
    - Stemmy and lots of seed heads = mature
    - Soft and no seed heads = immature
    - Forages with a low leaf-to-stem ratio (ie, relatively stemmy hays) are more appropriate for the overweight equine than for the underweight equine.
- Nutrient analysis is a more precise method for determining forage quality but often is the responsibility of the consumer versus the producer.
  - Methods of nutrient analysis include near-infrared spectroscopy and wet chemistry. Wet chemistry is ideally conducted using proximate analysis and Van Soest methods. The Van Soest analytical method better identifies cell wall components, that is, structural fibers. Near-infrared spectroscopy could be a cheaper alternative for wet chemistry (except potentially for water-soluble sugars and starch) if proper calibration curves are provided and if pre-dried samples are used.[61]
- When sampling forage for nutrient analysis, each batch of forage (ie, first cutting orchard grass and second cutting orchard grass) must be sampled and nutritionally analyzed separately.
- Guidelines for sampling a forage for nutrient analysis
  - Hay: the sample should be representative (generally 10% of bales in a batch should be sampled) and as random as possible. The authors typically sample approximately 10 bales of those available to sample (on the outside of the stack). A forage corer ideally is needed (vs hand-grab). Hay corers may be purchased or borrowed. In the United States, generally, veterinarians or owners may either borrow a hay corer from a local extension office or request that an extension agent come to the farm to sample the hay.
  - Haylage: care should be taken to only sample bales that will be used within the next 1 day to 2 days to prevent unhygienic conditions like molding.
  - Pasture: forage continues to respire if moisture concentration is greater than 40%. Fresh forages should be immediately frozen and shipped on ice to best capture the nutrient content of the forage as when sampled.
- Evaluating the nutrient analysis
  - DM concentration is an indication of proper hay preservation. Target DM for hay is greater than 85% (<15% moisture); see Harris and Shepherd's article, "What Would Be Good for all Veterinarians to Know About Equine Nutrition," in this issue.
  - Energy content
    - Based on forage data, an adult equine at maintenance (ie, not growing, breeding, pregnant, lactating, or working) easily could overconsume

calories relative to requirements when fed a moderate-quality to good-quality forage-free choice.[62]

○ Neutral detergent fiber (NDF) represents how bulky or filling the forage is; analytically, NDF represents the structural cell wall constituents, cellulose, hemicellulose, and lignin. Generally, NDF correlates negatively with intake.[59]

○ Acid detergent fiber (ADF) represents total tract digestibility; analytically, ADF represents hemicellulose and lignin; lignin negatively influences digestibility; ADF trends in parallel with NDF. See Harris and Shepherd's article, "What Would Be Good for all Veterinarians to Know About Equine Nutrition," and Shepherd and colleagues' article, "Nutritional Considerations When Dealing with an Obese Adult Equine," in this issue.

○ Protein
  ■ CP—9% to 13% CP and 18% to 20% CP on a DM basis generally are considered good quality for grass and alfalfa, respectively. CP requirements are dependent, however, on findings in the Patient Assessment section.
  ■ Digestible protein takes into account the digestibility of the protein source in horses.[63] When available, these data are preferred over CP data.

○ Water-soluble carbohydrates represent sugars plus fructan. See Harris and Shepherd's article, "What Would Be Good for all Veterinarians to Know About Equine Nutrition," and Shepherd and colleagues' article, "Nutritional Considerations When Dealing with an Obese Adult Equine," in this issue regarding water-soluble carbohydrates.

• See Harris and Shepherd's article, "What Would Be Good for all Veterinarians to Know About Equine Nutrition," in this issue regarding the forage type and hygiene.

How much forage is fed?

• Ideally, forage is fed at a minimum of 1.5% of BW in DM. Forage always should make up greater than 50% of total daily DM offered. Energy requirement/demand, however, should be considered. For example, a 100:0 forage-to-concentrate ratio may work for the equine in 1 hour of light work daily; a 50:50 forage-to-concentrate ratio may work for the equine exercising intensively or for a long duration. The highest possible forage-to-concentrate ratio should be strived for while meeting energy and macronutrient needs and not exceeding the maximum DM intake. For maintenance, light excercise and ealry gestation the anticipated dry matter intake is 2% of the BW. For moderate excercise and heavy/very heavy excercise, lactation and growth the anticipated dry matter intake increases to 2.25 and 2.5% BW respectively.[11]

• Complete feeds may be fed in absence of forage in that they are formulated to be relatively high in fiber. Feeding complete feeds without long-stem forage, however, should be reserved for specific situations (eg, severe dental disease, right dorsal colitis, and acute typhlocolitis).

• When there is an indication to feed less than 1.5% of BW (obesity treatment or intensive care nutrition), monitoring for colic and behavioral issues becomes increasingly important; see Shepherd and colleagues' article, "Nutritional Considerations When Dealing with an Obese Adult Equine," in this issue (obese). Traditionally and commonly, forage is fed by volume (eg, flake or bale). There is no weight standard, however, for a flake or bale. Feeding by weight allows for greater precision, and veterinarians should insist on weighing the amounts at least for evaluation of the ration.

- See Harris and Shepherd's article, "What Would Be Good for all Veterinarians to Know About Equine Nutrition," in this issue regarding how much equines eat.

How is the forage offered?

- Pasture
  - For how many hours per day is the equine on pasture?
  - As pasture access increases, the amount of preserved forage (eg, hay or hay-lage) should be reduced.
  - Are toxic plants present?
  - Is a grazing muzzle used? If there is current trouble in using a grazing muzzle (eg, equine successfully removes muzzle), then the approach to using a grazing muzzle needs to be reassessed. See Shepherd and colleagues' article, "Nutritional Considerations When Dealing with an Obese Adult Equine," in this issue (obese) regarding grazing muzzles.
- Processed forage (eg, hay)
  - Is the forage fed on the ground, in a trough, or in a hay net or a slow feeder?
    - Does the hay net look safe to use; is it intact; and could an equine stick a hoof through it? See Shepherd and colleagues' article, "Nutritional Considerations When Dealing with an Obese Adult Equine," in this issue regarding the use of slow feeder hay nets.
    - Keeping a horse on a sand lot can increase the risk of sand colic, especially if feeding hay directly of the ground, and keeping a horse on a dry lot may increase the risk of dermatologic problems like scratches (also known as mud fever).
  - How often is forage fed and how much time does the equine spend between meals? Ideally, the equine should not be fasted for more than 5 hours, except possibly a period over overnight.

Consider Feeds Other than Forage (eg, Grain and Commercial/Complementary Feeds)

- Nonforage feeds should make up less than 50% of total daily DM and, as discussed previously (How much forage is fed?), the highest forage-to-concentrate ratio considering the energy requirement should be strived for. See Harris and Shepherd's article, "What Would Be Good for all Veterinarians to Know About Equine Nutrition," in this issue regarding the importance of maximizing forage
- Is an energy-dense feed fed? And is it really needed?
- Are straight grains (eg, oats) fed? If corn or barley is fed, is it heat treated? When feeding straight grains, a ration balancer may be required to correct the inverse calcium-to-phosphorus ratio/low lysine/low vitamin content in grains.
  - Is a commercial textured or sweet feed fed?
    - If a commercial complementary feed is fed below manufacturer guidelines, then essential nutrient requirement may not be met and a commercial vitamin mineral supplement should be added.
  - Is a life-stage commercial feed provided (eg, mare and foal, senior, or creep feed to the suckling foal formulated for preweanling/suckling foals) and is it appropriate (eg, feeding a performance feed to a nonperforming equine)? Senior feeds still can be appropriate for a nonsenior equine in need of a feed with

such an energy/protein/fiber profile, and many seniors can be fed a suitable nonsenior feed.

- o How much is fed per meal and what is the starch content? A healthy equine should not receive more than 2 g of starch and sugar/kg BW/meal[4,10,64]; no more than 1 g/kg BW/meal,[65] if a horse is sensitive to starch. See also Harris and Shepherd's article, "What Would Be Good for all Veterinarians to Know About Equine Nutrition,", Hesta and Costa's article, "How Can Nutrition Help with Gastrointestinal Tract-Based Issues," and Shepherd and colleagues' article, "Nutritional Considerations When Dealing with an Obese Adult Equine," in this issue regarding limiting dietary starch and maximizing forage.
- o Is enough fed to meet all essential nutrient requirements?
  - ▪ Ration balancing software may be purchased or some feed companies offer free ration balancing software to veterinarians. This can be a useful tool when the limitations are fully appreciated and the interpretation of the output is done carefully.[66]
- Is a ration or forage balancer fed? If daily energy requirements are met with forage alone, a complementary feed is not needed for energy purposes. Forage alone, however, typically does not meet all essential nutrient requirements, especially sodium, chloride, trace mineral, and vitamins requirements. Therefore, a ration balancer often is needed.
  - o Vitamin E is needed in a ration balancer when processed forage is fed because it is not an adequate source of vitamin E unlike most fresh pasture. Vitamin E requirements increase with sport activity but also when supplementing vegetable oil.[67] See also Richards and colleagues' article, "Nutritional and Non-Nutritional Aspects of Forage," and Urschel and McKenzie's article, "Nutritional Influences on Skeletal Muscle and Muscular Disease," in this issue
  - o A trace mineral salt block/fortified lick stone generally is not a good replacer for a balancer because trace element concentrations generally are low and intake is very variable (from zero to excessive intake).
- Evaluate feed quality
  - o Any evidence of mold, foreign objects, dead animals, or toxic plants?
  - o What is the likely nutrient content? For noncommercial feeds, feed analysis laboratories can be good resources because some publish statistics on the feeds they analyze.[68] For commercial feeds, what information do they have available on a Web site and on the feed label? If more information is needed, then the manufacturer should be contacted. Asking about nutrient content is appropriate; the recipe likely is proprietary, but the nutrient content and ingredient list should not be.
  - o What is the starch and sugar content? See Harris and Shepherd's article, "What Would Be Good for all Veterinarians to Know About Equine Nutrition," in this issue regarding the importance of limiting starch to promote gastrointestinal health. See Shepherd and colleagues' article, "Nutritional Considerations When Dealing with an Obese Adult Equine," in this issue regarding feeding the obese horse.
  - o What is the manufacturer/company's reputation and adherence to quality systems (eg, Good Manufacturing Practice and Hazard Analysis and Critical Control Points)? Does the company have a properly trained team with a knowledge of equine physiology and nutrition, engineering, and food safety? Do their scientists publish in peer-reviewed scientific journals?

- Is a salt lick block available? Is it equine-specific? Is it molasses (If so, is it considered when evaluating sugar intake?)? Is it consumed? Some animals do not use the salt lick it at all, whereas others may overconsume. An electrolyte supplement could be more effective than a salt lick in correcting deficiencies after excessive sweating.
- Is there an item/product in the ration the veterinarian is unfamiliar with? Are supplements/nutraceuticals fed? Is there evidence of efficacy and safety? For the large majority, there is not. Could the nutraceutical result in a positive doping analysis? See Bishop and Dzanis's article, "Staying on the Right Side of the Regulatory Authorities," and Vervuert and Stratton-Phelps's article, "The Safety and Efficacy in Horses of Certain Nutraceuticals That Claim to Have Health Benefits," in this issue.
- Are treats fed (fruit, vegetables, commercial treats, and candy)? What is fed and how much? Are they safe?
- With all feeds factored in, especially forage and complementary feeds/energy-dense feeds, what is the total daily DM provision?

COMMUNICATION

Effective communication enhances history taking, compliance, and overall connection with equine owners/trainers/managers/caregivers. Effective implementation of currently available tools maximizes success. Effective communication is key to effective implementation and compliance. For example, taking a diet history with close-ended questions (eg, yes/no or what) likely limits the information gathered.[69] Without a clear view of the equine's current diet/ration, the recommended ration is based, at least in part, on speculation. Diet history taking and analysis are time-consuming. Spending a little extra time up-front, however, can save time in the long run.[70] For example, if what is practical and available to the owner is not considered, then the owner is not able to be compliant. If an equine is to be fed every 6 hours for an illness, it first should be determined if this is possible, given the current resources. Furthermore, feed accessibility to the caregiver should be considered; for example, a feed that is not practical should not be recommended; increasing turnout should not be recommended, if that is not an option where currently kept.

Care should be taken to not judge the owner during the assessment (eg, embarrassing the owner for overfeeding their obese equine or making an owner feel like they have made an obvious mistake that caused an illness). Judgment and guilt are barriers to communication, limit information gathered, and prevent effective care.

Consider all barriers to effective communication. Connection built through effective communication likely will foster compliance. Serve as a guide, rather than an authoritarian, center the owner in the dialogue versus talking at the owner.[71–74] Provide options, identify obstacles for the owner, provide solutions. Be cognizant about wording and nonverbal communication, give clear recommendations, avoid ambiguity, use first person versus "you".[75–77] Ensure that the owner understands why the recommendations/suggestions matter and what the rationale and follow-up are.[72] Provide a written summary of the to-do's and take-home messages, which includes details about whom to contact in cases of questions/problems with applying the advice.

Incorporating nutritional assessment into daily practice; some tips from companion animal nutrition[78,79]:

- Request owners to complete the nutritional history form prior to the visit and evaluate it.
- Place it in the medical record.
- Include muscle and body condition evaluation in your clinical examination.
- Make written recommendations.
- Provide informational handouts, brochures, and specific measuring cups, if needed.

ESTABLISH GOALS AND REASSESS

Establish goals; what does the diet/ration need to accomplish?

- Maintain current or achieve healthy weight; see Shepherd and colleagues' article, "Nutritional Considerations When Dealing with an Obese Adult Equine," in this issue.
- Maintain current or enhance athletic performance (eg, replace starch calories with fat calories to help reduce reactivity); see Urschel and McKenzie's article, "Nutritional Influences on Skeletal Muscle and Muscular Disease," and Vervuert and Stratton-Phelps's article, "The Safety and Efficacy in Horses of Certain Nutraceuticals That Claim to Have Health Benefits," in this issue.
- Maintain current or enhance reproductive performance; See Robles and colleagues' article, "Nutrition of Broodmares," in this issue.
- Reduce risk of disease (eg, developmental orthopedic disease, equine gastric ulcer syndrome, colic, or laminitis). See Harris and Shepherd's article, "What Would Be Good for all Veterinarians to Know About Equine Nutrition," and Hesta and Costa's article, "How Can Nutrition Help with Gastrointestinal Tract-Based Issues," in this issue.
- Manage nutrition-related diseases (eg, recurrent colic, gastric ulcers, laminitis, recurrent exertional rhabdomyolysis, polysaccharide storage myopathy, dental disease, and liver disease). See Hesta and Costa's article, "How Can Nutrition Help with Gastrointestinal Tract-Based Issues,", Jarvis and McKenzie's article, "Nutritional Considerations When Dealing with an Underweight Adult or Senior Horse," and Shepherd and colleagues' article, "Nutritional Considerations When Dealing with an Obese Adult Equine," in this issue.

Once the nutrition assessment is complete, recommendations may be drawn. Reassessment is critical for determining if the original recommendations are appropriate and the frequency of reassessment should be adapted individually. Conducting nutrition assessments should be an iterative process as the diet/ration should be adjusted as needed.

SUMMARY

A nutrition assessment includes evaluating the patient and the current diet/ration/feeds and feeding management. Effective history taking, using more open-ended questions, may take a bit more time but provides a clearer picture of the equine, the diet, and the owner's resources. Consider the role of effective communication and connection with the owner throughout the process. Finally, when in doubt, consultat with an equine nutritionist, preferably one who is experienced and up to date with training.

REFERENCES

1. Horseman S. The four priority welfare challenges. Equine Vet Educ 2017;29: 415–6.
2. Harris P. Feeding management of elite endurance horses. Vet Clin North Am Equine Pract 2009;25:137–53, viii.
3. Harris PA, Geor RJ. 36 - Nutrition for the equine athlete: nutrient requirements and key principles in ration design. In: Hinchcliff KW, Kaneps AJ, Geor RJ, editors. Equine sports medicine and surgery. 2nd edition. W.B. Saunders; 2014. p. 797–817. Available at: http://www.sciencedirect.com/science/article/pii/B9780702047718000363. Accessed August 31, 2020.
4. Vergnano D, Bergero D, Valle E. Clinical nutrition counselling service in the veterinary hospital: retrospective analysis of equine patients and nutritional considerations. J Anim Physiol Anim Nutr (Berl) 2017;101(Suppl 1):59–68.
5. Caloni F, Cortinovis C. Plants poisonous to horses in Europe. Equine Vet Educ 2015;27:269–74.
6. World Small Animal Veterinary Association Nutritional Assessment Guidelines Task Force. 2011 nutritional assessment guidelines. J S Afr Vet Assoc 2011;82: 254–63.
7. Becvarova I, Pleasant RS, Thatcher CD. Clinical assessment of nutritional status and feeding programs in horses. Vet Clin North Am Equine Pract 2009;25:1–21.
8. American College of Veterinary Nutrition. Nutrition Competencies of Equine Veterinarians. Available at: http://acvn.org/wp-content/uploads/2016/01/ACVN-Competencies-Equine.pdf. Accessed June 22, 2020.
9. Mastellar SL, Rosenthal EJ, Carroll HK, et al. Assessment of Equine Feeding Practices and Knowledge of Equine Nutrition in the Midwest. J Equine Vet Sci 2018;62:109–15.
10. NRC. Nutrient requirements of horses. 6th edition. Washington DC: The National Academies Press; 2007.
11. Jarvis N, Paradis MR, Harris P. Nutrition considerations for the aged horse. Equine Vet Educ 2019;31:102–10.
12. Cox R, Burden F, Gosden L, et al. Case control study to investigate risk factors for impaction colic in donkeys in the UK. Prev Vet Med 2009;92:179–87.
13. Siard-Altman MH, Harris PA, Moffett-Krotky AD, et al. Relationships of inflammaging with circulating nutrient levels, body composition, age, and pituitary pars intermedia dysfunction in a senior horse population. Vet Immunol Immunopathol 2020;221:110013.
14. Salem SE, Scantlebury CE, Ezzat E, et al. Colic in a working horse population in Egypt: Prevalence and risk factors. Equine Vet J 2017;49:201–6.
15. Jacob SI, Geor RJ, Weber PSD, et al. Effect of age and dietary carbohydrate profiles on glucose and insulin dynamics in horses. Equine Vet J 2018;50:249–54.
16. Giles SL, Rands SA, Nicol CJ, et al. Obesity prevalence and associated risk factors in outdoor living domestic horses and ponies. PeerJ 2014;2:e299. Available at: https://www.ncbi.nlm.nih.gov/pmc/articles/PMC3970797/. Accessed May 29, 2020.
17. Bamford NJ, Potter SJ, Harris PA, et al. Breed differences in insulin sensitivity and insulinemic responses to oral glucose in horses and ponies of moderate body condition score. Domest Anim Endocrinol 2014;47:101–7.
18. Burden FA, Bell N. Donkey Nutrition and Malnutrition. Vet Clin North Am Equine Pract 2019;35:469–79.

19. Smith, DG, Burden, FA. Practical donkey and mule nutrition. In: Equine applied and clinical nutrition. vol. 1. 2013. p. 304–316. Available at: https://doi.org/10.1016/C2009-0-39370-8.

20. Nicholas F. Equine Metabolic Syndrome. J Equine Vet Sci 2009;29:259–67.

21. Thatcher CD, Pleasant RS, Geor RJ, et al. Prevalence of Overconditioning in Mature Horses in Southwest Virginia during the Summer. J Vet Intern Med 2012;26:1413–8.

22. Martinson KL, Coleman RC, Rendahl AK, et al. Estimation of body weight and development of a body weight score for adult equids using morphometric measurements. J Anim Sci 2014;92:2230–8.

23. Rodríguez C, Rojas H, Briones M, et al. New formula for bodyweight estimation of thoroughbred foals. Vet Rec 2007;161:165–6.

24. Staniar WB, Kronfeld DS, Hoffman RM, et al. Weight prediction from linear measures of growing Thoroughbreds. Equine Vet J 2004;36:149–54.

25. Peugnet P, Mendoza L, Wimel L, et al. Longitudinal Study of Growth and Osteoarticular Status in Foals Born to Between-Breed Embryo Transfers. J Equine Vet Sci 2016;37:24–38.

26. Staniar, William B. Feeding the growing horse. In: Equine applied and clinical nutrition. 2013. p. 243–60.

27. Austbo D. The Scandinavian adaptation of the French UFC System. In: 3rd European Workshop equine nutrition, vol. 111. The Netherlands: EAAP Wageningen Academic Publishers; 2004. p. 69–78.

28. Coenen M. German feeding standards. In: 2000 Equine Nutr. Conf. for Feed Manufacturers. Versailles, KY, 2000;159–173.

29. Henneke DR, Potter GD, Kreider JL, et al. Relationship between Condition Score, Physical Measurements and Body-Fat Percentage in Mares. Equine Vet J 1983;15:371–2.

30. Burkholder WJ. Use of body condition scores in clinical assessment of the provision of optimal nutrition. J Am Vet Med Assoc 2000;217:650–4.

31. Dugdale AH, Grove-White D, Curtis GC, et al. Body condition scoring as a predictor of body fat in horses and ponies. Vet J 2012;194(2):173–8. Available at: http://www.ncbi.nlm.nih.gov/pubmed/22578691.

32. E. Kienzle, Schramme, S.C. Body condition scoring and prediction of body weight in adult warm blooded horses. Pferdeheilkunde 20:517–524.

33. Harris PA, Ellis AD, Fradinho MJ, et al. Review: Feeding conserved forage to horses: recent advances and recommendations. animal 2017;11:958–67.

34. Ringmark S, Roepstorff L, Essén-Gustavsson B, et al. Growth, training response and health in Standardbred yearlings fed a forage-only diet. Animal 2013;7:746–53.

35. Willing B, Voros A, Roos S, et al. Changes in faecal bacteria associated with concentrate and forage-only diets fed to horses in training. Equine Vet J 2009;41:908–14.

36. Varloud M, de Fombelle A, Goachet AG, et al. Partial and total apparent digestibility of dietary carbohydrates in horses as affected by the diet. Anim Sci 2004;79:61–72.

37. Kienzle E, Pohlenz J, Radicke S. Morphology of Starch Digestion in The Horse. J Vet Med Ser A 1997;44:207–21.

38. Jarvis NG. Nutrition of the Aged Horse. Vet Clin North Am Equine Pract 2009;25:155–66.

39. Nicholls VM, Townsend N. Dental disease in aged horses and its management. Vet Clin North Am Equine Pract 2016;32:215–27.

40. Potter SJ, Bamford NJ, Harris PA, et al. Prevalence of obesity and owners' perceptions of body condition in pleasure horses and ponies in south-eastern Australia. Aust Vet J 2016;94:427–32.
41. Morrison PK, Harris PA, Maltin CA, et al. Perceptions of obesity and management practices in a UK population of leisure-horse owners and managers. J Equine Vet Sci 2017;53:19–29.
42. Smith DG, Mayes RW, Hollands T, et al. Validating the alkane pair technique to estimate dry matter intake in equids. J Agr Sci 2007;145:273–81.
43. Longland AC, Ince J, Harris PA. Estimation of pasture intake by ponies from live-weight change during six weeks at pasture. J Equine Vet Sci 2011;31:275–6.
44. Longland AC, Barfoot C, Harris PA. Effects of grazing muzzles on intakes of dry matter and water-soluble carbohydrates by ponies grazing spring, summer, and autumn swards, as well as autumn swards of different heights. J Equine Vet Sci 2016;40:26–33.
45. Longland AC, Barfoot C, Harris PA. The effect of wearing a grazing muzzle vs not wearing a grazing muzzle on pasture dry matter intake by ponies. J Equine Vet Sci 2011;31:282–3.
46. Fitzgerald DM, Anderson ST, Sillence MN, et al. The cresty neck score is an independent predictor of insulin dysregulation in ponies. PLoS One 2019;14: e0220203.
47. Carter R, Geor R, Staniar W, et al. Apparent adiposity assessed by standardised scoring systems and morphometric measurements in horses and ponies. Vet J 2009;204–10.
48. Anon. Global Nutrition Guidelines | WSAVA Global Veterinary Community. Available at: https://www.wsava.org/Guidelines/Global-Nutrition-Guidelines. Accessed January 13, 2020.
49. Argo CM. Nutritional Management of the Older Horse. Vet Clin North Am Equine Pract 2016;32:343–54.
50. Duncan C. Equine Pathology and Laboratory Diagnostics. Veterinary Clinics of North America: Equine Practice 2015;31. Available at: https://www.elsevier.com/books/equine-pathology-and-laboratory-diagnostics-an-issue-of-veterinary-clinics-of-north-america-equine-practice/duncan/978-0-323-39362-1. Accessed October 12, 2020.
51. CVB. Chemische samenstelling, verteerbaarheid en voederwaarde van voeder-middelen. The Netherlands: Veevoedertabel. Lelystad; 2000.
52. Martin-Rosset W. Alimentation des chevaux. Paris: INRA Editions; 1990.
53. Ebert M, Moore-Colyer M. The energy requirements of performance horses in training. Transl Anim Sci 2020;4:569–88.
54. Giles SL, Nicol CJ, Harris PA, et al. Dominance rank is associated with body condition in outdoor-living domestic horses (Equus caballus). Appl Anim Behav Sci 2015;166:71–9.
55. Dunnett C. Dunnett C., 2013, Ration evaluation an formulation, E. 2013. p. 405–24.
56. Kamhues J. Feed hygiene and related disorders in horses. In: Equine applied and clinical nutrition. 2013. p. 375–6.
57. Cymbaluk N. 4 - Water. In: Geor RJ, Harris PA, Coenen M, editors. Equine applied and clinical nutrition. W.B. Saunders; 2013. p. 80–95. Available at: http://www.sciencedirect.com/science/article/pii/B9780702034220000031. Accessed October 2, 2020.
58. Ellis A. Biological basis of behaviour in relation to nutrition and feed intake in horses. EAAP Sci Ser 2010;128:53–74.

59. Cuddeford D. 3 - Factors affecting feed intake. In: Geor RJ, Harris PA, Coenen M, editors. Equine applied and clinical nutrition. W.B. Saunders; 2013. p. 64–79. Available at: http://www.sciencedirect.com/science/article/pii/B9780702034 220000031. Accessed October 2, 2020.

60. Julliand S, Dacremont C, Omphalius C, et al. Association between nutritional values of hays fed to horses and sensory properties as perceived by human sight, touch and smell. Animal 2019;13:1834–42.

61. Harris PA, Nelson S, Carslake HB, et al. Comparison of NIRS and Wet Chemistry Methods for the Nutritional Analysis of Haylages for Horses. J Equine Vet Sci 2018;71:13–20.

62. Anon. Common Feed Profiles | Equianalytical. Available at: https://equi-analytical.com/common-feed-profiles/. Accessed December 11, 2019.

63. Anon. CVB tabellenboek voeding paarden en pony's : voederbehoeften en waardering van voedermiddelen | Groenekennis. Available at: https://library.wur.nl/WebQuery/groenekennis/2060009. Accessed June 30, 2020.

64. Hoffman R. 8 - Carbohydrates. In: Geor RJ, Harris PA, Coenen M, editors. Equine applied and clinical nutrition. W.B. Saunders; 2013. p. 156–67. Available at: http://www.sciencedirect.com/science/article/pii/B9780702034220000031. Accessed October 2, 2020.

65. Durham A. 35 - Intestinal Disease. In: Geor RJ, Harris PA, Coenen M, editors. Equine applied and clinical nutrition. W.B. Saunders; 2013. p. 568–81. Available at: http://www.sciencedirect.com/science/article/pii/B978070203422000016X. Accessed October 12, 2020.

66. Dunnett C. Ration evaluation an formulation. In: Equine applied and clinical nutrition. , 2013;405–424.

67. Harris PA, Schott HC. 14 - Nutritional management of elite endurance horses. In: Geor RJ, Harris PA, Coenen M, editors. Equine applied and clinical nutrition. W.B. Saunders; 2013. p. 272–88. Available at: http://www.sciencedirect.com/science/article/pii/B9780702034220000146. Accessed October 12, 2020.

68. Anon. Feed Composition Library | Dairy One. Available at: https://dairyone.com/services/forage-laboratory-services/feed-composition-library/. Accessed May 29, 2020.

69. MacMartin C, Wheat HC, Coe JB, et al. Effect of question design on dietary information solicited during veterinarian-client interactions in companion animal practice in Ontario, Canada. J Am Vet Med Assoc 2015;246:1203–14.

70. Coe JB, O'Connor RE, MacMartin C, et al. Effects of three diet history questions on the amount of information gained from a sample of pet owners in Ontario, Canada. J Am Vet Med Assoc 2020;256:469–78.

71. Jessica Vogelsang. The irresistible magic of story. In: Hill's Global Symposium Proceedings. Toronto, Canada, 2019.

72. MacMartin C, Wheat HC, Coe JB, et al. Conversation analysis of veterinarians' proposals for long-term dietary change in companion animal practice in Ontario, Canada. J Vet Med Educ 2018;45(4):514–33.

73. Cornell KK, Kopcha M. Client-veterinarian communication: skills for client centered dialogue and shared decision making. Vet Clin North Am Small Anim Pract 2007;37:37–47.

74. Abood SK. Increasing adherence in practice: making your clients partners in care. Vet Clin North Am Small Anim Pract 2007;37:151–64.

75. Carson CA. Nonverbal communication in veterinary practice. Vet Clin North Am Small Anim Pract 2007;37:49–63.

76. Fitzpatrick SL, Wischenka D, Appelhans BM, et al. An evidence-based guide for obesity treatment in primary care. Am J Med 2016;129:115.e1-7.

77. Murphy M. Obesity treatment: environment and behavior modification. Vet Clin North Am Small Anim Pract 2016;46:883–98.

78. Rollins AW, Murphy M. Nutritional assessment in the cat: Practical recommendations for better medical care. J Feline Med Surg 2019;21:442–8.

79. Shepherd M. How to Feed the Overweight Performance Horse. In: Proceedings, Am Assoc Equine Pract. Vol 66. virtual, 2020;55–60.

.

Nutritional and Non-nutritional Aspects of Forage

Nerida Richards, PhD, RAnNutr[a],*, Brian D. Nielsen, PhD, PAS[b],
Carrie J. Finno, DVM, PhD[c]

KEYWORDS

- Forage • Roughage • Pasture • Fiber • Nonstructural carbohydrate • Mycotoxins
- Nitrate • Vitamins • Minerals • Grasses • Legumes • Supplementation

KEY POINTS

- Forages comprise an important part of the equine diet, often providing most of the nutrients fed to horses. By weight, forages should form the bulk of a horse's ration.
- Forages can vary widely in terms of digestible energy, protein, minerals, and vitamin content and forage(s) chosen for a particular horse should suit that individual's needs.
- However, forages alone may not be able to meet the full amino acid, mineral, and/or vitamin requirements of horses, particularly broodmares, horses in work and young, growing horses.
- Testing of forages for nutrient content enables rations to be designed that appropriately meet requirements.
- Non-nutritional factors can influence forage quality including, but not limited to, weeds, mold, mycotoxins, nitrates, and other noxious factors.

INTRODUCTION

Forages play a crucial role in the diet of horses. The inclusion of adequate forage promotes both physical and mental health.[1] An insufficient daily intake of forages can result in weight loss, nutrient deficiency, compromised fore and hindgut health, and dysbiosis, as well as the development of behavioral abnormalities. Although the mantra "forage first"—implying one should start by evaluating the forage portion of the diet and then provide a concentrate or complementary feed or ration balancer to meet nutrient requirements—is a wise approach, often this is misinterpreted to

[a] Equilize Horse Nutrition Pty Ltd, PO Box 11034, Tamworth, New South Wales 2340, Australia;
[b] Department of Animal Science, Michigan State University, 1287D Anthony Hall, 474 S. Shaw Lane, East Lansing, MI 48824-1225, USA; [c] Population Health and Reproduction, University of California Davis School of Veterinary Medicine, One Shields Avenue, Davis, CA 95616, USA
* Corresponding author.
E-mail address: nerida@equilize.com.au

Vet Clin Equine 37 (2021) 43–61
https://doi.org/10.1016/j.cveq.2020.12.002   vetequine.theclinics.com

mean "forage only." Although many horses survive and seem to thrive on a forage only diet, forage amino acid, vitamin, and/or mineral deficiencies, which are impossible to visually diagnose, and can be expensive to determine analytically, frequently exist. Without thoroughly evaluating the type and quantity of forage fed, one cannot be assured that all dietary requirements are met (and not fed to excess). Further, a forage that is appropriate for one class of horse (or individual) may not be appropriate for another. For instance, a hay that is harvested while immature and is high in energy may be considered "good hay" for a heavily exercising athletic horse, but it might prove to be too good for a sedentary horse with equine metabolic syndrome. Hence, having an understanding of the factors that differentiate various forages is critical for designing or evaluating what should be the foundation of any equine diet. Veterinarians should also consider the various non-nutritional forage factors that are outside the scope of this article, for example, the presence of poisonous weeds,[2] mycotoxins such as slaframine, or bacterial toxins (botulism). Hygienic aspects are mentioned in Patricia Harris and Megan Shepherd's article, "What Would Be Good for All Veterinarians to Know About Equine Nutrition," in this issue.

The importance of having forages analyzed for nutritional content cannot be overemphasized. Forages should constitute the majority of the diet, and thus be the primary source of the majority of nutrients consumed by horses. Therefore, not knowing what is provided by the forage is a major limitation in determining whether nutritional requirements are being met or if there are any concerns that need to be addressed in the diet. However, it is recognized that often forages are bought in small batches and the source of the forage may change frequently—in which case sending in a sample for analysis is of limited use, because the results from the analysis may not be back before the forage has been consumed. The ideal situation for conserved forges would be that all forage producers provide an analysis. Although this does happen in some parts of the world, it is not yet commonplace. As an industry, we need to start asking for prepurchase analyses to encourage this practice to become the standard. With pasture, given that the nutrient content of pastures can change dramatically over time, it is recognized that pasture analysis gives only an indication of what was being consumed at the time of sampling and the results may, therefore, have limited usefulness. However, with consistent sampling over time, a useful database of pasture nutrient values through various seasons can be developed. In any case, where an analysis is not possible, relying instead on typical nutrient values for the specific type of forage may give a reasonable estimate.

This article is designed to inform veterinarians on the various attributes of different types of forages so that this knowledge, in combination with a visual assessment of the forage,[3] can aid in forage selection and provide guidance even in the absence of a forage analysis.

WHICH FORAGE IS BEST?

When determining which forages to use in a specific horse's diet, it helps to understand some of the basic characteristics of each of the forage choices available. Broadly, forages can be divided into 3 categories; cool season grasses, warm season grasses, and legumes. Each of these forage categories has its own unique attributes in calorie, protein, amino acid, carbohydrate fractions and non-nutritional factors, which lend themselves either for or against a specific purpose in equine nutrition. Although forage species within each category are similar, they will also vary and have their own unique traits as described in more detail elsewhere.[4,5] A practical overview of the forage categories is provided in this article.

Cool Season Grasses

Cool season grasses include the cereal forage crops oat, wheat, rye, and barley, as well as perennial and annual pasture species such as orchard grass, fescue, bluegrass, and ryegrass. Cool season grasses, also known as C3 grasses or temperate grass species, typically have a higher energy and protein content at a comparable stage of maturity compared with the warm season grasses (see **Table 2**). The higher calorie characteristic is due to the lower cell wall content,[6] measured on analysis as neutral detergent fiber and a typically higher nonstructural carbohydrate (NSC) content than the warm season grasses.[7,8]

The forage maturity at the time of grazing or harvest for conserved forage, however, will ultimately determine the final calorie value.[9] It is possible to have low-calorie cool season forages, for example, mature orchard grass. Forage analysis is useful in determining the actual digestible energy (DE; calorie) content. However, a visual assessment may provide an estimate of likely DE content. Recent research[3] has shown that untrained people can differentiate hays with the highest DE from those with the lowest DE using only visual assessment. Hays with the highest DE were described as being dark green, thin, soft, and flexible. Hays with the lowest DE were described as being yellow, dry, rigid, prickly, and straw. Although not reported in this study, a similar visual assessment of pasture is possible. With very leafy and green pastures (**Fig. 1**) typically having a higher energy value than pastures with seed heads present (**Fig. 2**), which are higher in energy value than completely browned off pastures.

The higher energy characteristic of relatively immature cool season grasses mean they generally are well-suited to horses with higher caloric requirements, including late-pregnant and lactating broodmares as well as performance horses[10] (**Fig. 3**). Conversely for the same reason relatively immature, higher energy cool season grasses may be problematic for horses prone to obesity and their inclusion in a diet can hamper attempts at weight loss.[11]

Recent research has shown that barley straw, technically a form of cool season grass forage, fed 50/50 with cool season grass hay promoted significant weight loss in native, unrugged/nonblanketed ponies in the UK over winter.[12] As such, straw

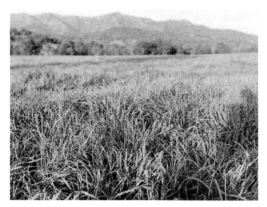

Fig. 1. Annual ryegrass in mid to late vegetative growth phase. Cool season grasses in vegetative growth are typically high in energy, protein, and vitamins with variable mineral content. This pasture was analyzed by Equi-Analytical Laboratories at 24.9% crude protein, 1.2 MCal/lb digestible energy, 0.29% calcium, 0.4% phosphorus, with a calcium phosphorus ratio of 0.7:1.0 on a dry matter basis.

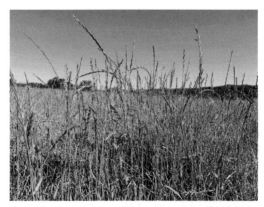

Fig. 2. Italian ryegrass in its reproductive phase of growth. Once grasses produce flowers and seed heads, their energy, protein, and vitamin content decrease. Mineral levels continue to be variable.

may form a useful part of an equine ration where weight loss is required, provided it is gradually introduced and is of good hygienic quality. Straw may increase the risk of impaction colics in some individuals, so caution is warranted. Care must be taken to also provide a nutritionally balanced diet when feeding straw or other low-quality forage. Straw, as the only forage, is not recommended (other than for donkeys) owing to the potential increased risk of gastric ulceration.[13]

Crude protein in cool season grasses is variable and depends heavily on nitrogen fertilizer application.[14] Some grasses, for example, specific varieties of ryegrass, can accumulate high levels of crude protein (eg, ≥20%).[14–17] The ryegrass pasture shown in **Fig. 1** was tested at 24.9% crude protein on a dry matter basis. Conversely, cereal forages and other cool season grasses, particularly in low-nitrogen soils or at later stages of maturity, can be low in protein (<10%).[18] At similar stages of maturity, cool season grasses (orchard grass and Kentucky bluegrass) will typically have a higher essential amino acid content (more similar to that found in alfalfa[17]) than the warm season grasses (eg, Teff). There will be some interspecies variation with ryegrass typically having lower lysine levels (on a percent of crude protein basis) compared with alfalfa.[19] The higher crude protein and essential amino acid

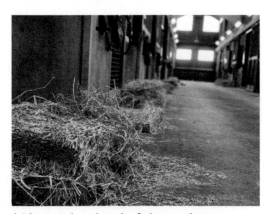

Fig. 3. Timothy hay laid out and ready to be fed to racehorses.

characteristics of certain cool season grasses are useful for supporting the increased protein and amino acid demands of lactating mares. Conversely, a high protein content could present a challenge for performance horses, especially those undergoing prolonged exercise in hot conditions.[20]

Nonstructural carbohydrates in cool season grasses

Owing to the C3 metabolism of cool season grasses, their primary storage carbohydrates are sucrose and fructans.[21] Concentrations of NSC (the sum of starch, simple sugars, and fructan) can be highly variable from day to day and even within a day and across a field or pasture[22] (see **Table 2**). The NSC concentration can reach as high as 40% dry matter under the right environmental conditions, for example, in regions that experience sunny days but cold overnight temperatures.[22,23] The potentially high concentrations are, in part, because the amount of fructan that can be stored by cool season grasses is relatively unlimited.

These potentially high concentrations of NSC are relevant when managing horses with or at risk of diseases where insulin dysregulation may be present, for example, laminitis,[22] equine metabolic syndrome, or pituitary pars intermedia dysfunction.[24,25] Additionally, high NSC forages may not be suitable for horses with polysaccharide storage myopathy owing to the increased insulin sensitivity and abnormal glycogen storage (see Kristine L. Urschel and Erica C. McKenzie's article, "Nutritional Influences on Skeletal Muscle and Muscular Disease," in this issue).[26] Many ryegrass varieties have been developed to accumulate high levels of water-soluble carbohydrates (simple sugars and fructan) to allow ruminants to maximize protein digestion and uptake.[27] This property makes ryegrass potentially particularly problematic for equines requiring a low NSC diet.

It is important to note that the NSC level of any forage can vary depending on the climate, time of day, soil nutrient and water status, and stage of growth. For detailed guidance on factors that affect the NSC content and assistance with selecting lower NSC forages where required, see Longland and Byrd,[28] particularly the section on pastures for laminitis-prone equidae.

Non-nutritional aspects of cool season grasses

Mycotoxins. Some species of cool season grasses, specifically perennial ryegrass and tall fescue, can cause mycotoxicosis in horses. To give the plant some resistance to environmental stressors, perennial ryegrass may be deliberately infected with an endophyte fungi[29] (*Epichloë festucae* var. *lolii*, previously known as *Neotyphodium lolii*) that produces lolitrem B. In horses, lolitrem B causes neuromuscular and neurosensory dysfunction in a condition commonly known as ryegrass staggers.[30,31] Ryegrass may also be infected with other *Epichloë* endophytes that produce a variety of ergot alkaloids, including ergovaline.[32] Ryegrass mycotoxicosis causes a change in animal behavior,[33] and it is the author's personal experience (N.R.) that "anxiousness" and hyperactivity are often the initial signs. Perennial ryegrass hay, if harvested from an endophyte infected sward, can pose the same risks. It should be noted that not all perennial ryegrass contains mycotoxin; however, it is impossible to know if a particular pasture or hay is infected without an analysis, which unfortunately can be difficult to obtain. Alternatively, asking the forage producer whether the seed used had been endophyte infected may help in determining if the forage is safe.

Tall fescue can also be infected with endophyte fungi that produce alkaloid mycotoxins (especially the ergopeptines), which affect mainly pregnant mares and their foals.[34] Pregnant mares grazing infected tall fescue pasture in the period leading up to foaling are likely to experience decreased mammary gland development, prolonged gestation, and dystocia, among other serious issues, which may include retained placenta and laminitis. Foals may be aborted or born dead or weak and oversized but underdeveloped.[35,36] The removal of mares from endophyte-infected tall fescue pastures at or before day 300 of gestation seems to eliminate the clinical abnormalities associated with endophyte-infected fescue pastures.[35]

Nitrates. Cool season grasses may also contribute to excessive consumption of nitrates. Although not widely reported in horses, excess consumption and acute toxicity of nitrates in horses is capable of damaging the gastrointestinal lining, causing diarrhea or gastrointestinal perforation, abortion, and death.[37] Chronic consumption of nitrate is suspected to contribute to mare reproductive loss syndrome and congenital limb deformity.[38,39] It is the author's experience (NR) that consumption of conserved forages with a nitrate content of greater than 3000 ppm can lead to abortion in Thoroughbred broodmares and limb deformities in foals, as well as potentially laminitis. Nitrate-induced abortion is reported more in cattle[40] than horses, perhaps owing to an under-recognition of this condition. Nitrate can be assessed by forage testing laboratories. Although not established in the literature, it is the author's (NR) experience that keeping nitrate in forages for horses to less than 1000 ppm, and ideally less than 500 ppm, is advisable. Care must be taken to ensure that the report provides the nitrate content and not nitrate–nitrogen. If nitrate–nitrogen is reported, it can be converted to nitrate by multiplying by 4.43. Forages are at an increased risk of high nitrate levels when they have been fertilized with nitrogen, after prolonged drought conditions, under 1 or more soil nutrient deficiencies that restrict the use of nitrogen taken up by the plant as nitrate (eg, sulfur deficiency) and during very cold, overcast, or windy conditions.[41]

Warm Season Grasses

Warm season grasses include bermudagrass, teff, and bahia. These grasses, also known as C4 or subtropical grasses, typically have a higher cell wall content and increased lignification making them generally the lowest energy group of the commonly available forages (see **Table 2**).[6,42] They are typically also lower in NSC, protein and essential amino acids than cool season grasses at a similar stage of maturity.[17]

With equine obesity affecting up to 70% of horses in some populations, the lower energy and NSC characteristics of the warm season grasses lend themselves well to horses not in work or in low to moderate intensity work with lower caloric requirements.[11] To maintain a healthy weight, or encourage weight loss, forage intakes often have to be restricted, which increases the risk of certain health (eg, gastric ulceration) and potential welfare issues.[1] Using warm season forages allows greater amounts of forage to be fed while still controlling calorie intake (see also Megan Shepherd and colleagues' article, "Nutritional Considerations When Dealing with an Obese Adult Equine," in this issue). In addition, personal observations (NR) suggest warm season grasses are less palatable than the often sweeter cool season grasses, which is helpful in situations where forage intake is being deliberately restricted because intake is slower and times without forage availability are therefore decreased. However, the lesser palatability may be problematic for horses in work with high energy requirements.

The lower caloric content and crude protein value of warm season grasses may present some challenges for horses with high calorie or protein and amino acid requirements, such as performance horses and broodmares. A careful dietary assessment should be made for these horses and additional calories or protein added to the diet as needed. Legume forages, such as alfalfa, with their high energy and crude protein characteristics (as discussed elsewhere in this article), for example, may compliment warm season grasses in these situations.

Nonstructural carbohydrates in warm season grasses

Owing to the C4 metabolism of warm season grasses, their primary storage carbohydrates are starch and sucrose.[21] Owing to the storage of starch being limited by space, warm-season grasses typically cannot store NSC to the same degree cool season (C3) grasses can.[43] As such, they tend be comparatively lower in NSC content (see **Table 2**).[7]

This lower NSC characteristic means they can be useful where low NSC feed ingredients are required. However, it is still possible for warm season forages to accumulate levels of NSC above the suggested 10% to 12% NSC on a Dry Matter (DM) basis to manage conditions like laminitis, Equine Metabolic Syndrome (EMS), and pituitary pars intermedia dysfunction. As such, analytical testing to determine NSC content and, therefore, the applicability of a specific forage is strongly recommended.

Non-nutritional aspects of warm season grasses

An important issue for some warm season grasses is oxalate content.[44,45] Oxalates bind calcium, potentially creating long-term calcium deficiency resulting in nutritional secondary hyperparathyroidism.[46] Based on the few reports of oxalate concentrations in teff straw[42] and bermudagrass,[40] it is the author's opinion (NR) that care must be taken to correctly supplement calcium to horses being fed large quantities of these forages to maintain the established calcium to oxalate ratio of at least 0.5:1.0.[47]

Mature, coastal bermudagrass hay reportedly increases the risk of ileal impaction colic.[48] Although it is likely that other factors, including hydration, are involved, ileal impaction colic seems to be relatively common in the Southeastern United States, where coastal bermudagrass is commonly fed. However, this issue is almost nonexistent in the Western United States, where legume hay and cool season grasses like timothy are used more commonly.[48]

Some horses on teff grass hay in Australia have experienced changes in behavior similar to that seen in horses affected by ryegrass mycotoxicosis. Most commonly, aggression and heightened reactivity to normal daily handling have been observed by this author (NR). There are no records of this behavior in the literature, but it is worth considering for horses on teff hay with unexpected changes in behavior. Finally, like cool season grasses, warm season grasses also have the ability to accumulate nitrates at toxic levels.

Legumes

Like grasses, legumes can be divided into cool and warm season varieties. The most widely used cool season legumes are alfalfa and various clovers, including white clover. Warm season legumes, like perennial peanut hay, can be used, but this practice is not common and the discussion here will be limited to the common cool season legumes.

As a forage category, legumes in general contain less fiber than cool season or warm season grasses making them typically the highest energy forage.[49] Legumes typically contain higher levels of protein at a similar stage of maturity than both cool and warm season grasses, owing to a symbiotic relationship with root microbes that fix nitrogen (**Table 1**). However, nitrogen fertilized and/or immature cool season grasses can have equal amounts of crude protein to legumes.[14,17]

These high energy, high protein features make legumes a useful part of the forage base of diets for horses with high energy and/or protein and amino acid requirements. However, care must be taken not to exceed protein requirement by too much (>160%

Table 1
Summary of typical energy, protein, and nonstructural carbohydrate (NSC) characteristics of cool season grasses, warm season grasses, and legumes when in their late vegetative to early reproductive stage of growth, as well as common toxicities and situations where each forage type is useful or may need to be restricted in the diet

Trait[a]	Cool Season Grasses	Warm Season Grasses	Cool Season Legumes
Energy/calorie content	Moderate to high	Low to moderate	Moderate to high
Protein	Moderate to high	Low to moderate	Moderate to high
Neutral detergent fiber	Moderate	High	Low to moderate
Primary storage carbohydrates	Sucrose and fructan	Sucrose and starch	Starch
NSC levels[b]	Variable, potentially high (>15%)	Moderate (15%) to low (<12%)	Moderate (15%) to low (<12%)
Potential major toxicities or issues	Mycotoxicities, nitrates	Oxalate, ileal impaction colic, nitrates	Enteroliths, blister beetle, nitrates
Useful for	Horses with moderate to high calorie and protein requirements Horse not sensitive to NSC	Horses on restricted calorie diets or horses requiring restricted NSC diets (eg, laminitics)	Horses with high calorie and protein requirements. Horses on high oxalate pastures Horses requiring a restricted NSC diet (eg, laminitics)
May need to be restricted for	Overweight or obese horses and horses requiring a low NSC diet If the grasses are high in protein, restrictions may be required for horses in hard work in hot and/ or humid climates	When fed as part of a balanced diet, can be used for all classes of horse and pony May not be capable of meeting a hard-working horse or broodmare's need for energy or protein so may need to be combined with other forage	Overweight or obese horses Horses in hard work, especially in hot and/or humid climates, young, growing horses where additional phosphorus is not supplemented Equines prone to enteroliths.

[a] The stage of growth of any forage species ultimately determines its nutrient content. Characteristics described in this table assume traits for late vegetative to early reproductive phases of growth. As plants mature, energy and protein decrease, whereas neutral detergent fiber increases, meaning even a cool season grass, when harvested or grazed at a late stage of maturity, can be low in energy and protein and high in neutral detergent fiber, which then changes the class of horse it is potentially most suitable for.
[b] Also see **Table 2**. Note that region and climate affect NSC level. Not all cool season grasses are high in NSC. Not all legumes are lower in NSC. Testing strongly recommended.

of requirement) in performance horses, and particularly those undertaking endurance type activities, or where water intake might be limited and especially in hot and/or humid environments.[20] In the author's experience (NR), racing Standardbreds and Thoroughbreds fed alfalfa as their only forage are particularly prone to tying up during hot and humid weather.

Table 2
The energy, crude protein, starch, water soluble carbohydrate (WSC), and nonstructural carbohydrate (NSC) characteristics of some common cool season grass, warm season grass and legume forages

	Energy (MCal/lb)		Protein (%)		Starch (%)		WSC (%)		NSC (%)	
	Average	Range	Average	Range	Average	Range	Average	Range	Average	Range
Cool season grasses										
Oat—fresh	1.0	0.9–1.1	17.5	11.3–23.8	2.9	0–5.9	12.0	5.2–18.8	13.0	6.6–19.5
Oat—hay	1.0	0.9–1.1	8.2	5.5–10.9	3.9	0.9–6.9	17.8	10.1–25.6	22.1	14.8–29.4
Rye—fresh	1.0	0.9–1.2	21.0	11.2–30.8	2.0	0.0–3.9	14.5	7.6–21.4	14.6	8.8–20.4
Rye—hay	1.0	0.9–1.1	11.0	5.4–16.6	2.1	0.4–3.8	15.0	8.9–21.3	17.8	11.8–23.8
Warm season grasses										
Bermudagrass—fresh	0.9	0.8–0.9	16.5	11.8–21.1	1.8	0.2–3.4	5.8	3.5–8.1	9.2	6.2–12.2
Bermudagrass—hay	0.9	0.8–1.0	11.3	8.5–14.1	4.0	1.1–7.1	7.3	5.2–9.3	13.0	8.9–17.1
Legumes										
Legume—fresh	1.1	1.0–1.2	23.0	19.3–26.6	2.4	0.3–4.5	7.4	5.0–9.8	9.9	6.4–13.5
Legume—hay	1.1	1.0–1.2	21.4	18.8–24.0	1.5	0.6–2.3	9.0	7.0–11.0	10.9	8.8–12.9

Data presented on a dry matter basis from Dairy-One Laboratory Services Interactive Common Feed Profiles Library from May 2000 through April 2019. Data from https://dairyone.com/services/forage-laboratory-services/feed-composition-library/.

Legumes typically have a higher calcium and magnesium content than grasses (**Table 3**), making them useful in the diets of growing horses and broodmares. However, this high mineral content combined with the high protein content may also predispose horses to enteroliths and associated colic.[48] Magnesium and protein are both components of the actual enteroliths themselves.[50] Additionally, the high calcium content and the tendency to maintain a more alkaline environment in the gastrointestinal tract likely contributes to the increased predisposition of some horses on high alfalfa ($\geq$50% of the diet) rations.[51,52] The exact reason why some horses are prone and others are not is not yet fully understood.[53] Alfalfa from different geographic regions may also have specific nutrient characteristics (eg, higher magnesium in alfalfa from southern California) that increase the risk of enteroliths (see also Myriam Hesta and Marcio Costa's article, "How Can Nutrition Help with Gastrointestinal Tract-Based Issues," in this issue).

Nonstructural carbohydrates in legumes

Legumes do not accumulate fructan as a storage carbohydrate,[54,55] and instead use starch as their storage carbohydrate.[55] This means, like warm season grasses, legumes are somewhat limited in their ability to accumulate NSC (see **Table 2**). However, under certain climatic or environmental conditions, legumes, particularly clovers, are able to accumulate higher levels of NSC than shown in **Table 2** which may make them unsuitable for horses sensitive to dietary NSC content as discussed elsewhere in this article.[55] Testing is again strongly recommended.

Non-nutritional aspects of legumes

Alfalfa hay may be contaminated with blister beetles[56] (*Epicauta spp*), which harbor the defensive poison cantharidin. If the beetles are eaten, they lead to cantharidin toxicity, which can be fatal.[57] Using first cut alfalfa, cut before the appearance of any flowers and purchased from reputable suppliers, decrease this risk in many cases. The poison is found in the beetles whether they are dead or alive; thus, using harvesting techniques in which the alfalfa is not crimped (thus allowing the beetles to fly away unharmed) can help to avoid killing and capturing the beetles in the hay. Within the United States, blister beetles are more common in hays grown in the southwest, but they have been found across many parts of the United States and other countries. Thus, owners should be advised to always check their alfalfa hay for potential contamination with beetles.[56]

Last, similar to cool and warm season grasses, legumes are able to accumulate nitrates at levels that are toxic for horses.

AT A GLANCE

Table 1 summarizes key characteristics of each of the forage types when harvested or grazed between late vegetative and early reproductive stages of growth. Note that when harvested or grazed at later stages of growth the energy and protein content of all types of forage will be lower. **Table 2** shows some typical nutrient values for some common species within each forage group. Data for UK forages for comparison can be found in the work by Harris and colleagues.[1]

Key points

- Cool season grasses, warm season grasses, and legumes all have unique characteristics that should be considered when determining which forages are most suitable for a particular horse.
- Where possible, and where availability within a region allows, a variety of forages should be used.

Table 3
The concentration (average and normal range) of minerals (DM basis) in legume and grass hays and pastures and the requirements for a maintenance horse consuming 2% of body weight on a DM basis[60]

	Legume Hay		Grass Hay		Mostly Grass Pasture		Grass Pasture		NRC Requirements Maintenance
	Average	Range	Average	Range	Average	Range	Average	Range	
Ca %	1.50	0.0–3.8[a]	0.49	0.27–0.71	0.58	0.30–0.85	0.52	0.27–0.77	0.20
P %	0.27	0.22–0.32	0.24	0.15–0.33	0.32	0.18–0.46	0.31	0–0.70	0.14
Mg %	0.32	0.25–0.40	0.21	0.13–0.29	0.23	0.14–0.32	0.24	0.14–0.35	0.075
K %	2.35	1.82–2.88	1.85	1.20–2.49	2.28	1.19–3.37	2.06	0.92–3.20	0.25
Na %	0.15	0.02–0.28	0.07	0–0.21	0.10	0–0.28	0.10	0–0.37	0.10
Fe ppm	401	3–799	198	0–487	407	0–1032	335	0–916	40
Zn ppm	27	0–858	30	0–1085	33	6–60	35	0–88	40
Cu ppm	9	4–14	8.5	0–17.4	9.3	3.5–15.2	9.3	3.9–14.7	10
Mn ppm	38	20–55	83	16–150	96	11–181	93	9–177	40
Co ppm	0.46	0–0.94	0.56	0–1.87	0.88	0.08–1.68	0.57	0–1.16	0.05
S %	0.29	0.16–0.41	0.18	0.11–0.25	0.25	0.18–0.35	0.23	0.13–0.34	0.15
Chloride %	0.72	0.39–1.05	0.60	0.17–1.03	0.96	0.43–1.49	0.82	0.20–1.44	0.40

[a] Although it is recognized that when no mineral was detected in a sample, such as when a legume hay was found to contain no Ca, reanalyzing the sample would be warranted. Data reproduced with kind permission from Equi-Analytical Laboratory Services Interactive Common Feed Profiles Library from May 2000 through April 2018. https://equi-analytical.com/common-feed-profiles/interactive-common-feed-profile/.

From NRC, *Nutrient Requirements of Horses.* 6th ed. ed. 2007, Washington, DC; with permission.

FORAGE MINERAL CONTENT

Forage analysis is critical to assess mineral concentrations. Often, horses will require supplementation on a forage-only diet to meet the requirements.[58] Although mineral digestibility does not seem to differ between adult horses and aged horses, geriatric aged horses or those with infirmities may require additional supplementation.[59]

When a forage analysis is not available, Equi-Analytical, for example, has a public database listing the averages and ranges of minerals for common forages analyzed by their laboratory, as illustrated in **Table 3** (which also provides the requirements of a horse at maintenance consuming 2% of its body weight in forage on a DM basis).[60] This clearly shows requirements often would not be met by the forage alone for some minerals, in particular, for all the forages shown, Zn and Cu. Low Cu can increase the risk of osteochondrosis and osteodysgenesis, with accompanying lameness, and insufficient Zn intake can result in a lack of appetite, a decreased growth rate, and parakeratosis.[60] At least one of the forage types would not meet the requirements for Na and Mn and only Mg and K requirements would have been met by all forages shown. Many minerals are required in greater amounts at more demanding life-stages (eg, growing, lactating, or exercising) and therefore in these circumstances it is increasingly unlikely that mineral requirements would be met on an all forage diet.[60]

There are also potential concerns with excess or imbalanced intakes of minerals. For instance, it is possible to have a forage-based diet high in P relative to Ca leading to nutritional secondary hyperparathyroidism.[61] Further, as discussed elsewhere in this article, some warm season grasses contain oxalates, which interfere with Ca absorption and can create nutritional secondary hyperparathyroidism even when both Ca and P are provided in seemingly appropriate amounts. Although most forages contain more Ca than P, studies have shown this to not always be the case.[8] An imbalance in Ca:P is particularly prevalent in young, rapidly growing pastures, especially where there is a history of phosphorus fertilizer and pasture improvement (see **Fig. 1**). Ratios as low as 0.3:1.0 have been observed by one author (NR).

Most forages are rich in iron (Fe); thus, iron supplementation is not warranted for most horses.[62] Furthermore, forages are high in K and normally far exceed requirements,[63] which is typically not a concern unless feeding a horse with hyperkalemic periodic paralysis (see Kristine L. Urschel and Erica C. McKenzie's article, "Nutritional Influences on Skeletal Muscle and Muscular Disease," in this issue). Owing to cost, forage analyses do not typically include selenium (Se) and iodine (I), although both can be requested. Concentrations of both minerals are influenced heavily by concentrations in the soils in which the forages are grown[60,64] and, thus, there can be important regional variations which it is important to recognize. Both Na and Cl concentrations in forages can be low and often insufficient, especially for exercising horses prone to sweating. Salt should always be provided if horses are maintained on a forage-only diet.

For a comprehensive review of equine mineral nutrition including excesses or deficiencies see the NRC report[60] and Argo and associates.[19]

Key points

- Unless a forage is analyzed to know what the mineral concentrations are, it is not possible to guarantee a horse is receiving adequate and appropriate amounts of dietary minerals.

- In a large majority of cases, horses left unsupplemented on forage-only diets will be deficient in 1 or more minerals and these deficiencies have the potential to adversely impact their health.

- Most horses on a forage-only diet therefore will need a ration balancer, fortified concentrate, commercial feed, or mineral supplement to ensure all mineral requirements are met.

FORAGE VITAMIN CONTENT

Vitamins can be broadly classified as water soluble (B complex vitamins and vitamin C) and fat soluble (vitamins A, D, E, and K). In this section, we focus on vitamin concentrations of A, D, and E in forage. Although not the focus of this section, ensuring adequate B complex vitamin intake is also important. B complex vitamins are generally provided through good-quality forage and via natural production by a healthy fiber fermenting microbial population within the horses' own gastrointestinal tract.

Vitamin A and β-Carotene

Vitamin A is the name of a group of fat-soluble retinoids, including retinol, retinal, and retinyl esters. In human diets, 2 forms of vitamin A are available; preformed vitamin A (retinol and retinyl ester), found in foods from animal sources including dairy, fish, and meat, and provitamin A carotenoids (β-carotene), derived from plant pigments. Both provitamin A and preformed vitamin A must be metabolized to retinal and retinoic acid, the active forms of vitamin A, to support biologic functions. Vitamin A plays an important role in vision, adaptive immunity and fertility. Horses convert β-carotene to vitamin A at an average conversion rate of about 33%.[60] Vitamin A accumulates in the liver and grazing animals generally obtain more than adequate liver reserves of vitamin A to last 3 to 6 months.

Grazing horses meet their vitamin A requirements from β-carotene in forage. Vitamin A concentrations range from 15 to 606 mg β-carotene/kg DM in fresh green forages to 1 to 162 mg/kg DM in hays.[65] Fresh pasture often exceeds the vitamin A requirement in horses. Fortunately, with downregulation of the conversion of β-carotene to vitamin A when requirements are met, vitamin A toxicity is not a concern. Additional sources of β-carotene include carrots, yellow maize, and legume seeds. Apart from the yellow corn found in many commercial feeds, most ingredients used to produce horse feed have negligible quantities of β-carotene. The majority of commercial feeds are, therefore, fortified with synthetic vitamin A.

Fresh grass and high-quality leafy hay are the most important natural sources of vitamin A for horses.[66] Other factors affect the content of β-carotene in pasture, including the plant species, climatic conditions, and stage of maturity. In particular, β-carotene concentrations are affected by the leaf to stem ratio, because the stems contain much less β-carotene than the leaves (eg, mean values of around 278 mg/kg DM have been published for vegetative, leafy, or immature grasses compared with a mean of 59 mg/kg DM for mature grasses[65]).

Beta-carotene is one of the most difficult nutrients within forage to preserve.[66] There are, furthermore, differences in the availability of β-carotene between different forage species and also between different hays,; for example, the availability of β-carotene in alfalfa is better than in grass hays. Sun-cured hay has lower concentrations than fresh forage. The process of conserving forages can destroy around 80% of the β-carotene present and then biological oxidation continues at a rate of 6% to 7% per month during hay storage.[65,67] This point means that hay would have close to zero β-carotene present after only 3 to 4 months of storage. Rapid dehydration, such as occurs in drier climates, can help to preserve the β-carotene content of alfalfa.

Vitamin D

Vitamin D is a fat-soluble vitamin that is, obtained from sun exposure or diet. Vitamin D has 2 forms, vitamin D_2 (ergocalciferol) in plants and vitamin D_3 (cholecalciferol) in animal tissue. In plants, ergosterol is converted to vitamin D_2 after exposure to ultraviolet radiation, yet measurable amounts are only found in sundried and dead leaves of forage.[68] Ultraviolet rays from sunlight convert 7-dehydrocholesterol, which is synthesized by the liver, to vitamin D_3 (cholecalciferol) in the skin of horses. Vitamin D, either ingested or produced in the skin, is transported bound to a specific plasma transport protein to the liver, where it is stored and converted to 25-hydroxyl vitamin D (25-OH-D). Bound to the same specific transport protein, 25-OH-D is transported to the kidney, where it is hydroxylated to either the most active form, calcitrol (1,25(OH)$_2$D) if needed or, if not, the less active form 24,25(OH)$_2$D is produced. Calcitrol helps to maintains plasma calcium concentrations by working in conjunction with parathyroid hormone at the level of the bone (resorption) and intestine (absorption).

In naturally exposed forages, some vitamin D_2 will be synthesized from ergosterol if the forage is exposed, after cutting, to UV light.[67,68] Levels range from 31 to 1800 IU/kg DM in fresh green forages to 90 to 5560 IU/kg DM in hays.[65] Therefore, barn-dried hay will contain much less vitamin D_2 (470 IU/kg DM) than sun-dried material (around 971 IU/kg DM).[65] Furthermore, the proportion of dead leaves will affect the vitamin D level in the final preserved forage regardless of sunlight levels. Thus, poor handling of hay resulting in a loss of leaves can decrease the natural intake of vitamin D from sun-cured forages.

It should be noted that some plants, particularly from the Solanaceae family, contain glycosides that are biologically active analogues of vitamin D_3 and are capable of causing vitamin D toxicity and enzootic calcinosis, even after the plants may be baled into hay.[69]

Vitamin E

There are 8 forms of naturally occurring vitamin E; however, RRR-α-tocopherol is the most active form in the body. Vitamin E is absorbed across the intestine and travels bound to chylomicron to the liver, where the RRR-alpha-tocopherol stereoisomer is selected for transport to the other body tissues, bound to very low-density lipoproteins. Vitamin E is essential for normal neuromuscular function by acting as a potent antioxidant, but can also modulate the expression of certain genes and inhibit platelet aggregation. A review of vitamin E and associated equine disorders (for example, neuroaxonal dystrophy/equine degenerative myeloencephalopathy, vitamin E–deficient myopathy and equine motor neuron disease) is suggested for further reading[70] (see also Kristine L. Urschel and Erica C. McKenzie's article, "Nutritional Influences on Skeletal Muscle and Muscular Disease," in this issue).

Vitamin E, unlike vitamin A, is not stored in the body in large amounts for any length of time; therefore, a regular dietary source is important. The richest sources of vitamin E are the oils of green plants. Factors that promote the production of lush green plants also tend to promote higher vitamin E content. Fresh green forage can be rich, but also highly variable in vitamin E (eg, 9–400 mg/kg DM).[65] Young grass is a better source of vitamin E than mature herbage, with leaves containing 20 to 30 times as much vitamin E as the stems.[68] Wheat germ oil is one of the richest sources, containing approximately 20 milligrams per tablespoon of RRR-α-tocopherol.[71] Commonly sold vegetable oils may contain vitamin E, but the vitamin E is primarily used to protect polyunsaturated fatty acids and thus may not be available for use when ingested by horses.

Vitamin E content varies markedly among equine dietary constituents, with the highest levels in fresh grass and decreasing concentrations with processing and storage.[67] A significant decrease in vitamin E occurs between the first and fifth cutting of alfalfa hay[72] and storage losses can reach 50% in 1 month, even under good storage conditions.[67] Concentrations in hay can decrease by up to 90% with processing.[68] Therefore, any horse that is not maintained on an adequate pasture should be supplemented with vitamin E. For further information on types and amount of supplementation, readers are referred to this review[70] and Kristine L. Urschel and Erica C. McKenzie's article, "Nutritional Influences on Skeletal Muscle and Muscular

Disease," in this issue. A seasonal variation in plasma vitamin E concentrations occurs with increased plasma vitamin E in the summer in grazing horses fed fresh forage compared with the winter, when horses were fed hay and oats.[73,74] Haylage and silage may contain 60% of initial α-tocopherol content after ensiling.[75]

Assessing Vitamin Content in Forage

The methods of analysis used to assess forage vitamin concentrations have a tendency to overestimate concentrations.[76] All geometric isomers of all-trans-β-carotene have less biological activity yet are assessed when determining β-carotene concentrations.[65] Similar caution applies when estimating vitamin D content in forage owing to sensitivity of various analytical techniques and effects on biologic availability.[67]

With these caveats delineated, it is worthwhile to note that many timothy hays, when analyzed, will have less than 700 IU vitamin A and vitamin E concentrations ranging from undetectable to 9 to 45 IU.[77] Sampling from alfalfa hays typically identify higher vitamin A and E concentrations, ranging from 900 to 1410 IU/kg and 25 to 47 mg/kg DM, respectively (personal communication, Dr Frank McGovern, 2020). Because vitamin A can be stored in the liver, feeding high-quality forage that includes alfalfa leaves may provide adequate vitamin A, but vitamin E needs cannot be met with feeding hay alone. Additionally, it is more useful to measure an individual horse's serum α-tocopherol concentration than it is to base estimates on feed analyses, as individual absorption varies widely[70,78] (see also Kristine L. Urschel and Erica C. McKenzie's article, "Nutritional Influences on Skeletal Muscle and Muscular Disease," in this issue).

SUMMARY

Forage is the single most important feed component of a horse's diet and often determines a horse's overall long-term health. With differences between commonly available forage types, suitable forages must be carefully selected based on a horse's nutrient and physiologic requirements. The selection of an inappropriate forage can have dire consequences, particularly in cases where high NSC forages are selected for laminitis-prone individuals. Often, a combination of forages works to meet requirements. For example, warm season grasses and legumes may combine well to control calorie intake but also to ensure protein and amino acid requirements can be met.

Within all forage categories, there are issues that must be considered and managed. Additionally, a majority of forages are unable to meet a horse's full mineral and vitamin requirements, so additional supplementation is almost always required. Although a forage analysis is the gold standard in determining the nutrient content of a forage, it is not always practical or possible. However, reliable estimates of the nutrient content of various forages are available and it is these values that should be used in the absence of an analysis as the basis of sound diet formulation, aided by appropriate diet analysis software. Asking advice from a nutritionist experienced in the forages available in the area can also be very beneficial.

DISCLOSURE

There are no commercial or financial conflicts of interest or any funding source for any of the authors.

REFERENCES

1. Harris PA, Ellis AD, Fradinho MJ, et al. Review: feeding conserved forage to horses: recent advances and recommendations. Animal 2017;11(6):958–67.

2. Barr AC, Reagor JC. Toxic plants: what the horse practitioner needs to know. Vet Clin North Am Equine Pract 2001;17(3):529–46.

3. Julliand S, Dacremont C, Omphalius C, et al. Association between nutritional values of hays fed to horses and sensory properties as perceived by human sight, touch and smell. Animal 2019;13(9):1834–42.

4. Collins M, Nelson CJ, Moore KJ, et al. Forages, volume 1: an introduction to grassland agriculture. Hoboken, New Jersey: Wiley; 2017.

5. Abaye AO. Common grasses, legumes and forbs of the eastern United States: identification and adaptation. Cambridge, Massachusetts: Academic Press; 2019.

6. Wilson JR. Cell wall characteristics in relation to forage digestion by ruminants. J Agric Sci 1994;122(2):173–82.

7. DeBoer ML, Hathaway MR, Kuhle KJ, et al. Glucose and insulin response of horses grazing alfalfa, perennial cool-season grass, and teff across seasons. J Equine Vet Sci 2018;68:33–8.

8. Fulkerson WJ, Slack K, Hennessy DW, et al. Nutrients in ryegrass (<emph type="2">Lolium</emph> spp.), white clover (<emph type="2">Trifolium</emph> repens) and kikuyu (<emph type="2">Pennisetum clandestinum</emph>) pastures in relation to season and stage of regrowth in a subtropical environment. Aust J Exp Agr 1998;38(3):227–40.

9. Särkijärvi S, Sormunen-Cristian R, Heikkilä T, et al. Effect of grass species and cutting time on in vivo digestibility of silage by horses and sheep. Livestock Science 2012;144(3):230–9.

10. Jansson A, Lindberg JE. A forage-only diet alters the metabolic response of horses in training. Animal 2012;6(12):1939–46.

11. Rendle D, McGregor Argo C, Bowen M, et al. Equine obesity: current perspectives. UK-Vet Equine 2018;2(Sup5):1–19.

12. Dosi M, Kirton R, Hallsworth S, et al. Inducing weight loss in native ponies: is straw a viable alternative to hay? Vet Rec 2020;187(8):e60.

13. Luthersson N, Nielsen KH, Harris P, et al. Risk factors associated with equine gastric ulceration syndrome (EGUS) in 201 horses in Denmark. Equine Vet J 2009;41(7):625–30.

14. Loaiza PA, Balocchi O, Bertrand A. Carbohydrate and crude protein fractions in perennial ryegrass as affected by defoliation frequency and nitrogen application rate. Grass Forage Sci 2017;72(3):556–67.

15. Tas B. Perennial ryegrass for dairy cows: intake, milk production and nitrogen utilization. Wageningen. The Netherlands: Ph.D.Thesis, Wageningen Institute of Animal Sciences,Wageningen University; 2005.

16. Wilson GF, Dolby RM. Ryegrass varieties in relation to dairy cattle performance. New Zeal J Agr Res 1969;12(3):489–99.

17. DeBoer ML, Martinson KL, Kuhle KJ, et al. Plasma amino acid concentrations of horses grazing alfalfa, cool-season perennial grasses, and teff. J Equine Vet Sci 2019;72:72–8.

18. Tinsley SL, Brigden CV, Barfoot C, et al. Nutrient values of forage grown in the UK in 2012 -2013. In proceedings of the 7th European Workshop on Equine Nutrition Leipzi 28 September – 2 October 2014, Leipzig, Germany: p. 82–3.

19. Argo CM, Bishop R, Burden FA, et al. Contributors. In: Geor RJ, Harris PA, Coenen M, editors. Equine applied and clinical nutrition. Philadelphia: W.B. Saunders; 2013. p. xiii–xiv.

20. Connysson M, Muhonen S, Lindberg JE, et al. Effects on exercise response, fluid and acid-base balance of protein intake from forage-only diets in Standardbred horses. Equine Vet J Suppl 2006;36:648–53.
21. White LM. Carbohydrate reserves of grasses: a review. Journal of Range Management 1973;26.13-8.
22. Longland AC, Byrd BM. Pasture nonstructural carbohydrates and equine laminitis. J Nutr 2006;136(7):2099S–102S.
23. Kagan IA, Kirch BH, Thatcher CD, et al. Seasonal and diurnal variation in simple sugar and fructan composition of orchardgrass pasture and hay in the piedmont region of the United States. J Equine Vet Sci 2011;31(8):488–97.
24. Morgan R, Keen J, McGowan C. Equine metabolic syndrome. Vet Rec 2015; 177(7):173–9.
25. Durham AE, Frank N, McGowan CM, et al. ECEIM consensus statement on equine metabolic syndrome. J Vet Intern Med 2019;33(2):335–49.
26. Borgia L, Valberg S, McCue M, et al. Glycaemic and insulinaemic responses to feeding hay with different non-structural carbohydrate content in control and polysaccharide storage myopathy-affected horses. J Anim Physiol Anim Nutr (Berl) 2011;95(6):798–807.
27. Capstaff NM, Miller AJ. Improving the yield and nutritional quality of forage crops. Front Plant Sci 2018;9:535.
28. Longland AC. Pastures and pasture management. In: Harris P, Geor RJ, Coenen M, editors. Equine clinical and applied nutrition. London: Elsevier; 2013. p. 332–50.
29. Wiewióra B, Żurek G, Żurek M. Endophyte-mediated disease resistance in wild populations of perennial ryegrass (Lolium perenne). Fungal Ecology 2015; 15:1–8.
30. Prestidge RA. Causes and control of perennial ryegrass staggers in New Zealand. Agric Ecosyst Environ 1993;44(1):283–300.
31. Johnstone LK, Mayhew IG, Fletcher LR. Clinical expression of lolitrem B (perennial ryegrass) intoxication in horses. Equine Vet J 2012;44(3):304–9.
32. Hovermale J, Craig A. Correlation of ergovaline and lolitrem B levels in Endophyte-Infected Perennial Ryegrass (Lolium Perenne). J Vet Diagn Invest 2001;13:323–7.
33. Reddy P, Rochfort S, Read E, et al. Tremorgenic effects and functional metabolomics analysis of lolitrem B and its biosynthetic intermediates. Sci Rep 2019; 9(1):9364.
34. Klotz JL, McDowell KJ. Tall fescue ergot alkaloids are vasoactive in equine vasculature. J Anim Sci 2017;95(11):5151–60.
35. Boosinger TR, Brendemuehl JP, Schumacher J, et al. Effects of short-term exposure to and removal from the fescue endophyte acremonium coenophialum on pregnant mares and foal viability1. Biol Reprod 2018;52(monograph_series1):61–7.
36. Rohrbach BW, Green EM, Oliver JW, et al. Aggregate risk study of exposure to endophyte-infected (Acremonium coenophialum) tall fescue as a risk factor for laminitis in horses. Am J Vet Res 1995;56(1):22–6.
37. Oruc HH, Akkoc A, Uzunoglu I, et al. Nitrate poisoning in horses associated with ingestion of forage and alfalfa. J Equine Vet Sci 2010;30(3):159–62.
38. Swerczek TW. An alternative model for fetal loss disorders associated with mare reproductive loss syndrome. Anim Nutr 2020;6(2):217–24.
39. Swerczek T. Effects of nitrate and pathogenic nanoparticles on reproductive losses, congenital hypothyroidism and musculoskeletal abnormalities in mares and

other livestock: New Hypotheses. Animal and Veterinary Sciences 2019;7. 10.11648/j.avs.20190701.11.

40. Nitrates or nitrites and abortion in cattle. Nutr Rev 1960;18(6):175–7.
41. Sidhu PK, Bedi GK, Meenakshi, et al. Evaluation of factors contributing to excessive nitrate accumulation in fodder crops leading to ill-health in dairy animals. Toxicol Int 2011;18(1):22–6.
42. Giordano A, Liu Z, Panter SN, et al. Reduced lignin content and altered lignin composition in the warm season forage grass Paspalum dilatatum by down-regulation of a Cinnamoyl CoA reductase gene. Transgenic Res 2014;23(3): 503–17.
43. Chatterton NJ, Harrison PA, Bennett JH, et al. Carbohydrate partitioning in 185 accessions of gramineae grown under warm and cool temperatures. J Plant Physiol 1989;134(2):169–79.
44. Rahman MM, Kawamura O. Oxalate accumulation in forage plants: some agronomic, climatic and genetic aspects.(Report). Asian-Australas J Anim Sci 2011; 24(3):439.
45. Skerman PJ, Riveros F. Tropical grasses. Rome: Food and Agriculture Organization of the United Nations; 1990.
46. McKenzie RA, Gartner RJ, Blaney BJ, et al. Control of nutritional secondary hyperparathyroidism in grazing horses with calcium plus phosphorus supplementation. Aust Vet J 1981;57(12):554–7.
47. Blaney BJ, Gartner RJW, McKenzie RA. The effects of oxalate in some tropical grasses on the availability to horses of calcium, phosphorus and magnesium. J Agric Sci 1981;97(3):507–14.
48. Fleming K, Mueller POE. Ileal impaction in 245 horses: 1995-2007. Can Vet J 2011;52(7):759–63.
49. Buxton DR, Redfearn DD. Plant limitations to fiber digestion and utilization. J Nutr 1997;127(5):814S–8S.
50. Rouff AA, Lager GA, Arrue D, et al. Trace elements in struvite equine enteroliths: concentration, speciation and influence of diet. J Trace Elem Med Biol 2018;45: 23–30.
51. Hassel DM, Rakestraw PC, Gardner IA, et al. Dietary risk factors and colonic pH and mineral concentrations in horses with enterolithiasis. J Vet Intern Med 2004; 18(3):346–9.
52. Hassel DM, Aldridge BM, Drake CM, et al. Evaluation of dietary and management risk factors for enterolithiasis among horses in California. Res Vet Sci 2008;85(3): 476–80.
53. Kelleher ME, Puchalski SM, Drake C, et al. Use of digital abdominal radiography for the diagnosis of enterolithiasis in equids: 238 cases (2008-2011). J Am Vet Med Assoc 2014;245(1):126–9.
54. Jenkins C, Snow A, Simpson R, et al. Fructan formation in transgenic white clover expressing a fructosyltransferase from Streptococcus salivarius. Funct Plant Biol 2002;29:1287–98.
55. Kagan IA, Anderson ML, Kramer KJ, et al. Seasonal and diurnal variation in water-soluble carbohydrate concentrations of repeatedly defoliated red and white clovers in Central Kentucky. J Equine Vet Sci 2020;84:102858.
56. Schmitz DG. Cantharidin toxicosis in horses. J Vet Intern Med 1989;3(4):208–15.
57. Helman RG, Edwards WC. Clinical features of blister beetle poisoning in equids: 70 cases (1983-1996). J Am Vet Med Assoc 1997;211(8):1018–21.
58. Elzinga S, Nielsen B, Schott Ii H, et al. Comparison of nutrient digestibility between three diets for aged and adult horses. J Equine Vet Sci 2017;52:89.

59. Elzinga S, Nielsen BD, Schott HC, et al. Comparison of nutrient digestibility between adult and aged horses. J Equine Vet Sci 2014;34(10):1164–9.
60. NRC. Nutrient requirements of horses. 6th edition. Washington, DC: The National Academies Press; 2007.
61. Stewart J, Liyou O, Wilson G. Bighead in horses-not an ancient disease. Aust Equine Vet 2010;29:55–62.
62. Richards N, Nielsen B. Comparison of equine dietary iron requirements to iron concentrations of 5,837 hay samples. Comp Exer Phys 2018;14.
63. Coenen M. Exercise and stress: impact on adaptive processes involving water and electrolytes. Livest Prod Sci 2005;92(2):131–45.
64. Survey, U.S.G. Selenium in Counties of the Conterminous States. Available at: https://mrdata.usgs.gov/geochem/doc/averages/se/usa.html. Accessed July, 2020.
65. Ballet N, Robert JC, Williams PEV. Vitamins in forages. In: Givens DJ, Owne E, Axford RFE, et al, editors. Forage evaluation in ruminant nutrition. Oxfordshire, England: CABI Publishing; 2000. p. 399–432.
66. Fonnesbeck PV, Symons LD. Utilization of the carotene of hay by horses. J Anim Sci 1967;26(5):1030–8.
67. McDowell LR. Vitamins in animal and human nutrition. In: McDowell LR, editor. 2nd edition. Ames (IA): Iowa State Press; 2000. p. 155–217.
68. McDonald P, Edwards RA, Greenhalgh JFD. Animal nutrition. 7th edition. Harlow (England): Pearson Education Ltd; 2010.
69. Odriozola E, Rodriguez A, Micheloud J, et al. Enzootic calcinosis in horses grazing Solanum glaucophyllum in Argentina. J Vet Diagn Invest 2018;30(2):286–9.
70. Finno CJ, Valberg SJ. A comparative review of vitamin E and associated equine disorders. J Vet Intern Med 2012;26(6):1251–66.
71. U.S. Department of Agriculture, A.R.S. FoodData Center. 2019. Available at: https://fdc.nal.usda.gov/. Accessed July, 2020.
72. Bruhn JC, Oliver JC. Effect of storage on tocopherol and carotene concentrations in alfalfa hay. J Dairy Sci 1978;61:980–2.
73. Maenpaa PH, Koskinen T, Koskinen E. Serum profiles of vitamins A, E and D in mares and foals during different seasons. J Anim Sci 1988;66(6):1418–23.
74. Maenpaa PH, Lappetelainen R, Virkkunen J. Serum retinol, 25-hydroxyvitamin D and alpha-tocopherol of racing trotters in Finland. Equine Vet J 1987;19(3): 237–40.
75. Muller CE, Moller J, Jensen SK, et al. Tocopherol and carotenoid level in baled silage and haylage in relation to horse requirements. Anim Feed Sci Technol 2007;137:182–97.
76. Ullrey DE. Biological availability of fat-soluble vitamins: vitamin A and carotene. J Anim Sci 1972;35(3):648–57.
77. Finno CJ, Estell KE, Katzman S, et al. Blood and cerebrospinal fluid alpha-tocopherol and selenium concentrations in neonatal foals with neuroaxonal dystrophy. J Vet Intern Med 2015;29(6):1667–75.
78. Brown JC, Valberg SJ, Hogg M, et al. Effects of feeding two RRR-alpha-tocopherol formulations on serum, cerebrospinal fluid and muscle alpha-tocopherol concentrations in horses with subclinical vitamin E deficiency. Equine Vet J 2017;49(6):753–8.

How Can Nutrition Help with Gastrointestinal Tract– Based Issues?

Myriam Hesta, DVM, PhD[a],*, Marcio Costa, DVM, PhD[b]

KEYWORDS

- Horses • Intestinal diseases • Intestinal microbiota • Dysbiosis • Nutrition • Equines
- Colic • EGUS

KEY POINTS

- Changing away from natural feeding behavior can lead to gastrointestinal (GI) issues in horses.
- Nutritional strategies can be used to help prevent and manage GI issues.
- Nutrition has a direct impact on the GI microbiota of horses.
- Microbiota manipulation might be used in the future to aid in the prevention and treatment of GI issues.

INTRODUCTION

The herbivorous horse is a hind gut fermenter because the gastrointestinal (GI) tract is characterized by a well-developed cecum and colon, which, together with the GI microorganisms. allows it to retrieve enough energy on a grass-based diet. Horses, however, are prone to the development of GI disease. The diet and dietary management of many horses today are quite different from that of their wild ancestors. Under natural circumstances, horses spend most of their time foraging whereas today horses may be confined in stables and fed preserved forage and concentrates, often rich in starch and sugars, sometimes in only 2 meals per day. In some cases, this may disturb the microbial balance and lead to GI disease. Therefore, this article starts with a brief overview on the role of the microbiome and the effect of diet. Afterward, the focus is on nutrition as a cause as well as treatment of GI disease.

[a] Department of Veterinary Medical Imaging and Small Animal Orthopedics, Faculty of Veterinary Medicine, Ghent University, Salisburylaan 133, Merelbeke B9820, Belgium; [b] Department of Veterinary Biomedical Sciences, University of Montreal, Saint-Hyacinthe, Canada
* Corresponding author.
E-mail address: myriam.hesta@ugent.be

Vet Clin Equine 37 (2021) 63–87
https://doi.org/10.1016/j.cveq.2020.12.007

Advances in Microbiota Characterization

The advent of molecular technologies largely has improved understanding of the interaction between nutrition, the intestinal microbiota, and the host. The vast majority of bacteria fails to grow in conventional culturing media[1] and the use of DNA sequencing allows for a broader characterization of the intestinal microorganisms, also referred to as *microbiota* or *microbiome* (if all their genetic material rather than just taxonomic genes is considered). Next-generation sequencing (NGS) technologies are able to sequence millions of DNA strands concomitantly, decreasing sequencing costs and increasing data yield. Studies using previous DNA sequencing technologies have passed from a few hundred to many millions of sequences after NGS.[2] Accordingly, the number of publications indexed under the search, "equine microbiota", in the PubMed database (https://pubmed.ncbi.nlm.nih.gov/) increased from 1 in 2006 to 44 in 2019, highlighting the increasing interest in this field.

The intestinal microbiota is constantly interacting with the host and heavily influences host homeostasis. The intestinal microbiota plays a major role in the pathophysiology of many conditions across species, such as obesity, diabetes, immune-mediated diseases, and behavioral abnormalities.[3] Much work, however, remains to be performed to elucidate how changes in the microbiota can influence the horse's health and the occurrence of diseases. Unfortunately, many assumptions are extrapolated from studies performed in laboratory animals, especially considering the mechanistic nature of those interactions. Nevertheless, many descriptive studies using NGS now are available, providing vital information regarding the importance of nutrition on the horse intestinal microbiota.

Although NGS has been considered a revolution in science, it has many limitations.[4] The most used technologies are not able to read long sequences of DNA, which decreases the ability to classify organisms at the species level. For example, a sequence classified as Clostridium can be any of the hundreds of species of *Clostridium*. Most of the current studies are descriptive, and the detection of microbiota shifts do not imply causality (eg, an increase in specific bacteria might be the cause or the consequence of the disease). Also, taxonomic changes do not necessarily imply functional changes, because many species may be able to play the same functional role (eg, carbohydrate digestion). Inconsistent results can be obtained by using different methodologies (eg, different primers or reference databanks). Finally, feces are used as a proxy of the distal gut microbiota,[5–7] but specific changes found in the colon of horses with intestinal diseases might not be detected in feces,[8] and differences between the mucosal and luminal microbiota might be relevant.[9]

Therefore, although understanding on the interaction between horses and their intestinal microbiota largely has improved, much work remains to be done before this knowledge can be used to improve health and prevent diseases in horses.

Importance of Intestinal Microbiota in Horses

Horses are monogastric herbivores that rely on their intestinal microbiota to break down complex plant carbohydrates by fermentation, producing volatile fatty acids (VFAs) that are used as a major energy source.[10] Therefore, changes in the normal microbiota composition, frequently referred to as *dysbiosis*, are normally present in horses with intestinal diseases.[8,11]

Many factors can affect the intestinal microbiota of horses, including age,[12–16] pregnancy,[17] level of physical activity,[18] and environment.[19] Of especial interest is the potential of diet and nutritional supplements to modify and modulate specific bacterial populations beneficial to horses.[16,20]

Factors affecting early life microbiota of foals

The intestinal colonization of foals starts at the moment of delivery, when they get in contact with the bacteria present in the birth canal and environment.[21] In humans, the vaginal microbiota of the mother heavily influences composition of their newborn's microbiota,[22] and the vaginal microbiota of mares also might be important for shaping the foal's first colonizers. Considering the horse anatomy, it is likely that fecal bacteria greatly influence the vaginal environment, and because diet has an impact on fecal bacteria of horses,[20,23] it can be hypothesized that nutrition of the mare can contribute indirectly to the colonization of foals.

Specific microbiota profiles have been selected in each animal species during evolution,[24] and colonization with "abnormal" microbiota might have negative effects on their general health. The concept, however, of "normal" microbiota might be difficult to establish, because domesticated horses already might harbor an altered microbiota.[25] In general, wild animals have a more diverse microbiota compared with their domesticated related species.[26] It has been shown in other species that germ-free animals have poor development of the intestinal mucosa and might present abnormal immune response against commensal bacteria.[27] Furthermore, the (often exaggerated) use of antimicrobials decreases the intestinal bacterial diversity in horses,[6,28] which may impair the immune response against infection.[29]

The microbiota of foals is unique during the first month of life,[13–15,30] likely because of colostrum ingestion[31,32] and the comparatively high concentrations of IgA in the mare's milk.[33] This could be an interesting period for microbiota manipulation before their microbiota becomes stable. Foals harboring 2 different GI microbial communities differed in microbial VFA production, parasite egg load, and cortisol levels after weaning.[34] There might be a relationship between the intestinal microbiota and parasitic infections.[35,36] The descriptive nature of microbiota studies (rather than mechanistic), however, preclude major conclusions regarding the cause(s) or consequence(s) of microbiota alterations.

Therefore, further attention to the impact of current feeding recommendations, housing, and other stressors on the intestinal microbiota of mares and foals is required.

Impact of diet on the intestinal microbiota of horses

As monogastric herbivores, horses were selected in nature to ingest small amounts of forage and walk during most of the day. Domestication, however, has greatly changed those feeding habits in order to fulfill energy requirements, especially by the introduction of starch and lipids into their diet. It currently is well established that diet is one of the major factors influencing the intestinal microbiota of horses.[16,19,23,37,38] Even the frequency that meals are fed can affect specific populations,[39] and, due to interindividual variability, each horse's microbiota may respond differently to each type of diet.[23]

The main influence of modern nutritional management is the use of readily fermentable carbohydrates (ie, starch), which have been shown to increase lactic acid–producing bacteria and to decreased bacterial diversity.[40,41] Reduced diversity commonly is associated with higher predisposition to pathogens.

Fig. 1 summarizes the main intestinal bacteria (at different taxonomic levels) associated with different diets in horses. In foals, weaning might increase fibrolytic bacteria, such as *Fibrobacter* and *Prevotella* spp.[8,34,42]

Future Perspectives for Microbiota Manipulation

The advance of NGS has launched a new era in science as it revealed the close interaction of the host and its microbiota. Therefore, microbiota manipulation, in theory, can be

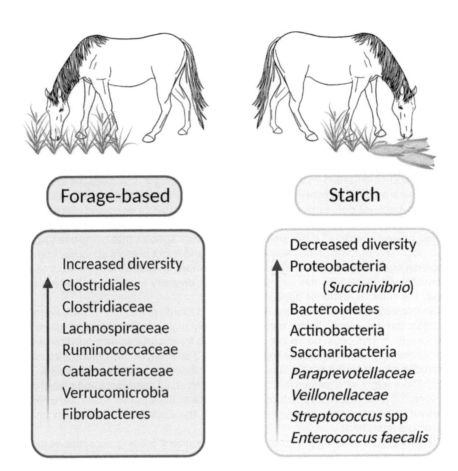

Fig. 1. Intestinal bacteria associated with different types of diets in horses. Diet composition varied widely between studies. In general, forage-based refers to pasture or hay-only diets and starch refers to supplementation with 2-g starch/kg BW/d. (*Data from* Refs.[16,20,23,38,40,41,43]; and Created with BioRender.com.)

used to achieve better health, but, to date, there are no clear and objective guidelines that could be recommended for horses.

The use of dietary supplements in gastrointestinal disease

Probiotics. Probiotics are live bacteria given to improve gut health. The use of probiotics to treat intestinal dysbiosis is of great interest for equine practitioners, but, comparatively, research performed in horses is only in its infancy. It is beyond the scope of this article to extensively review the previous literature but, in summary, there is no agreement between studies,[44] and, unfortunately, many of them used small sample sizes or no control groups and/or were performed outside the equine body (adding probiotics to feces). Furthermore, studies sometimes reported numerical (but not statistical) differences and tendencies toward significance. **Table 1** summarizes the data of recent studies evaluating the use of prebiotics and probiotics in horses.

Lactobacillus, Bifidobacterium, Enterococcus, and Saccharomyces spp are the main organisms found in commercial products marketed for horses. Although those

Table 1
Description of recent studies using prebiotics and probiotics to modulate the microbiota of horses

Product	Age	Method	Outcome	Study
Probiotics				
Lactobacillus plantarum LUHS135, *L paracasei* LUHS244	34 adult horses	Culture	Increased lactic acid bacteria and decreased enterobacteria in feces and decreased lactate in blood	Zavistanaviciute et al,[45] 2019
L rhamnosus, *Enterococcus faecium*	34 healthy foals	DGGE and qPCR	No effect in the fecal microbiota	Urubschurov et al,[46] 2019
L rhamnosus SP1, *L rhamnosus* LHR19, *L plantarum* LPAL, *L plantarum* BG112, *Bifidobacterium animalis*	38 healthy foals	NGS	None or very limited effect in the fecal microbiota	Schoster et al,[47] 2016
L acidophilus, *L buchneri*, *L reuteri*	Feces from 3 adult horses	Ex vivo	Avoided decrease in pH, increased lactate-utilizers and decreased amylolytics	Harlow et al,[48] 2017
Prebiotics				
Oligofructose	5 canulated adult horses overloaded with oligofructose for induction of laminitis	FISH	Increased *Streptococcus* spp in cecum	Milinovich et al,[49] 2008
Short-chain fructooligosaccharides	4 canulated adult horses	Culture	Avoided increases of *Lactobacillus*, *Streptococcus* and D-lactate after barley intake	Respondek et al,[50] 2008
Fructooligosaccharides and inulin	12 adult horses	NGS	Increased diversity. Increased *Lactobacillus* and reduced *Streptococcus* in the stomach. Increased *Lactobacillus* and reduced Lachnospiraceae and Ruminococcaceae in the distal gut. Increased *Ruminococcus* in the cecum and colon transversum	Glatter et al,[51] 2019

(continued on next page)

Table 1
(continued)

Product	Age	Method	Outcome	Study
Fructooligosaccharides and inulin	6 adult horses	N/A	Tendency to faster decrease of glucose and insulin levels after feeding	Glatter et al,[52] 2017
Fructooligosaccharides and Inulin	Content from stomach, cecum and colon from 12 adult horses	Ex vivo	Accelerated gas production in gastric contents. No impact on hindgut fermentation	Bachmann et al,[53] 2020
Exposure of gastric mucosa to butyric acid at same concentrations produced by fructooligosaccharides	Gastric tissue from 3 adult horses	In vitro	Impaired functional integrity and severe pathohistologic changes in the glandular mucosa	Cehak et al,[54] 2019
Cellobiose	8 adult horses and 2 ponies	NGS	Increased Coriobacteriales and Clostridium, reduced Bacteroidetes	Passlack et al,[55] 2020
Salacinol	35 healthy foals (14 for microbiota analysis)	T-RFLP	Increased Clostridium cluster XIVa and decreased number of days with fever	Iida et al,[56] 2020

Abbreviations: DGGE, denaturing gradient gel electrophoresis; FISH, fluorescence in situ hybridization; qPCR, quantitative polymerase chain reaction; T-RFLP, terminal restriction fragment length polymorphism.

strains have shown benefits in vitro, they are not the most abundant species found in the distal gut of horses and foals,[13,57] and normally they fail to permanently colonize the gut because it is difficult to compete with species already well stablished. Commensal species of clostridia, which are a majority in horses, have been used to correct dysbiosis in humans[58] and are important in healthy dogs,[59] but the use of *Clostridium* spp has not been reported in horses. In theory, probiotics would be more efficient when intestinal dysbiosis is present (eg, diarrhea and treatment with antimicrobials). Furthermore, microbiota manipulation might be more efficient during a foal's first month of life, before the microbiota become more stable. Feeding yogurt to foals is practiced, but more information is needed before further recommendations to treat intestinal diseases can be made. One novel approach, yet to be used in horses, is the use of complex ecosystems, which are probiotics containing many organisms (sometimes more than 25 different species of bacteria and yeasts) to reestablish intestinal homeostasis.[58]

Prebiotics. Prebiotics are compounds nondigestible for the host that can be used as a food source by certain beneficial bacteria. A summary of recent studies is presented in **Table 1**. Prebiotics, when giving in combination with probiotics, are called symbiotics, but studies evaluating this combination in horses are rare.

Postbiotics. Postbiotics are metabolites produced by bacteria (ie, butyrate), that can promote intestinal health directly or serve as a dietary source for other beneficial bacteria. The potential of metabolites to modulate the intestinal microbiota has been demonstrated.[60] Treatment with microencapsulated sodium butyrate might be beneficial in horses,[61] but further research is required.

Fecal microbiota transplantation

Among the different options available to manipulate the intestinal microbiota, fecal microbiota transplantation (FMT) is likely the most efficient method to correct a dysbiosis, as demonstrated in humans[62] and dogs.[63,64] FMT consists of the transfer of the whole ecosystem (microorganisms and metabolites) present in feces of a healthy donor into a dysbiotic patient. The restoration of the microbiota is believed to break the cycle of inflammation caused by dysbiosis.[63,65] Controlled studies demonstrating the benefits of FMT in horses, however, remain to be performed. One study demonstrated that the microbiota of 3 out of 5 horses with diarrhea was similar to the microbiota of healthy horses after FMT,[66] but results should be interpreted with caution considering the small sample size and that a control group with animals not receiving FMT was not included.

In humans, the rectal administration of FMT is more efficient than the oral route because the acidic gastric pH and digestive enzymes decrease bacterial viability.[62,67] In horses, bacterial viability by oral delivery may be further hindered by the length of the small intestine and a well-developed cecum. Unfortunately, the long small colon in horses is a barrier for FMT, administrated via enema, to reach the large colon. Therefore, FMT needs to be delivered via nasogastric tube in horses. It is possible that more proximal changes, not detectable in feces, might occur, but more scientific based evidence is necessary before FMT can be recommended to treat intestinal diseases in horses.

NUTRITION AS CAUSE OR TREATMENT OF GASTROINTESTINAL DISEASE
Equine Gastric Ulcer Syndrome

Introduction
Equine gastric ulcers may be classified as equine squamous gastric disease (ESGD) or equine glandular gastric disease (EGGD). Lesions in ESGD are the consequence of an

increased exposure to aggressive factors, such as HCl, VFAs, and possibly bile acids and lactic acid.[68] Conversely, in EGGD, the mucosal defense mechanisms might need to be damaged before HCl and a low pH can contribute to the lesions.[68] To prevent ESGD recurrence, nutritional and management changes are needed in addition to pharmacologic treatment.[69–71] Nutrition plays a clearer role in ESGD prevention and management but it is thought that these principles also may apply for EGGD.

Nutritional risk factors

Nutritional risk factors and dietary treatment of equine gastric ulcer syndrome (EGUS) have been discussed and reviewed,[68,69] although a systematic meta-analysis is missing. Briefly, horses at pasture generally have a decreased risk for ESGD. Moving horses, however, from low-quality pasture to individually controlled stalls improved overall ulcer scores possibly due to an improved nutritional quality and/or decreased feeding stress and highlighting the importance of an individual evaluation of nutritional and management changes.[72] Intermittent feeding (>6 hours between meals) compared with continuous feeding increases the risk for ESGD due to the drop in the gastric pH.[68,69] Feeding more than 1 g of starch/kg body weight (BW)/meal significantly increases the risk for ESGD,[73] in part because of the fast consumption rate with a reduced buffering effect of saliva. Furthermore, VFA produced by microbial fermentation also decreases gastric pH. Often, a combination of factors resulting in a reduction of chewing time, salivation, and buffering may cause a cumulative negative effect. Although feeding more than 1 g starch/kg BW/meal when a fiber-based feed is fed with a slow consumption rate may not cause any problem, compliance with the general recommendations stated throughout this session is advised.

Alfalfa hay compared with grass hay may have a protective effect on ESGD, potentially due to the buffering effect of the higher calcium and protein content.[74] The form in which alfalfa is fed, however, seems to be important. Alfalfa chaff (short chopped forage) and molasses alfalfa chaff significantly increased lesions at the pylorus in weanling foals compared with grass hay or a total mixed ration.[75,76] The sharp structure of the alfalfa chaff used in these studies might have mechanically injured the pylorus, making it more vulnerable to further injuries. This may lead to pylorus stenosis with delayed gastric emptying. These negative effects were not noted when feeding alfalfa pellets even with their decreased particle size.[76] Adult horses fed only alfalfa chaff (fed at 1.5% of BW on dry matter [DM] basis) tended (did not reach significance) to have more severe glandular lesions, which healed after being on pasture for 16 days.[77] Fecal particle size was higher in adult horses fed alfalfa hay compared with meadow hay, but negative effects on the glandular mucosa were not noted. Furthermore, mild squamous lesions disappeared after feeding alfalfa hay for 3 weeks.[78] In conclusion, alfalfa hay is beneficial for the squamous gastric region in both adults and foals. Large amounts of sharp alfalfa chaff, however, should be avoided, especially in foals.[78] Feeding straw, which is very high in NDF (cell wall), as the sole source of forage increases the risk for ESGD probably due to physical effects and lower buffering (low protein and calcium).[68,69,73] Also, intermittent access to water might increase the risk for EGUS.[73]

The gastric microbiota of horses is complex and presents great interindividual variability,[6,57] with many factors likely influencing its composition, including the bacteria ingested with the diet and type of bedding.[57,79,80] The gastric microbiota is important in the pathophysiology of human gastric ulcers, mainly *Helicobacter pylori*, but not in horses.[79,80] *Streptococcus equi* was present in EGUS lesions[79] and lower bacterial diversity was found in the stomach of horses with EGUS,[81] but a causation effect remains to be demonstrated.

Nutritional management

The recurrence rate of ESGD is high; thus, medical and nutritional management strategies should be applied together to achieve long-term beneficial effects.[69–71] The nutritional recommendations are summarized in **Fig. 2**. Pasture turnout is preferred, even if feeding grass hay ad libitum is possible.[71] Stressors (eg, competition for feed and bullying) and feeding feedstuff high in nonstructural carbohydrates (NSCs) should be avoided.[69,70] When pasture grazing is not possible, forage (alfalfa hay and good quality grass hay) should be fed ad libitum, but if not possible, forage should be fed in an amount of at least 1.5% of the BW on a DM basis in 4 meals to 6 meals per day.[68–70] The small meals should be divided equally during daylight hours and the last meal late in the evening should provide enough forage to eat during night-time. Feeding time can be maximized by using slow feeders or double hay nets.[82] Care should be taken to reduce the NSC intake (<20%).[70] Grain, grain-based, and molasses feeds with high amounts of starch and sugar should be avoided or fed in limited amounts. Vegetable oil may be preferred over starch and sugars in case of high energy needs.

Feeding a grain-free, high-fiber, high-vegetable oil/fat concentrate with alfalfa as first ingredient improved incidence and severity of gastric ulcers compared with usual concentrates.[83] Reducing starch intake in horses with an ESGD score of 2/4 showed no significant benefit in 1 field study.[84] In those horses with an ESGD score greater than or equal to 3/4 and whose diets were not changed, however, there was no longer any significant improvement 6 weeks after ceasing omeprazole treatment, whereas there remained a significant improvement for those whose diet was changed. This

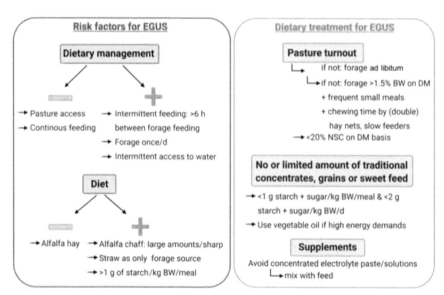

Fig. 2. Most common risk factors and dietary treatments currently recommended for EGUS. The green line indicates a reduced risk for EGUS whereas the red cross represents an increased risk for EGUS. It needs to be stressed that the complete individual situation needs to be evaluated before identifying the risk factors and making any nutritional recommendations. For example, pasture access may increase the risk for EGUS if stress is increased by feed competition or bullying. On top, EGUS can be caused by a high NSC intake on pasture, especially when the time of grazing is limited (high intakes in a limited time period and thus in contrast to the natural trickle feeding). (Created with BioRender.com.)

highlights the importance of combining medical with nutritional treatment (especially reducing the NSC intake).[84]

A plethora of supplements for gastric ulcers is available; however, most have not been tested under field conditions.[69,71] Herbal products, magnesium oxide, and others did not differ from placebo to prevent nonglandular gastric ulcers.[69,85,86] Some mixtures (sea buckthorn, pectin, lecithin, antacids, *Saccharomyces cerevisiae*, and salts of organic acids), however, showed promising results and may be an alternative to long-term medical treatment. Corn oil supplementation may have potential as an adjunct treatment in glandular ulcers but did not prevent the formation of squamous ulcers.[69,87] See also Ingrid Vervuert and Meri Stratton-Phelps' article, "The Safety and Efficacy in Horses of Certain Nutraceuticals that Claim to Have Health Benefits," in this issue.

Concentrated electrolyte pastes and solutions may increase the number and severity of squamous ulcers,[88] but mixing them in the feed might avoid these negative effects.

Colic

Introduction
Colic is one of the most frequent and serious conditions in equine practice,[89] with an incidence varying between 3.5 to 10.6 episodes per 100 horses per year.[90,91] The multifactorial nature makes it difficult to investigate the role of nutrition, because covariables may be associated (eg, breed, level of activity, feed, and season).[92] Change in feed and housing management is the most evident risk factor for colic.[89] Prospective nutritional studies with control groups mostly are lacking[93] and needed because colic prevention is based mainly on avoiding risk factors.

Prevention and treatment of colic in general by nutrition
The current recommendations for dietary management to prevent and aid in colic treatment are summarized in **Fig. 3**. In most cases, spasmodic/gas colic (42.9%) or colic with unknown cause (26.4%) is diagnosed.[94] Furthermore, a history of colic is a strong risk factor for future episodes[91] and a prevalence of 36.5% for recurrent colic has been shown.[95] Although some risk factors (eg, breed, age, and season) cannot be changed, nutritional management often can be adapted more easily.

Changes in feeding practices. Any change in concentrates/complementary feeds (amount, source, and frequency) as well as forage, including changing to a new batch, can increase the risk of colic.[94,96–101] Dietary changes within 2 weeks prior to the episode of colic often are reported,[94,96,99,100] stressing the importance of gradual adaptation (at least 2 weeks),[102] including transition to a new batch of forage.[93]

Concentrates. Frequency of feeding, type, and especially amount of concentrates/complementary feeds rich in starch and sugars are important in the etiopathogenesis of colic.[99,103] Feeding high (>5 kg/d) but also moderate (2.5–5 kg/d) amounts of high-starch/sugar concentrates substantially increases the risk for colic,[94,101] likely because of incomplete prececal starch digestion. Adaptation to higher starch levels by increasing levels of α-amylase is limited and slow in horses. As a consequence, feeding a high-starch/sugar concentrate can lead to intraluminal colonic lactic acidosis and decreased fibrolytic and increased acidophilic microbial species.[92] Marked divergences in genes involved in starch digestibility have been shown for different breeds, suggesting a relationship between genetics and nutritional management.[104] Inclusion of germinated barley (0.5 kg/100 kg BW/d; 34.7% starch and sugar) may reduce the incidence of colic in horses at pasture (stabled overnight),[105] possibly

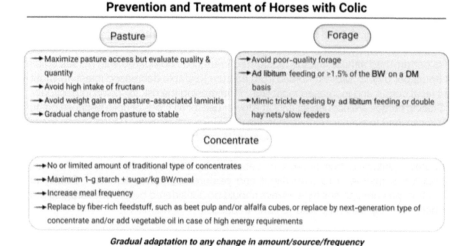

Fig. 3. Dietary recommendations for equine colic prevention and treatment. (Created with BioRender.com.)

as consequence of the prebiotic properties of this feed. A confounding effect could have influenced the results, however, because the supplement was only fed in 1 of the 2 periods. Also, the high NSC content and hygienic quality of any such germinated product require attention and further research is required.

The guideline to limit starch feeding to 2 g/kg BW/meal[106] is likely too high for horses prone to developing colic and, therefore, needs to be lowered to a maximum of 1 g of starch/kg BW/meal, and preferably even lower intakes are warranted.[92,107] In addition, the source of starch may be important because corn and oats have different effects on fecal microbiota.[38] Increasing meal frequency or (partly) replacing starch-rich concentrates by highly digestible fiber sources (eg, soya hulls, sugar beet, and alfalfa cubes) and/or vegetable oil/fat-rich feeds all may be solutions to overcome the limited capacity of the equine small intestine to hydrolyze starches in individuals with high energy requirements.[92] Low-starch concentrates often combine those characteristics and are preferred over high-starch concentrates.

Preserved forage and management. The type of dried forage might not influence the risk for colic.[91] Some hays, however, have been associated with an increased risk, likely due to their lower digestibility.[94]

Preserved forage should be applied in amounts equal to at least 1.5% of the BW on a DM basis,[102] with gradual change to the new forage/batch. Simulation of the natural trickle feeding behavior by giving free access to forage is encouraged.[92] Care should be taken, however, to not induce weight gain in animals prone to obesity and to not increase the risk of colic through changes instigated when managing or preventing obesity. Animals prone to weight gain may benefit from a more mature cut, while avoiding a too low digestible forage, using slow feeders or double hay nets to slow down ingestion time and avoiding prolonged periods of fasting (see Nerida Richards and collegaues' article, "Nutritional and Non-Nutritional Aspects of Forage"; Megan Shepherd and colleagues' article, "Nutritional Considerations When Dealing with an Obese Adult Equine," in this issue).

Pasture. A decreased exposure to pasture both in time and space had a 3-fold increased risk for colic,[94] but type and quality (percent of edible vegetation) of pasture were not nor was stock density.[91] Mild forms of colic, however, may not be noted on pasture in contrast to closely monitored stabled horses.[90,103] Horses with 12 hours of pasture access per day had almost half the risk for recurrent colic compared with horses stabled 24 hours per day.[108] Moving horses from pasture to stable decreased intestinal motility and fecal output and increased fecal DM,[109] increasing the risk for colon impaction.

Grazing horses are not necessarily at a lower risk for all types of colic because pasture NSCs can lead to similar colonic changes to high-starch intakes. Typical trickle feeding of grass sugars/fructans during 14 hours to 18 hours of grazing, however, may have a different effect on the microbiota compared with the bolus feeding of starch-rich concentrates.[92] Allowing free access to pasture may limit variable consumption rates, although this may lead to overweight and pasture-associated laminitis. Quality and quantity of pasture and soil type always should be considered before encouraging grazing because they also may lead to sand impaction or duodenitis.[92]

Nutritional advice for specific forms of colic

Impaction. In general, changing from pasture to stable may increase the risk for colon impaction. Feeding coarse (low-digestibility) roughage, eating straw bedding, and feeding coastal Bermuda grass hay are associated with impaction.[110,111] Warm season grass types of forages, such as Bermuda grass (see Nerida Richards and collegaues' article, "Nutritional and Non-Nutritional Aspects of Forage," in this issue), especially the coastal variety, are assumed to be of lower quality due to the higher fiber content. Furthermore, due to the fine and soft texture, they might contribute to ileal impaction due to improper chewing.[112,113] Forage digestibility decreases by 0.5% per 1% increase in NDF concentration in horses.[114] Apart from fiber concentration, fiber composition (insoluble and soluble fiber fractions, cellulose, hemicellulose, and lignin) can affect fiber digestibility. Digestibility of Bermuda grass decreased with increasing maturity; however, fiber digestibility of alfalfa and orchard grass was similar to the early-cut Bermuda grass hay, and retention time of Bermuda grass hay was longer compared with the 2 other types of hay.[113] Consequently, hay (or straw) that is less digestible and of poorer quality may predispose horses to impaction.[96] When feeding coastal Bermuda hay, it is advised to use only the best quality and to introduce it slowly.[112] Also, meal feeding and large concentrate meals might increase the risk of impactions due to increased flux of colonic fluids, which could be avoided by frequent small feedings (up to 6 equal meals).[112]

In general. Withholding food is recommended initially to prevent the impaction getting worse, even though GI motility is likely to decrease.[110] Refeeding, with small but frequent amounts of forage, can be started when there is evidence of resolution of the impaction,[93] increasing feed amounts over a 2-day to 4-day period. Traditional types of concentrates should be avoided for at least 3 days to 7 days, depending on the severity of the impaction, with slow reintroduction.[93] Water intake should be stimulated by providing an additional bucket with water with small amounts of sweetening agents, such as fruit juice, molasses, or isotonic electrolytes.[110] A mash rich in fiber and low in starch and sugar is an additional palatable option that may increase hydration.

Impaction with sand/sand colic Horses fed directly from the ground where there is short or no grass have increased risk for developing sand colic in sandy soil areas. Consequently, horses should be fed from bins or racks or the ground should be covered with a rubber mat or a concrete slab.[93]

Adding psyllium (500 g, twice daily, or 1 g/kg BW/d) to mineral oil (2 L/d) or magnesium sulfate (1 g/kg BW/d) significantly increased sand clearance compared with the medical treatment without psyllium.[115–118] Giving 4 times the recommended dose of pelleted psyllium, however, resulted in obstructing bezoars composed of psyllium.[119] Psyllium combined with a probiotic showed no advantage in sand clearance compared with the control group.[120]

Epiploic foramen entrapment. Crib-biting and wind-sucking behavior increases the risk of epiploic foramen entrapment (EFE), with an odds ratio of 72.[121] Studies have suggested a link between gastric health and stereotypical behavior, although results are not consistent.[122] Access to salt blocks may decrease the risk of EFE perhaps due to increased licking and consequent salivation, increasing the buffering effect in the stomach.[121] Increased licking in crib-biting horses otherwise healthy compared with normal horses also could be a coping strategy when confined in stables.[123] Being fed at the same time as the other horses also was found a risk factor for EFE and may point to the role of food anticipation.[121] The authors refer to Sarrafchi and Blokhuis[124] for prevention of stereotypical behavior, which is based mainly on mimicking the natural feeding behavior as closely as possible: pasture access or free-choice hay; as much turnout as possible; or, when pasture access is not possible, encourage foraging enrichment and increased feeding time (see Megan Shepherd and colleagues' article, "Nutritional Considerations When Dealing with an Obese Adult Equine," in this issue). Increasing meal frequency, however, has been shown to have contradictory results in oral stereotypical behavior.[124]

Duodenitis-proximal jejunitis. A strong association with pasture grazing and a modest association with feeding a large amount of concentrates have been reported in horses with duodenitis-proximal jejunitis.[125] It is unclear if it is pasture per se or the type of pasture that is important because the majority of forage in this study was Bermuda grass. Nutritional recommendations to treat ileus are discussed later.

Inflammatory bowel disease (malabsorption syndrome/impaired glucose absorption). The dietary advice for horses with inflammatory bowel disease (IBD) is challenging because these horses often are underweight and consequently need more energy and nutrients to gain weight. Furthermore, IBD may lead to malassimilation, which could lead to more GI disturbances. A customized diet with small and frequent meals (at least 4/d), therefore, is preferred.[126,127]

If obstruction is a concern (eg, secondary to intestinal wall thickening), a complete pelleted diet may be helpful, preferably fed soaked. Beet pulp and other feeds high in digestible fiber (easily fermented) may provide extra energy due to the production of VFA.[93,128] Feeding enough fiber is important because it may reduce the reliance on the small intestine to provide energy from starch and sugars.[129] Considering the enteric protein loss and malabsorption of nutrients, protein intake should be increased by providing alfalfa and/or complementary feeds with at least 14% protein.[93,128]

High-starch/sugar concentrates should be avoided in cases of glucose malabsorption. The starch and sugar intake should be lower than 1 g/kg BW/meal. Although there is a lack of knowledge on the prevalence of fat malabsorption, corn oil can be supplemented gradually (10–14 days) to increase energy density (up to 5.5% crude fat on DM basis in the total diet).[126,127] A positive outcome was noted in 13/15 horses with malabsorption syndrome by combining medical and nutritional treatment (ie, reduced starch/sugar, added oil, and improved protein intake/quality) and including vitamin E (1–1.5l U/mL oil), a general vitamin mineral supplement, and S cerevisiae.[126,127]

Food allergies may be associated with IBD. A monodiet composed of oats, oil, and grass hay sometimes is proposed to eliminate potential inciting antigens.[129] Diagnosis of food allergies, however, is challenging. An IgE-based test for food allergy was not reliable in healthy ponies, generating many false-positive and inconsistent results over a short time period.[130] Small intestinal mucosal samples from healthy and IBD horses did not show a different expression of a specific cytokine receptor, which plays a role in human celiac disease and gluten allergy.[131] Similarly, blood levels of antibodies known to be important in human celiac disease did not differ between control horses on a gluten-rich diet and horses with inflammatory small bowel disease.[132] However, 1 horse with high concentrations of some of these antibodies clinically recovered (including duodenal histopathology) after being on a wheat gluten–free diet. Another horse with case of tentative diagnosis of inflammatory small bowel disease combined with a generalized skin reaction completely recovered after a 3-month gluten-free diet.[133] Although there currently is limited scientific evidence to support feeding a monodiet or a hypoallergenic diet in IBD, it may result in clinical recovery in exceptional case and needs further investigation.

Right dorsal colitis. The dietary treatment of right dorsal colitis is challenging because appetite may be decreased. Furthermore, the diet should not contain long-stem roughage in order to decrease the physiologic and mechanical load on the colon.[134] Changing to a diet without long-stem roughage should be done gradually over a period of 5 days to 10 days and should last for 3 months to 6 months or well beyond resolution of clinical signs.[134] A commercial complete pelleted diet and other fiber sources, such as beet pulp and alfalfa pellets, can be used to meet the forage requirements. Vegetable oil may be used to increase calories. Furthermore, psyllium mucilloid (100 g daily for 3–6 months) may increase microbial production of VFAs, such as butyrate, that are beneficial for colonic mucosal repair, but further studies in horses are required.[61,134–136]

Acute typhlocolitis. Hypophagia and anorexia are common in acute typhlocolitis. Horses should consume at least 60% to 70% of the resting digestible energy requirement after 1 day to 3 days. The ideal diet should be highly digestible and low in bulk, thus relatively low in insoluble fiber (eg, NDF). Immature/high-quality grass and alfalfa hay and/or a complete pelleted diet may be helpful.[134] Small amounts of fresh grass may stimulate the appetite; however, large amounts of lush grass and conserved forage high in NSCs should be avoided. Grains and high-starch/sugar concentrates also should be avoided.[137]

Enteroliths. Feeding greater than 50% alfalfa and less than 50% of oat or grass hay may increase the risk of enterolithiasis. Higher colonic pH and calcium, magnesium, phosphorus, and sulfur have been shown in horses with enteroliths (8–14 weeks after the initial enterolith surgery) compared with healthy controls.[138] Similar findings (except for sulfur) and a decreased colonic sodium and potassium concentration have been noted in horses fed alfalfa compared with grass hay. Although the sample size was small, this study suggests that horses with susceptibility for enteroliths are characterized by true physiologic distinctions or that prior existence of an enterolith results in permanent colonic physiologic changes.[138]

The lack of daily access to pasture also has been associated with an increased risk of enteroliths.[139–141] Eliminating alfalfa from the diet and feeding oat or grass hay instead and providing daily access to pasture are recommended to animals at risk.[140] The addition of apple cider vinegar sometimes is suggested to decrease the colonic pH[141]; however, this has not been studied in horses with enteroliths and potentially can be harmful.

When patients present poor appetite postoperatively, completely avoiding alfalfa is not needed because ingestion of energy and nutrients is more important at that time point[137] (discussed later).

Large colon volvulus. Being fed hay (compared with haylage or grass) or sugar beet, a change in pasture over the past 28 days, and an alteration in the amount of forage in the past week all were identified as risk factors for large colon volvulus.[142] These factors not only may relate to the typical peculiarities of managing broodmares in the peripartum period, which have a higher risk for large colon volvulus, but also may relate to microbiota changes altering motility and gas production.[17,112] Also, quidding behavior and having more than 2 caretakers were associated with an increased risk, possibly due to inconsistency in feeding management.[142]

Postoperative feeding after surgical treatment of colic. Proper dietary management can improve postoperative recovery. Higher percent of DM as forage and reaching the minimal DM intake faster were associated with shorter recovery time in 37 horses subjected to surgical colic.[143] Also, time to the first feeding was associated positively with recovery length, which stresses the importance of introducing feed as soon as clinical parameters allow it. Feeding amounts that meet 70% of the digestible resting energy requirements can be used initially,[134] but, depending on the GI function, a more conservative approach could be warranted. Small but frequent amounts of grass or grass hay are recommended postoperatively for large bowel disorders unless reflux or ileus is present.[134] Good hygienic quality, immature/high-quality hay is the best choice, which may be combined with a complete feed.

Ileus and dysmotility are more common after small intestinal surgery, and feeding should be postponed until ileus and gastric reflux have subsided. More digestible feeds (such as alfalfa, fresh grass, and complete pellets) in small but frequent servings then can be started. Bulky and coarse feed (eg, straw/very mature hay) should be avoided.[137] In humans, the use of chewing gum as a form of sham feeding has been shown to decrease the time for resolution of postoperative ileus probably by increasing vagal stimulation.[144] Therefore, suspending a hay net outside the stable but visible for the patient has been proposed somehow as a form of sham feeding in horses where early postoperative feeding is not possible but efficacy has not been evaluated. Inflammation plays a key role in the pathophysiology of postoperative ileus; thus, feeds and supplements with anti-inflammatory properties (rich in n-3 fatty acids) might be useful in preventing postoperative ileus.[145] Supplements to modulate the intestinal microbiota might be useful because dysbiosis may contribute to the development of postoperative diarrhea.[8]

Nutritional Treatment of Horses with Diarrhea

Foals and foal heat diarrhea

Diarrhea is common in foals, with 50% of them experiencing 1 or more bouts of diarrhea.[146] Within the group of noninfectious causes of diarrhea, foal heat diarrhea probably is the most important one, affecting 75% to 80% of 5-day to 15-day old foals. Although changes in milk composition have been speculated as a cause, orphaned foals on milk replacers[136,147] also are affected; maturational changes in intestinal microbiota, therefore, might play a role.[148]

Foals that develop pica and ingest large amounts of sand can develop diarrhea and colic. Mare's milk has a relatively higher concentration of lactose, but although primary lactose intolerance is rare, secondary lactose intolerance, due to rotavirus or *Clostridioides difficile* infection, may occur and be treated with lactase supplementation.

Dietary intolerances in foals receiving milk replacers also are described, stressing the importance of correct preparation and choosing high-quality appropriate products. Diarrhea also can develop secondary to over-administration of lactose and/or electrolytes, particularly in high milk-producing mares.[136,147,149]

Foals with mild to moderate diarrhea without signs of colic are allowed to suckle, because ingesting as little as 60 mL of milk every few hours provides energy to the enterocytes. Severe cases can benefit from a 12-hour to 24-hour period of fasting, but parenteral support is needed in neonates fasted for 4 hours to 6 hours and with fasting for 12 hours to 24 hours in older foals.[147]

Adult horses with chronic diarrhea and fecal water syndrome

In adult horses, chronic diarrhea often is a sign of large intestinal or colonic disease.[135] Unfortunately, the scientific information on dietary treatment of diarrhea is scarce (discussed previously).

Fecal water syndrome. Horses with fecal water syndrome (FWS) produce normal feces in addition to liquid feces that are defecated separately. Several nutritional factors anecdotally have been suggested as potential causes, including increased amounts of alfalfa hay, feeding haylage or silage, and drinking very cold water. In 1 study, none of these nutritional factors could be related to a predisposition to FWS.[150] Social stress, however, might be important because 40% of the affected horses were the last or second last in the hierarchy, and 62% did not defend their food against other horses, which could lead to changes in peristalsis and cause FWS.[150] Several commercial dietary supplements to improve FWS are available; however, there is little scientific evidence for their efficacy.

A reduction in particle size has been postulated as a potential treatment of FWS. Smaller particles reduce passage rate (ie, shorten transit time, such that particles pass at the same rate as liquid), lower the free water content, and result in more homogenous digesta. A pelleted diet also could induce mechanical rest by decreasing bulk.[151] The correct ratio between pellet and long hay may be important because the safe upper limit for ground and pelleted meadow hay inclusion in 1 study was 4 kg (BW: 620 kg; body condition score 7/9) for achieving an acceptable fecal consistency.[151] Inclusion of beet pulp or grass cobs did not appear to be helpful.[150] Clinical signs improved when the diet was changed from wrapped forage to hay or pasture, but 25% of the cases also improved when the batch of wrapped forage was changed, making it hard to generalize that FWS is attributed to feeding wrapped forage.[152] In addition, the microbiota of horses with FWS are similar to healthy individuals, precluding more specific recommendations.[153]

SUMMARY

In summary, nutrition is intimately related to the pathophysiology of GI-related diseases. Standard nutritional evaluation is warranted because of its important role in prevention but also in the treatment and management of these diseases. When medical and nutritional treatment are combined, success rates will be higher e.g. in gastric ulcers. A new field of research that integrates the impact of diet on the GI microbiota and its consequences on gut health has become available and might be used in the future for prevention and treatment of those diseases in horses.

ACKNOWLEDGMENTS

Rebecca DiPietro for creating the Figures (BioRender.com).

DISCLOSURE

The authors have nothing to disclose.

REFERENCES

1. Eckburg PB, Bik EM, Bernstein CN, et al. Diversity of the human intestinal microbial flora. Science 2005;308(5728):1635–8.
2. Costa MC, Weese JS. Understanding the Intestinal Microbiome in Health and Disease. Vet Clin North Am Equine Pract 2018;34(1):1–12.
3. Thursby E, Juge N. Introduction to the human gut microbiota. Biochem J 2017; 474(11):1823–36.
4. Costa M, Weese JS. Methods and basic concepts for microbiota assessment. Vet J 2019;249:10–5.
5. Dougal K, de la Fuente G, Harris PA, et al. Identification of a core bacterial community within the large intestine of the horse. PLoS One 2013;8(10):e77660.
6. Costa MC, Silva G, Ramos RV, et al. Characterization and comparison of the bacterial microbiota in different gastrointestinal tract compartments in horses. Vet J 2015;205(1):74–80.
7. Grimm P, Philippeau C, Julliand V. Faecal parameters as biomarkers of the equine hindgut microbial ecosystem under dietary change. Animal 2017; 11(7):1136–45.
8. Salem SE, Maddox TW, Antczak P, et al. Acute changes in the colonic microbiota are associated with large intestinal forms of surgical colic. BMC Vet Res 2019;15(1):468.
9. Arroyo LG, Rossi L, Santos BP, et al. Luminal and mucosal microbiota of the cecum and large colon of healthy and diarrheic horses. Animals (Basel) 2020; 10(8):1403.
10. Merritt AM, Julliand V. 1 - Gastrointestinal physiology. In: Geor RJ, Harris PA, Coenen M, editors. Equine applied and clinical nutrition. W.B. Saunders; 2013. p. 3–32.
11. Costa MC, Arroyo LG, Allen-Vercoe E, et al. Comparison of the fecal microbiota of healthy horses and horses with colitis by high throughput sequencing of the V3-V5 region of the 16S rRNA gene. PLoS One 2012;7(7):e41484.
12. Morrison PK, Newbold CJ, Jones E, et al. The Equine Gastrointestinal Microbiome: Impacts of Age and Obesity. Front Microbiol 2018;9:3017.
13. Costa MC, Stampfli HR, Allen-Vercoe E, et al. Development of the faecal microbiota in foals. Equine Vet J 2016;48(6):681–8.
14. Lindenberg F, Krych L, Kot W, et al. Development of the equine gut microbiota. Sci Rep 2019;9(1):14427.
15. De La Torre U, Henderson JD, Furtado KL, et al. Utilizing the fecal microbiota to understand foal gut transitions from birth to weaning. PLoS One 2019;14(4): e0216211.
16. Dougal K, de la Fuente G, Harris PA, et al. Characterisation of the faecal bacterial community in adult and elderly horses fed a high fibre, high oil or high starch diet using 454 pyrosequencing. PLoS One 2014;9(2):e87424.
17. Weese JS, Holcombe SJ, Embertson RM, et al. Changes in the faecal microbiota of mares precede the development of post partum colic. Equine Vet J 2015; 47(6):641–9.
18. Almeida ML, Feringer WHJ, Carvalho JR, et al. Intense exercise and aerobic conditioning associated with chromium or l-carnitine supplementation modified the fecal microbiota of fillies. PLoS One 2016;11(12):e0167108.

19. Kaiser-Thom S, Hilty M, Gerber V. Effects of hypersensitivity disorders and environmental factors on the equine intestinal microbiota. Vet Q 2020;40(1):97–107.

20. Langner K, Blaue D, Schedlbauer C, et al. Changes in the faecal microbiota of horses and ponies during a two-year body weight gain programme. PLoS One 2020;15(3):e0230015.

21. Husso A, Jalanka J, Alipour MJ, et al. The composition of the perinatal intestinal microbiota in horse. Sci Rep 2020;10(1):441.

22. Dominguez-Bello MG, Costello EK, Contreras M, et al. Delivery mode shapes the acquisition and structure of the initial microbiota across multiple body habitats in newborns. Proc Natl Acad Sci U S A 2010;107(26):11971–5.

23. Morrison PK, Newbold CJ, Jones E, et al. Effect of age and the individual on the gastrointestinal bacteriome of ponies fed a high-starch diet. PLoS One 2020; 15(5):e0232689.

24. Ochman H, Worobey M, Kuo CH, et al. Evolutionary relationships of wild hominids recapitulated by gut microbial communities. PLoS Biol 2010;8(11): e1000546.

25. Metcalf JL, Song SJ, Morton JT, et al. Evaluating the impact of domestication and captivity on the horse gut microbiome. Sci Rep 2017;7(1):15497.

26. Gao H, Chi X, Li G, et al. Gut microbial diversity and stabilizing functions enhance the plateau adaptability of Tibetan wild ass (Equus kiang). Microbiologyopen 2020;9(6):1150–61.

27. Qian LJ, Kang SM, Xie JL, et al. Early-life gut microbial colonization shapes Th1/Th2 balance in asthma model in BALB/c mice. BMC Microbiol 2017;17(1):135.

28. Arnold CE, Isaiah A, Pilla R, et al. The cecal and fecal microbiomes and metabolomes of horses before and after metronidazole administration. PLoS One 2020;15(5):e0232905.

29. Pringle J, Storm E, Waller A, et al. Influence of penicillin treatment of horses with strangles on seropositivity to Streptococcus equi ssp. equi-specific antibodies. J Vet Intern Med 2020;34(1):294–9.

30. Bordin AI, Suchodolski JS, Markel ME, et al. Effects of administration of live or inactivated virulent Rhodococcccus equi and age on the fecal microbiome of neonatal foals. PLoS One 2013;8(6):e66640.

31. Song Y, Malmuthuge N, Li F, et al. Colostrum feeding shapes the hindgut microbiota of dairy calves during the first 12 h of life. FEMS Microbiol Ecol 2019;95(1). https://doi.org/10.1093/femsec/fiy203.

32. Zheng W, Zhao W, Wu M, et al. Microbiota-targeted maternal antibodies protect neonates from enteric infection. Nature 2020;577(7791):543–8.

33. Catanzaro JR, Strauss JD, Bielecka A, et al. IgA-deficient humans exhibit gut microbiota dysbiosis despite secretion of compensatory IgM. Sci Rep 2019; 9(1):13574.

34. Mach N, Foury A, Kittelmann S, et al. The effects of weaning methods on gut microbiota composition and horse physiology. Front Physiol 2017;8:535.

35. Peachey LE, Molena RA, Jenkins TP, et al. The relationships between faecal egg counts and gut microbial composition in UK Thoroughbreds infected by cyathostomins. Int J Parasitol 2018;48(6):403–12.

36. Clark A, Salle G, Ballan V, et al. Strongyle infection and gut microbiota: profiling of resistant and susceptible horses over a grazing season. Front Physiol 2018; 9:272.

37. Bulmer LS, Murray JA, Burns NM, et al. High-starch diets alter equine faecal microbiota and increase behavioural reactivity. Sci Rep 2019;9(1):18621.

38. Harlow BE, Lawrence LM, Hayes SH, et al. Effect of dietary starch source and concentration on equine fecal microbiota. PLoS One 2016;11(4):e0154037.

39. Venable EB, Fenton KA, Braner VM, et al. Effects of feeding management on the equine cecal microbiota. J Equine Vet Sci 2017;49:113–21.

40. Warzecha CM, Coverdale JA, Janecka JE, et al. Influence of short-term dietary starch inclusion on the equine cecal microbiome. J Anim Sci 2017;95(11): 5077–90.

41. Hansen NC, Avershina E, Mydland LT, et al. High nutrient availability reduces the diversity and stability of the equine caecal microbiota. Microb Ecol Health Dis 2015;26:27216.

42. Faubladier C, Julliand V, Beuneiche L, et al. Comparative fibre-degrading capacity in foals at immediate and late post-weaning periods. Animal 2017; 11(9):1497–504.

43. Fernandes KA, Kittelmann S, Rogers CW, et al. Faecal microbiota of forage-fed horses in New Zealand and the population dynamics of microbial communities following dietary change. PLoS One 2014;9(11):e112846.

44. Schoster A. Probiotic use in equine gastrointestinal disease. Vet Clin North Am Equine Pract 2018;34(1):13–24.

45. Zavistanaviciute P, Poskiene I, Lele V, et al. The influence of the newly isolated Lactobacillus plantarum LUHS135 and Lactobacillus paracasei LUHS244 strains on blood and faeces parametersin endurance horses. Pol J Vet Sci 2019;22(3):513–21.

46. Urubschurov V, Stroebel C, Gunther E, et al. Effect of oral supplementation of probiotic strains of Lactobacillus rhamnosus and Enterococcus faecium on the composition of the faecal microbiota of foals. J Anim Physiol Anim Nutr (Berl) 2019;103(3):915–24.

47. Schoster A, Guardabassi L, Staempfli HR, et al. The longitudinal effect of a multi-strain probiotic on the intestinal bacterial microbiota of neonatal foals. Equine Vet J 2016;48(6):689–96.

48. Harlow BE, Lawrence LM, Harris PA, et al. Exogenous lactobacilli mitigate microbial changes associated with grain fermentation (corn, oats, and wheat) by equine fecal microflora ex vivo. PLoS One 2017;12(3):e0174059.

49. Milinovich GJ, Burrell PC, Pollitt CC, et al. Microbial ecology of the equine hindgut during oligofructose-induced laminitis. ISME J 2008;2(11):1089–100.

50. Respondek F, Goachet AG, Julliand V. Effects of dietary short-chain fructooligosaccharides on the intestinal microflora of horses subjected to a sudden change in diet. J Anim Sci 2008;86(2):316–23.

51. Glatter M, Borewicz K, van den Bogert B, et al. Modification of the equine gastrointestinal microbiota by Jerusalem artichoke meal supplementation. PLoS One 2019;14(8):e0220553.

52. Glatter M, Bochnia M, Goetz F, et al. Glycaemic and insulinaemic responses of adult healthy warm-blooded mares following feeding with Jerusalem artichoke meal. J Anim Physiol Anim Nutr (Berl) 2017;101(Suppl 1):69–78.

53. Bachmann M, Glatter M, Bochnia M, et al. In vitro gas production from batch cultures of stomach and hindgut digesta of horses adapted to a prebiotic dose of fructooligosaccharides and inulin. J Equine Vet Sci 2020;90:103020.

54. Cehak A, Krageloh T, Zuraw A, et al. Does prebiotic feeding affect equine gastric health? A study on the effects of prebiotic-induced gastric butyric acid production on mucosal integrity of the equine stomach. Res Vet Sci 2019;124: 303–9.

55. Passlack N, Vahjen W, Zentek J. Impact of Dietary Cellobiose on the Fecal Microbiota of Horses. J Equine Vet Sci 2020;91:103106.

56. Iida A, Saito H, Amao A, et al. The effects of a nutritional supplement containing salacinol in neonatal Thoroughbred foals. J Equine Sci 2020;31(1):11–5.

57. Ericsson AC, Johnson PJ, Lopes MA, et al. A microbiological map of the healthy equine gastrointestinal tract. PLoS One 2016;11(11):e0166523.

58. Petrof EO, Gloor GB, Vanner SJ, et al. Stool substitute transplant therapy for the eradication of Clostridium difficile infection: 'RePOOPulating' the gut. Microbiome 2013;1(1):3.

59. Blake AB, Guard BC, Honneffer JB, et al. Altered microbiota, fecal lactate, and fecal bile acids in dogs with gastrointestinal disease. PLoS One 2019;14(10): e0224454.

60. Ott SJ, Waetzig GH, Rehman A, et al. Efficacy of sterile fecal filtrate transfer for treating patients with clostridium difficile Infection. Gastroenterology 2017; 152(4):799–811.e7.

61. Wambacq WA, van Doorn DA, Rovers-Paap PM, et al. Dietary supplementation of micro-encapsulated sodium butyrate in healthy horses: effect on gut histology and immunohistochemistry parameters. BMC Vet Res 2020;16(1):121.

62. Gough E, Shaikh H, Manges AR. Systematic review of intestinal microbiota transplantation (fecal bacteriotherapy) for recurrent Clostridium difficile infection. Clin Infect Dis 2011;53(10):994–1002.

63. Pereira GQ, Gomes LA, Santos IS, et al. Fecal microbiota transplantation in puppies with canine parvovirus infection. J Vet Intern Med 2018;32(2):707–11.

64. Chaitman J, Ziese AL, Pilla R, et al. Fecal microbial and metabolic profiles in dogs with acute diarrhea receiving either fecal microbiota transplantation or oral metronidazole. Front Vet Sci 2020;7:192.

65. Borody TJ, Khoruts A. Fecal microbiota transplantation and emerging applications. Nat Rev Gastroenterol Hepatol 2011;9(2):88–96.

66. McKinney CA, Oliveira BCM, Bedenice D, et al. The fecal microbiota of healthy donor horses and geriatric recipients undergoing fecal microbial transplantation for the treatment of diarrhea. PLoS One 2020;15(3):e0230148.

67. Ramai D, Zakhia K, Fields PJ, et al. Fecal Microbiota Transplantation (FMT) with colonoscopy is superior to enema and nasogastric tube while comparable to capsule for the treatment of recurrent Clostridioides difficile infection: a systematic review and meta-analysis. Dig Dis Sci 2020. https://doi.org/10.1007/s10620-020-06185-7.

68. Sykes BW, Hewetson M, Hepburn RJ, et al. European College of Equine Internal Medicine consensus statement—equine gastric ulcer syndrome in adult horses. J Vet Intern Med 2015;29(5):1288–99.

69. Andrews FM, Larson C, Harris P. Nutritional management of gastric ulceration. Equine Vet Educ 2017;29(1):45–55.

70. Camacho-Luna P, Buchanan B, Andrews FM. Advances in diagnostics and treatments in horses and foals with gastric and duodenal ulcers. Vet Clin North Am Equine Pract 2018;34(1):97–111.

71. Reese RE, Andrews FM. Nutrition and dietary management of equine gastric ulcer syndrome. Vet Clin North Am Equine Pract 2009;25(1):79–92, vi–vii.

72. Woodward MC, Huff NK, Garza F Jr, et al. Effect of pectin, lecithin, and antacid feed supplements (Egusin®) on gastric ulcer scores, gastric fluid pH and blood gas values in horses. BMC Vet Res 2014;10(Suppl 1):S4.

73. Luthersson N, Nielsen KH, Harris P, et al. Risk factors associated with equine gastric ulceration syndrome (EGUS) in 201 horses in Denmark. Equine Vet J 2009;41(7):625–30.

74. Nadeau JA, Andrews FM, Mathew AG, et al. Evaluation of diet as a cause of gastric ulcers in horses. Am J Vet Res 2000;61(7):784–90.

75. Fedtke A, Pfaff M, Volquardsen J, et al. Effects of feeding different roughage-based diets on gastric mucosa after weaning in warmblood foals. Pferdeheilkunde 2015;31(6):596–+.

76. Vondran S, Venner M, Vervuert I. Effects of two alfalfa preparations with different particle sizes on the gastric mucosa in weanlings: alfalfa chaff versus alfalfa pellets. BMC Vet Res 2016;12(1):110.

77. Vondran S, Venner M, Coenen M, et al. Effects of alfalfa chaff on the gastric mucosa in adult horses. Pferdeheilkunde Equine Med 2017;33:66–71.

78. Bäuerlein V, Sabban C, Venner M, et al. Effects of feeding alfalfa hay in comparison to meadow hay on the gastric mucosa in adult Warmblood horses. Equine Med 2020;35(1):29–36.

79. Perkins GA, den Bakker HC, Burton AJ, et al. Equine stomachs harbor an abundant and diverse mucosal microbiota. Appl Environ Microbiol 2012;78(8):2522–32.

80. Dong HJ, Ho H, Hwang H, et al. Diversity of the gastric microbiota in thoroughbred racehorses having gastric ulcer. J Microbiol Biotechnol 2016;26(4):763–74.

81. Erck-Westergren EV, Woort Ft. Diet-induced changes in gastric and faecal microbiota in horses: association with gastric ulcer healing. Equine Vet J 2019;51(S53):21.

82. Rochais C, Henry S, Hausberger M. "Hay-bags" and "Slow feeders": Testing their impact on horse behaviour and welfare. Appl Anim Behav Sci 2018;198:52–9.

83. Böhm S, Mitterer T, Iben C. The impact of feeding a high-fibre and high-fat concentrated diet on the recovery of horses suffering from gastric ulcers. Pferdeheilkunde 2018;34:237–46.

84. Luthersson N, Bolger C, Fores P, et al. Effect of changing diet on gastric ulceration in exercising horses and ponies after cessation of omeprazole treatment. J Equine Vet Sci 2019;83:102742.

85. Munsterman AS, Dias Moreira AS, Marqués FJ. Evaluation of a Chinese herbal supplement on equine squamous gastric disease and gastric fluid pH in mares. J Vet Intern Med 2019;33(5):2280–5.

86. Fedtke AFA, Venner M, Vervuert I. Effects of different neutraceutic supplements on the gastric mucosa of weanling foals. Pferdeheilkunde 2015;31:364–70.

87. Frank N, Andrews FM, Elliott SB, et al. Effects of dietary oils on the development of gastric ulcers in mares. Am J Vet Res 2005;66(11):2006–11.

88. Holbrook TC, Simmons RD, Payton ME, et al. Effect of repeated oral administration of hypertonic electrolyte solution on equine gastric mucosa. Equine Vet J 2005;37(6):501–4.

89. Curtis L, Burford JH, England GCW, et al. Risk factors for acute abdominal pain (colic) in the adult horse: A scoping review of risk factors, and a systematic review of the effect of management-related changes. PLoS One 2019;14(7):e0219307.

90. Kaneene JB, Miller R, Ross WA, et al. Risk factors for colic in the Michigan (USA) equine population. Prev Vet Med 1997;30(1):23–36.

91. Traub-Dargatz JL, Kopral CA, Seitzinger AH, et al. Estimate of the national incidence of and operation-level risk factors for colic among horses in the United States, spring 1998 to spring 1999. J Am Vet Med Assoc 2001;219(1):67–71.

92. Durham AE. The role of nutrition in colic. Vet Clin North Am Equine Pract 2009; 25(1):67–78, vi.

93. House AM, Warren LK. Nutritional management of recurrent colic and colonic impactions. Equine Vet Educ 2016;28(3):167–72.

94. Hudson JM, Cohen ND, Gibbs PG, et al. Feeding practices associated with colic in horses. J Am Vet Med Assoc 2001;219(10):1419–25.

95. Scantlebury CE, Archer DC, Proudman CJ, et al. Recurrent colic in the horse: incidence and risk factors for recurrence in the general practice population. Equine Vet J Suppl 2011;(39):81–8.

96. Cohen ND, Gibbs PG, Woods AM. Dietary and other management factors associated with colic in horses. J Am Vet Med Assoc 1999;215(1):53–60.

97. Cohen ND, Matejka PL, Honnas CM, et al. Case-control study of the association between various management factors and development of colic in horses. Texas Equine Colic Study Group. J Am Vet Med Assoc 1995;206(5):667–73.

98. Cohen ND, Peloso JG. Risk factors for history of previous colic and for chronic, intermittent colic in a population of horses. J Am Vet Med Assoc 1996;208(5): 697–703.

99. Hillyer MH, Taylor FG, Proudman CJ, et al. Case control study to identify risk factors for simple colonic obstruction and distension colic in horses. Equine Vet J 2002;34(5):455–63.

100. McCarthy HE, French NP, Edwards GB, et al. Equine grass sickness is associated with low antibody levels to Clostridium botulinum: a matched case-control study. Equine Vet J 2004;36(2):123–9.

101. Tinker MK, White NA, Lessard P, et al. Prospective study of equine colic risk factors. Equine Vet J 1997;29(6):454–8.

102. Harris PA, Ellis AD, Fradinho MJ, et al. Review: Feeding conserved forage to horses: recent advances and recommendations. Animal 2017;11(6):958–67.

103. Archer DC, Proudman CJ. Epidemiological clues to preventing colic. Vet J 2006; 172(1):29–39.

104. Coizet B, Nicoloso L, Marletta D, et al. Variation in salivary and pancreatic alpha-amylase genes in Italian horse breeds. J Hered 2014;105(3):429–35.

105. Troya L, Blanco J, Romero I, et al. Comparison of the colic incidence in a horse population with or without inclusion of germinated barley in the diet. Equine Vet Educ 2020;32(S11):28–32.

106. Raymond Geor PH, Manfred Coenen. Ration evaluation and formulation. 1st edition. In: Dunnett CE, editor. Equine applied and clinical nutrition. 2013. p. 412.

107. Raymond Geor PH, Manfred Coenen. Intestinal Diseases. 1st edition. In: Durham AE, editor. Equine applied and clinical nutrition 2013. p. 575.

108. Scantlebury CE, Archer DC, Proudman CJ, et al. Management and horse-level risk factors for recurrent colic in the UK general equine practice population. Equine Vet J 2015;47(2):202–6.

109. Williams S, Horner J, Orton E, et al. Water intake, faecal output and intestinal motility in horses moved from pasture to a stabled management regime with controlled exercise. Equine Vet J 2015;47(1):96–100.

110. Hallowell GD. Medical management of large colonic impactions. Equine Vet Educ 2017;29(7):385–90.

111. Little D, Blikslager AT. Factors associated with development of ileal impaction in horses with surgical colic: 78 cases (1986-2000). Equine Vet J 2002;34(5): 464–8.

112. Blikslager AT. Colic prevention to avoid colic surgery: a surgeon's perspective. J Equine Vet Sci 2019;76:1–5.

113. Hansen TL, Chizek EL, Zugay OK, et al. Digestibility and retention time of coastal bermudagrass (cynodon dactylon) hay by horses. Animals (Basel) 2019;9(12):1148.
114. Hansen TL, Lawrence LM. Composition factors predicting forage digestibility by horses. J Equine Vet Sci 2017;58:97–102.
115. Hotwagner K, Iben C. Evacuation of sand from the equine intestine with mineral oil, with and without psyllium. J Anim Physiol Anim Nutr (Berl) 2008;92(1):86–91.
116. Kaikkonen R, Niinistö K, Lindholm T, et al. Comparison of psyllium feeding at home and nasogastric intubation of psyllium and magnesium sulfate in the hospital as a treatment for naturally occurring colonic sand (geosediment) accumulations in horses: A retrospective study. Acta Vet Scand 2016;58:73.
117. Niinistö K, Hewetson M, Kaikkonen R, et al. Comparison of the effects of enteral psyllium, magnesium sulphate and their combination for removal of sand from the large colon of horses. Vet J 2014;202(3):608–11.
118. Niinisto KE, Ruohoniemi MO, Freccero F, et al. Investigation of the treatment of sand accumulations in the equine large colon with psyllium and magnesium sulphate. Vet J 2018;238:22–6.
119. Bergstrom TC, Sakai RR, Nieto JE. Catastrophic gastric rupture in a horse secondary to psyllium pharmacobezoars. Can Vet J 2018;59(3):249–53.
120. Hassel DM, Curley T, Hoaglund EL. Evaluation of fecal sand clearance in horses with naturally acquired colonic sand accumulation with a product containing probiotics, prebiotics, and psyllium. J Equine Vet Sci 2020;90:102970.
121. Archer DC, Pinchbeck GL, French NP, et al. Risk factors for epiploic foramen entrapment colic in a UK horse population: A prospective case-control study. Equine Vet J 2008;40(4):405–10.
122. Nicol CJ, Davidson HP, Harris PA, et al. Study of crib-biting and gastric inflammation and ulceration in young horses. Vet Rec 2002;151(22):658–62.
123. Moore-Colyer MJS, Hemmings A, Hewer N. A preliminary investigation into the effect of ad libitum or restricted hay with or without Horslyx on the intake and switching behaviour of normal and crib biting horses. Livestock Sci 2016;186:59–62.
124. Sarrafchi A, Blokhuis HJ. Equine stereotypic behaviors: Causation, occurrence, and prevention. J Vet Behav 2013;8(5):386–94.
125. Cohen ND, Toby E, Roussel AJ, et al. Are feeding practices associated with duodenitis-proximal jejunitis? Equine Vet J 2006;38(6):526–31.
126. Galinelli N, Wambacq W, Broeckx BJG, et al. High intake of sugars and starch, low number of meals and low roughage intake are associated with Equine Gastric Ulcer Syndrome in a Belgian cohort. J Anim Physiol Anim Nutr (Berl) 2019. https://doi.org/10.1111/jpn.13215.
127. Galinelli NC, Wambacq W, Lefère L, et al. Can the outcome of an impaired oral glucose absorption test in horses be improved with fat supplementation and dietary modifications? Vet Rec Case Rep 2019;7(3):e000844.
128. Fascetti A, Stratton-Phelps M. Clinical Assessment Of Nutritional Status And Enteral Feeding In The Acutely III Horse. Current Therapy in Equine Medicine: 5th edition. 2003:705-710.
129. Kalck KA. Inflammatory bowel disease in horses. Vet Clin North Am Equine Pract 2009;25(2):303–15.
130. Dupont S, De Spiegeleer A, Liu DJ, et al. A commercially available immunoglobulin E-based test for food allergy gives inconsistent results in healthy ponies. Equine Vet J 2016;48(1):109–13.

131. Van den Hove R. TD, Bankuti P. Chronic Inflammatory Bowel Disease (CIBD) and Celiac disease, are these linked in the horse? vol. 33. 1st edition. Pferdeheilkunde2017.

132. van der Kolk JH, van Putten LA, Mulder CJ, et al. Gluten-dependent antibodies in horses with inflammatory small bowel disease (ISBD). Vet Q 2012;32(1):3–11.

133. van Proosdij R, Mulder C, Reijm M, et al. Preliminary Notes On Equine Tissue Transglutaminase Serology And A Case Of Equine Gluten -Sensitive Enteropathy And Dermatitis In An 11-Year -Old Dutch Warmblood Horse. J Equine Vet Sci 2020;90:102999.

134. Magdesian KG, Bozorgmanesh R. Nutritional considerations for horses with colitis. Part 2: Parenteral nutrition, new nutritional considerations and specific dietary recommendations. Equine Vet Educ 2018;30(11):608–15.

135. Oliver-Espinosa O. Diagnostics and treatments in chronic diarrhea and weight loss in horses. Vet Clin North Am Equine Pract 2018;34(1):69–80.

136. Oliver-Espinosa O. Foal diarrhea: established and postulated causes, prevention, diagnostics, and treatments. Vet Clin North Am Equine Pract 2018;34(1): 55–68.

137. Magdesian KG. Nutrition for critical gastrointestinal illness: feeding horses with diarrhea or colic. Vet Clin North Am Equine Pract 2003;19(3):617–44.

138. Hassel DM, Spier SJ, Aldridge BM, et al. Influence of diet and water supply on mineral content and pH within the large intestine of horses with enterolithiasis. Vet J 2009;182(1):44–9.

139. Cohen ND, Vontur CA, Rakestraw PC. Risk factors for enterolithiasis among horses in Texas. J Am Vet Med Assoc 2000;216(11):1787–94.

140. Hassel DM, Aldridge BM, Drake CM, et al. Evaluation of dietary and management risk factors for enterolithiasis among horses in California. Res Vet Sci 2008;85(3):476–80.

141. Hassel DM, Rakestraw PC, Gardner IA, et al. Dietary risk factors and colonic pH and mineral concentrations in horses with enterolithiasis. J Vet Intern Med 2004; 18(3):346–9.

142. Suthers JM, Pinchbeck GL, Proudman CJ, et al. Risk factors for large colon volvulus in the UK. Equine Vet J 2013;45(5):558–63.

143. Valle E, Giusto G, Penazzi L, et al. Preliminary results on the association with feeding and recovery length in equine colic patients after laparotomy. J Anim Physiol Anim Nutr (Berl) 2019;103(4):1233–41.

144. Vásquez W, Hernández AV, Garcia-Sabrido JL. Is gum chewing useful for ileus after elective colorectal surgery? A systematic review and meta-analysis of randomized clinical trials. J Gastrointest Surg 2009;13(4):649–56.

145. Hudson NPH, Pirie RS. Equine post operative ileus: A review of current thinking on pathophysiology and management. Equine Vet Educ 2015;27(1):39–47.

146. Cohen ND. Causes of and farm management factors associated with disease and death in foals. J Am Vet Med Assoc 1994;204(10):1644–51.

147. Mallicote M, House AM, Sanchez LC. A review of foal diarrhoea from birth to weaning. Equine Vet Educ 2012;24(4):206–14.

148. Kuhl J, Winterhoff N, Wulf M, et al. Changes in faecal bacteria and metabolic parameters in foals during the first six weeks of life. Vet Microbiol 2011;151(3–4): 321–8.

149. Magdesian KG. Neonatal foal diarrhea. Vet Clin North Am Equine Pract 2005; 21(2):295–312, vi.

150. Kienzle E, Zehnder C, Pfister K, et al. Field study on risk factors for free fecal water in pleasure horses. J Equine Vet Sci 2016;44:32–6.

151. Valle E, Gandini M, Bergero D. Management of chronic diarrhea in an adult horse. J Equine Vet Sci 2013;33:130–5.
152. Lindroth KM, Johansen A, Båverud V, et al. Differential defecation of solid and liquid phases in horses—a descriptive survey. Animals 2020;10(1):76.
153. Schoster A, Weese JS, Gerber V, et al. Dysbiosis is not present in horses with fecal water syndrome when compared to controls in spring and autumn. J Vet Intern Med 2020;34(4):1614–21.

Nutritional Considerations when Dealing with an Underweight Adult or Senior Horse

Nicola Jarvis, BVetMed, CertAVP(EM), CertAVP(ESST)[a],
Harold C. McKenzie III, DVM, MS, MSc (VetEd)[b],*

KEYWORDS

- Weight loss • Decreased appetite • Underlying disease • Dental disorders • Horses

KEY POINTS

- Weight loss can be insidious and multifactorial, making it difficult to identify the primary cause.
- Although inadequate energy intake is often the cause of poor body condition, underlying disease conditions in multiple body systems may also play an important role.
- Thorough dental assessment is always indicated in horses with weight loss because dental disorders may impair a horse's ability to ingest and process feedstuffs appropriately.

INTRODUCTION

Weight loss occurs when there is an imbalance between the supply of energy and the expenditure of energy in an individual. Weight loss can be multifactorial (**Box 1**),[1] especially in older horses, so a methodical approach to weight-loss investigation and treatment is required. Repeated assessment is also indicated, because comorbidities are common and new conditions may arise as the initial problems are being treated or resolved.

ASSESSMENT OF UNDERWEIGHT HORSES

It is important to take an organized approach to assessing affected horses (**Box 2**). The first step is the collection of a thorough history, to include detailed dietary, housing

[a] Redwings Horse Sanctuary, Hapton, Norwich, Norfolk NR15 1SP, UK; [b] Department of Large Animal Clinical Sciences, Virginia Maryland College of Veterinary Medicine, Virginia Tech, 215 Duckpond Drive, Blacksburg, VA 24061, USA
* Corresponding author.
E-mail address: hmckenzi@vt.edu

Vet Clin Equine 37 (2021) 89–110
https://doi.org/10.1016/j.cveq.2020.12.003
0749-0739/21/© 2020 Elsevier Inc. All rights reserved.

Box 1
Potential causes of weight loss in adult and aged horses

Reduced consumption of feed
  Malnutrition (poor dietary design)
  Deliberate starvation (abuse)
  Dental disorders
  Social hierarchy issues
  Musculoskeletal disorders
  Winter-associated stress

Malabsorption
  Inadequate mastication (dental disorders)
  Gastrointestinal disorders
  Endoparasitism

Impaired nutrient use
  Hepatic insufficiency

Increased use of energy and nutrients
  Systemic or localized inflammatory or infectious disease
  Protein-losing enteropathy
  Chronic renal insufficiency
  Chronic musculoskeletal disease
  Hyperthyroidism
  Pituitary pars intermedia dysfunction
  Equine asthma
  Cardiac failure

Other
  Equine motor neuron disease

Adapted from Tamzali Y. Chronic weight loss syndrome in the horse: a 60 case retrospective study. *EVE.* 2006;18(6):289-296; with permission.

---

and management information, the presence of historical or concurrent disease, as well as the presence of other animals that compete for resources (food, shelter). The diet should be carefully evaluated (see Myriam Hesta and Megan Shepherd's article, "How to Perform a Nutritional Assessment in a First Line/General Practice," in this issue) in order to determine whether weight loss is the result of inadequate provision of feedstuffs, and/or caused by poor feed quality. Rather than relying on owner perception, care should be taken to personally assess the amounts fed, the quality of the feeds (including forages), and how they have been stored. A full clinical examination must be completed to help differentiate primary malnutrition from weight loss secondary to clinical disease. This examination should include subjective assessment of a body condition score (BCS) (see Myriam Hesta and Megan Shepherd's article, "How to Perform a Nutritional Assessment in a First Line/General Practice"; Megan Shepherd and colleagues' article, "Nutritional Considerations When Dealing with an Obese Adult Equine," in this issue), with a score of less than 4 out of 9 being of concern. It is important to ascertain the owner's perception of the patient's body condition, because it may differ substantially from the veterinarian's assessment of BCS. This assessment should include a determination of the owner's perception of changes in body condition over time, in order to ascertain whether a change in BCS is an acute or chronic change. A thorough dental examination is important to assess whether the horse is physically able to eat the feeds offered. Reasons for increased calorie demands such as pregnancy and lactation must be ascertained. Hematology and biochemistry testing are indicated in order to investigate underlying conditions such

---

Box 2
Diagnostic approach to underweight horse

- Collect historical information
- Thorough physical examination
- Diagnostic examination
  - ○ Systemic
    - ■ Complete blood count
    - ■ Serum chemistry
    - ■ Endocrine testing
  - ○ Gastrointestinal tract
    - ■ Oral examination
    - ■ Gastroscopic examination
    - ■ Abdominal ultrasonography examination
    - ■ Rectal examination
    - ■ Rectal mucosal biopsy
    - ■ Fecal floatation
    - ■ Fecal sedimentation
  - ○ Hepatic
    - ■ Serum chemistry
      - • Glucose
      - • Bilirubin
      - • Albumin
      - • Aspartate transaminase
      - • Lactate dehydrogenase
      - • Gamma-glutamyl transferase
      - • Alkaline phosphatase
    - ■ Serum bile acids
    - ■ Sorbitol dehydrogenase
    - ■ Glutamate dehydrogenase
  - ○ Renal
    - ■ Serum chemistry
      - • Creatinine
      - • Blood urea nitrogen
    - ■ Symmetric dimethylarginine (SDMA)

---

as hepatic disease, renal disease, or protein-losing enteropathy. Endocrine testing may be indicated in order to assess for underlying pituitary pars intermedia dysfunction (PPID) or hyperthyroidism.[2,3] Fecal floatation is a simple test that can be very useful in assessing for endoparasitism. A rectal examination is useful for assessment of structural abnormalities involving the gastrointestinal viscera and other caudal abdominal structures, such as the urinary bladder, left kidney, uterus, and ovaries. Additional diagnostics, such as gastroscopy, intestinal absorption studies, abdominal ultrasonography examination, or rectal biopsy may be indicated depending on the findings of the initial examination, as discussed later. In some situations, these diagnostics may not be available because of issues of access or financial concerns, and decisions regarding management and treatment may need to be made on physical examination alone.

Determining the most useful ordering of diagnostics in the evaluation of weight loss can be challenging. Using a detailed diagnostic approach to the evaluation of chronic weight loss, such as that described by Tamzali[1] (2006), can be helpful. In this mechanistic approach, the various diagnostic techniques are grouped into 3 classes. The first is simple first-intention tests, and includes collection of a thorough history; performance of a thorough physical examination, rectal examination, and routine hematology, to include fibrinogen and possibly serum amyloid A (SAA); routine serum biochemistry; and fecal floatation. The second group of tests includes intestinal absorption studies (glucose or D-xylose), abdominocentesis, rectal biopsy, detailed biochemistry analysis of renal or hepatic function; and testing for PPID. The third and final group of diagnostic tests are more specific and complex and include endoscopy (upper respiratory tract, esophagus, stomach, duodenum), abdominal and thoracic ultrasonography, echocardiography, biopsies (liver, kidney), laparoscopy, exploratory laparotomy, or postmortem examination.

CAUSES OF POOR CONDITION
Malnutrition

Malnutrition results from provision of a diet with a deficiency, excess, or imbalance of nutrients such as proteins, vitamins, and minerals or total energy intake. The term is most commonly used to describe dietary deficiencies alone and that is the focus here. Malnutrition can result from poor dietary design, caused by limited resources, inadequate awareness/education, or neglect (intentional or otherwise). Starvation is when an animal has severe malnutrition, which can occur acutely, such as when food has been abruptly and completely withdrawn, or chronically as a result of prolonged, but less severe, feed deprivation.[4] The determination of the cause of malnutrition is typically based on assessment of the individual's dietary needs and comparing these with the composition of the diet being provided. It is important to keep in mind that a malnourished animal may have other disease processes contributing to the loss of body condition, such as dental disease or endoparasitism, because these represent common comorbidities in animals with poor management.

It is important to consider each equine as an individual when evaluating a diet. A late pregnant or lactating mare (see Morgane Robles and colleagues' article, "Nutrition of Broodmares," in this issue), high-level competition or endurance horse, or a growing youngster requires a higher level of energy provision than an adult horse in light work (see Kristine L. Urschel and Erica C. McKenzie's article, "Nutritional Influences on Skeletal Muscle and Muscular Disease," in this issue). Recommended dietary levels of protein also vary throughout a horse's life, with foals and yearlings typically requiring higher-protein diets, compared with an adult horse at maintenance (see Kristine L. Urschel and Erica C. McKenzie's article, "Nutritional Influences on Skeletal Muscle and Muscular Disease," in this issue).[5] Even with attention to energy and protein requirements, vitamin and mineral deficiencies can result from long-term hay-only rations, lack of pasture access, grazing mineral-deficient soils, or restricted diets as part of obesity management. An example is vitamin E, which is typically found in high levels in fresh grass. Long-term restriction to a diet without green feeds can lead to a deficiency in vitamin E and may result in equine motor neuron disease,[6] giving the appearance of poor condition because of muscle wastage (see Kristine L. Urschel and Erica C. McKenzie's article, "Nutritional Influences on Skeletal Muscle and Muscular Disease," in this issue).

Deliberate Starvation/Abuse

A veterinary surgeon may be asked to attend a horse where acute or chronic starvation is suspected as part of a criminal prosecution case according to local law. For example, in England and Wales, the welfare of animals is currently safeguarded by the Animal Welfare Act 2006. Under Section 9 of the Act, those responsible for animals have a duty to ensure the animals' welfare needs are met, regardless of intention, which includes the provision of a suitable diet. The key to a successful prosecution for neglect is demonstrating that correct feeding and provision of adequate dental and veterinary care results in weight gain. Regular recording of weight, BCS, feed intake, anthelmintic provision, and medication should be accompanied by photographic evidence.[7]

Dental Disease

Horses are highly reliant on good dentition in order to reduce the fiber particle length of forage and increase feed surface area to facilitate enzymatic and bacterial processing within the digestive tract. In Tamzali's[1] report, 20% of horses presented for assessment of weight loss were diagnosed with dental abnormalities. Du Toit and colleagues[8] studied a large population of donkeys and found dental disease in 73.1% and concluded that dental disease was significantly associated with weight loss, poor BCS, and colic. A thorough dental examination should begin with observation of the horse eating both forage and processed feed to check for quidding (dropping feed), food pocketing (eg, feed residing in diastemas/periodontal pocket), or excessive salivation. The head should be assessed externally for facial symmetry, muscle mass, and abnormalities of the temporomandibular joints. Lateral excursion of the mandible, which reflects occlusal contact, should be symmetric and pain free. A Hausmann-type gag, bright light source, and mirror should be used to identify loss or reduction of the functional occlusal surfaces and potential sources of pain.[9]

The equine tooth is hypsodont, with an extensive reserve crown that gradually erupts to counter natural attrition at the occlusal surface. In younger horses, the cheek teeth abut squarely in each arcade and function as a single unit, but, in older horses, gaps appear between the teeth, known as senile diastemata. These gaps may be valvelike, where the diastema is wider at the gingival surface than the occlusal. Food becomes trapped and decomposes, leading to inflammation of the gingiva, which, if left untreated, extends to the deeper periodontal tissues and ultimately results in periodontitis, periodontal pocketing, and loss of alveolar bone and associated teeth (**Fig. 1**). Periodontal disease is exquisitely painful and can reduce appetite, particularly for chilled feeds and water in winter. The physical presence of trapped forage may also ulcerate the tongue and buccal mucosa, causing further discomfort (**Fig. 2**). Periodontal disease is increasingly prevalent in horses more than 15 years of age[10] and examination of 400 cadaver skulls at an abattoir showed a high

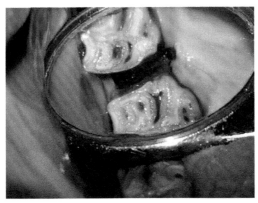

Fig. 1. Food packing within this diastema has resulted in painful periodontal disease and deep periodontal pocketing.

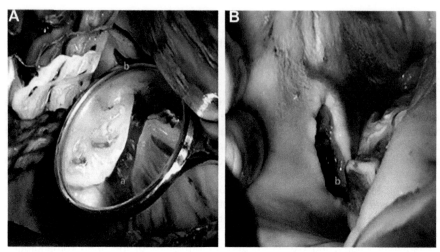

Fig. 2. Narrow or valve diastemata (*A*) can trap coarse forage and chopped fiber leading to excoriation and ulceration of the buccal mucosa (*B*) and tongue.

prevalence of diastemata (40%), mobile teeth (12.2%), and missing teeth (18.4%) in horses more than 15 years of age.[11]

Horses rely on the difference in attrition of enamel, dentine, and cementum to provide enamel ridges for grinding forage. In aged horses, these enamel ridges are gradually worn away until the horse is unable to masticate long fiber effectively (smooth mouthed).[9] Dental pain and conditions such as so-called wry nose can cause abnormal masticatory movements that lead to shear mouth, where the molar occlusal angle, normally between 12.5° and 30°, becomes exaggerated.[12] An abnormal molar occlusal angle has been reported to reduce digestibility of crude fiber and protein.[13]

Clinical signs of dental disease include quidding, food pocketing, hypersalivation (suggests pain), facial swelling, halitosis, weight loss, poor appetite, and an increased incidence of choke or colic.[14] Deterioration in a horse's ability to chew forage may result in more subtle signs, such as normal droppings/manure followed by a significant quantity of liquid, and increased fiber particle length (FPL) within the droppings/manure. An FPL greater than 3.6 mm may indicate dental disorder and may improve following routine dental rasping.[15] When owners notice quidding and weight loss, they may be tempted to reduce forage intake and increase the complimentary feed/concentrate ration without seeking treatment.[16] However, reduced lateral excursion of the mandible when eating a pelleting feed versus long fiber encourages further development of dental abnormalities.[17]

Equine odontoclastic tooth resorption and hypercementosis (EOTRH) is an extremely painful condition characterized by unregulated deposition of dental cementum and resorption of tooth apices diagnosed by radiography.[18] The incisors, canines, and premolars are typically affected. Clinical signs include severe gingival inflammation and recession (**Fig. 3**), hypersalivation, mobile incisors, halitosis, inappetence, weight loss, and difficulty in prehension of food.[19] Reluctance to bite down on a carrot can often be used to demonstrate incisor pain. Exodontia is frequently the only treatment option.

Endoparasitism

Endoparasites, most notably cyathostomes (small strongles) are a common cause of weight loss with or without diarrhea. The weight loss in these cases is often insidious,

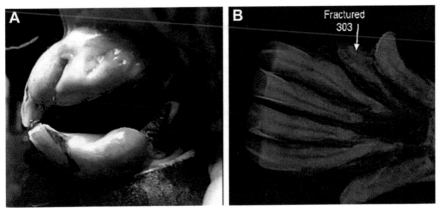

Fig. 3. (A) Painful gingival swellings and discharging tracts associated with the retained roots of 202, 203, and 303 following pathologic fracture of the incisors. (B) Ventrodorsal radiographic image of affected area. This pony was diagnosed with EOTRH and had been unable to eat forage. Extraction of the diseased incisors was performed. The pony began to eat forage the following day.

caused by long-term gastrointestinal malabsorption and protein-losing enteropathy.[20] Of 60 animals admitted to a referral hospital for chronic weight loss, larval cyathostominosis was the final diagnosis in 31% of cases.[1] Endoparasitism is of increased concern in horses with malnutrition, poor management, and overstocking.[21] Increasing age does not seem to be associated with an increased risk of endoparasitism, but horses with PPID have been shown to have higher parasite burdens.[22] The pathogenic larval stages of cyathostomes burrow into the mucosal and submucosal layers of the large intestine where development may be arrested (hypobiosis) for up to 2 years before emerging as fourth-stage larvae. Synchronized reactivation of hypobiotic larvae and mass reemergence causes severe inflammation and erosion of the intestinal wall.[23] Mass reemergence may result in a variety of potential clinical signs, including weight loss, diarrhea, dehydration, pyrexia, and subcutaneous edema caused by a protein-losing enteropathy and absorption of bacterial enterotoxins.[23] Mortalities of 40% to 70% have been reported, despite aggressive treatment.[24] Resistance to anthelmintics is of increasing concern, because this may result in a failure to respond to anthelmintic administration.[25] Common clinicopathologic findings include hypoalbuminemia, neutrophilia, hyperglobulinemia, and hyperfibrinogenemia.[26] A fecal worm egg count should be repeated once a day for 5 days with a wet smear or sedimentation used to check for larvae, because false-negative test results may occur and this approach improves the sensitivity of the test.[24] Adult cyathostomes and fourth-stage larvae may be seen in the feces or observed on a gloved arm following a rectal examination. A positive fecal floatation finding, or the observance of parasites, is a clear indication for larvicidal anthelmintic treatment. Because of the potential for false-negative results when performing fecal floatation tests,[27] larvicidal anthelmintic administration is sometimes performed empirically, and subsequent improvement in body condition may represent a positive response to this diagnostic test.

Anthelmintic protocols include 5 consecutive days of oral fenbendazole 7.5 mg/kg body weight (BW) or a single dose of moxidectin 0.4 mg/kg BW. However, when the larvicidal action of fenbendazole was investigated in horses naturally infected with cyathostomes, larval death was associated with severe tissue damage, inflammation, and ulceration mimicking larval cyathostominosis, whereas, with moxidectin, larvae appeared to disintegrate and be resorbed without adverse effects on the intestinal wall.[23] Subsequent work suggests that the inflammatory response following larvicidal therapy is not severe, and is comparable between treatment types.[28] However, this concern regarding possible secondary intestinal inflammation associated with the death of encysted larval organisms is sometimes addressed by accompanying anthelmintic therapy with corticosteroid administration, particularly in severely affected individuals.[21] Treatment protocols may include prednisolone (0.5–1.0 mg/kg BW, by mouth, every 24 h or every 12 h) or dexamethasone (0.02–0.05 mg/kg BW, intravenously, intramuscularly, or by mouth, every 24–48 h).[26]

Social Issues

Because weight loss may be multifactorial in origin, it is important to record any recent social and environmental changes. Hierarchy plays an essential role in access to food and shelter. It has been shown that higher-ranked horses improved condition over the winter months, whereas the opposite was true in lower-ranked animals.[29,30] With advancing age, an equine may fall lower in the field hierarchy,[29] become excluded from the group, and consume less food than the owner believes. Underlying musculoskeletal disease may exacerbate this problem (discussed later). Horses with poor dentition consume food more slowly and quidded forage is often eaten by herdmates, again presenting a false picture of energy intake for that individual. Loss of a close companion, introduction of a new horse to the group, or moving yards can cause stress and inappetence. If bullying is an issue, consider separating the affected individual from the herd, or removing the individuals responsible for the bullying behavior from the field. Alternatively, extra forage/feeds given individually in a stall, or a small corral on the pasture, can help ensure the horse receives adequate nutrition, prevent bullying, and can be very useful with a slow eater (**Fig. 4**).

Winter-Associated Stress

In areas where winter temperatures decrease substantially, there is an increase in energy demands in order to maintain body temperature, and these demands are likely further increased in windy, rainy, and snowy conditions.[31,32] In horses already underconditioned, there is little reserve capacity to meet energy demands.[33] For horses with low BCS, it is likely that they will lose further condition during these

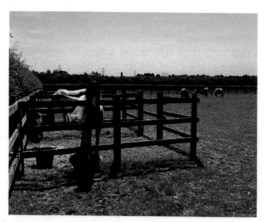

Fig. 4. Corrals with slip rails allow individual horses to receive supplementary feed and forage while remaining on pasture with herd mates.

periods of environmental stress unless additional steps are taken to ensure adequate nutrition is provided and consumed. Ongoing monitoring of BCS is also important in order to assess whether feed provision is adequate. Owners often blanket horses in these harsh conditions, which can be helpful, but obscures visual appreciation of changes in BCS. Thus, effort is needed to remove the blanket to regularly recheck BCS.

Water intake is often reduced, either because of the cold temperature of the water source or because access to water is impaired by freezing. Horses with cervical pain may have increasing difficulty accessing water or feedstuffs at ground level, especially during cold weather. Weak or lame horses may not be willing or able to ambulate in order to access feed or water sources, particularly when out at pasture in snowy or icy conditions. These problems can be exacerbated by loss of position within the social hierarchy, which may further decrease their access to food.[29,34] Weak or lame horses may also spend more time in recumbency, which, in cold conditions, can dramatically increase their heat losses, potentially resulting in the development of hypothermia. Harsh winter conditions often seem to exacerbate underlying health and malnutrition issues and can be associated with rapid clinical deterioration, especially in geriatric individuals. It is important that animals at risk are routinely monitored for changes in body condition, and this includes removing blankets periodically to allow thorough visual assessment.

Underlying Disease

Any underweight horse should be considered to potentially have underlying localized or systemic disease, even if 1 or more of the previously discussed conditions is present. Weight loss is often multifactorial; disease in almost any body system can be associated with weight loss, so clinicians must keep an open mind.

Gastrointestinal disorders

The gastrointestinal tract is of primary importance in maintaining body condition, from prehension through digestion to elimination, and should receive detailed attention. In addition to the conditions discussed earlier, clinicians must consider infectious conditions (equine proliferative enteropathy, enteritis, colitis), inflammatory conditions (gastric ulceration, colonic ulceration, inflammatory bowel disease), infiltrative bowel disease, as well as neoplasia. Although some of these conditions are discussed briefly here, please see Myriam Hesta and Marcio Costa's article, "How Can Nutrition Help with Gastrointestinal Tract-Based Issues," in this issue for a more thorough discussion of gastrointestinal conditions.

Gastric ulceration involving the squamous and/or glandular mucosa is a common cause of decreased appetite in adult horses, and as a result can contribute to loss of body condition.[35] Definitive diagnosis requires gastric endoscopic examination, and medical treatment relies on acid suppression, gastric mucosal protection, and enhancing gastric mucosal blood flow. The chronic or excessive administration of nonsteroidal antiinflammatory drugs to horses can cause injury to the intestinal mucosa, most commonly involving the stomach and right dorsal colon.[36,37] Right dorsal colitis can present acutely, with signs of colic, shock, and severe diarrhea, or chronically, with intermittent colic, mild diarrhea, weight loss, and protein-losing enteropathy.[38] Inflammatory or infiltrative bowel diseases can present with weight loss, often despite a good appetite, and also may show ventral edema caused by hypoalbuminemia resulting from protein-losing enteropathy.[39,40] Neoplasia in any body system can result in weight loss, but neoplasia within the abdominal cavity is particularly likely to have this result.[41]

Hepatic disease

Liver disease is common in horses and accounted for 10% of animals with weight loss admitted to a referral hospital.[1] Smith and colleagues[42] (2003) used liver biopsy and histopathology to classify the disease category in 88 horses referred for clinical or clinicopathologic signs of liver disease. Although 48.1% of cases remained unclassified, cholangiohepatitis accounted for 19.8% of cases, megalocytic hepatopathy caused by pyrrolizidine alkaloid toxicity in 13.6% of cases, and chronic active hepatitis in 9.9% of cases. Hepatic disease caused by consumption of ragwort (*Senecio jacobaea*; also known as tansy ragwort) is more common in starvation/welfare cases, because this prolific plant thrives on poorly managed and overgrazed pasture (**Fig. 5**). The fresh ragwort plant has a bitter taste but is readily consumed if grazing is sparse or the plant is inadvertently dried and baled in forage. Ragwort contains hepatotoxic pyrrolizidine alkaloids, which, when consumed over a period of time, cumulate to cause chronic liver disease.

Clinical signs associated with liver disease include depression, weight loss, anorexia, colic, jaundice, photosensitization, and diarrhea. However, many cases of liver disease are asymptomatic because of the large functional reserve of the liver. In a study of 61 horses with liver disease confirmed by biopsy, 44 horses were either clinically normal or showed mild, nonspecific signs of disease.[43] A review of diagnostic tests concluded that histologic evaluation of hepatic biopsies provided better prognostic information for horses with liver disease than the results of blood tests.[44] With regard to the commonly used blood tests for hepatic disease (total and direct bilirubin, gamma-glutamyl transferase, aspartate transaminase, alkaline phosphatase, sorbitol dehydrogenase, glutamate dehydrogenase, total bile acids, and serum ammonia), total bile acids and serum globulins have been shown to provide useful prognostic information for survival/nonsurvival.[44–46] Following diagnosis of liver disease in 1 individual, testing of other horses on the same premises is recommended even in the absence of clinical signs, and abnormal values of any of the blood tests mentioned earlier is an indication for further assessment of that animal.[47] Establishing the presence of more widespread disease implies a nutritional or toxic cause, and is a clear indication for evaluation of the environment for evidence of causal agents such

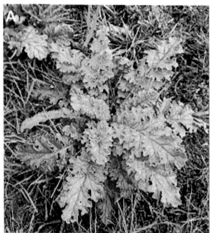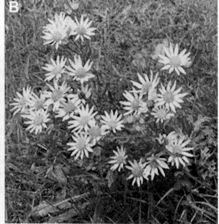

Fig. 5. Ragwort (*S jacobaea*). (*A*) Rosette stage before flowering. Removal is recommended at this stage to minimize further spread. (*B*) Flowering stage.

as hepatotoxic mycotoxins, toxic plants, or contamination of the environment or water source. Fusariotoxins are the most commonly occurring mycotoxins found in animal grain/cereal-based feeds.[48] Of particular note is fumonisin B1, which although associated with leukoencephalomalacia in horses, can cause liver damage and cardiovascular dysfunction.[49] *Aspergillus* spp are natural contaminants of many animal feedstuffs and, under stressful conditions, may produce aflatoxins, such as alfatoxin B1, a powerful hepatocarcinogen.[50] In a study of equines with hepatopathy caused by chronic iron toxicity, the source was found to be natural water supplies, so sampling and testing of water supplies may be justified.[51] Combining multiple propriety feed supplements and vitamin and mineral balancers with already fortified feeds also could lead to provision of excessive iron or copper.

Renal disease
Chronic renal disease frequently presents with clinical signs of weight loss, inappetence, and lethargy.[52] Chronic renal failure is uncommon in horses, with a reported incidence of less than 1%, but is insidious and is often not recognized until the condition has advanced to end-stage renal disease.[52] Conditions leading to chronic renal insufficiency include glomerulonephritis (immune mediated, idiopathic), toxic nephropathies (nonsteroidal antiinflammatory drugs, aminoglycosides, pigmenturia), leptospirosis, and bacterial pyelonephritis.[53] Although the presence of polydipsia or polyuria may be suggestive, definitive diagnosis of renal insufficiency is based on clinicopathologic assessment and the documentation of azotemia. Hypercalcemia and hypophosphatemia are common findings, as is persistent isosthenuria.[52]

Musculoskeletal disorders
Musculoskeletal disease is particularly common in older horses. One study showed that 24% of horses more than 20 years old had musculoskeletal disease, of which 40% were diagnosed with osteoarthritis.[54] Lameness or deterioration in existing lameness may be underdiagnosed in older horses, particularly once retired. One survey showed that although lameness was present in 50% of horses more than 15 years old examined by a veterinarian, only 23% of owners detected the lameness.[10] Clinical signs of osteoarthritis range from marked lameness, synovial effusion, new bone formation, a reduction in range of joint movement, and muscle wastage to more subtle signs of reluctance to flex a limb and stand still for the farrier. Many human and animal assessment scales to score pain feature loss of appetite as a criterion, so it is possible that chronic pain contributes to weight loss.[55] Pain management either by systemic use of analgesia and/or intra-articular medication combined with remedial farriery, controlled exercise, and management changes is essential to improve appetite. Chronic use of nonsteroidal drugs may lead to damage to the gastrointestinal tract in the form of gastric or right dorsal colon ulceration, as well as renal toxicity.[56]

When standing square, the center of gravity for a horse lies just caudal to the withers[57]; however, when the horse lowers the head to graze, the center of gravity moves forward over the forelimbs. A horse with osteoarthritis of the forelimbs may show reluctance to graze or eat from a bucket on the floor. Osteoarthritis of the cervical vertebrae may make pulling hay from a net or grazing difficult. A simple raised feeding manger, gate bracket, or stacked car tires (**Fig. 6**) can be used to raise feed and water to improve comfort and consumption.[58] Generalized osteoarthritis reduces the desire to ambulate and reduces grass intake, particularly if the pasture surface is poached or uneven or slippery because of mud or snow.[59] Although uncommon, osteoarthritis of the temporomandibular joint can lead to inability to masticate food and severe weight loss.[60]

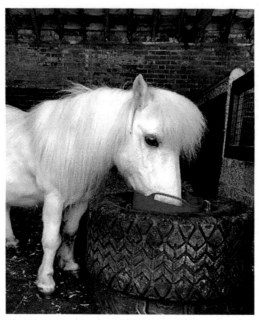

Fig. 6. Inexpensive raised feed and water stations can be made from stacking used tires.

MANAGEMENT OF UNDERWEIGHT HORSES
Feeding for Acute and Chronic Starvation

Dietary management of starved horses can be challenging and should be cautiously initiated to allow the affected animal to metabolically adapt to the reintroduction of nutrients and to prevent gastrointestinal disturbance.[34] Horses with a BCS less than 3 out of 9[61] are thought to be at risk of refeeding syndrome when feed is reintroduced.[34] When first exposed to starvation, the horse metabolizes stores of fat and carbohydrate, which are replaced when the horse is fed. If food deprivation continues, these stores become depleted and the body resorts to using protein as an energy source. Because protein is found in most body tissues, this process of catabolism affects not only skeletal muscle but also structures such as the heart and intestine. A sudden reintroduction of feeding leads to a rapid increase in serum glucose level followed by a surge in insulin level. Insulin drives glucose and potassium into the cells and promotes the synthesis of glycogen, protein, and fat. The production of ATP within the cells requires phosphorus and essential cofactors such as magnesium and thiamine. Starvation means the body already has depleted levels of electrolytes, minerals, and vitamins, and their sudden movement from the circulation into the intracellular space leads to hypokalemia, hypophosphatemia, hypomagnesemia, and acute thiamine deficiency, putting the horse at risk of neurologic disturbances; cardiac, respiratory, or renal failure; and death. This syndrome may manifest between days 3 and 7 after feeding.[21,34,62]

Predicting survival in horses with refeeding syndrome can be challenging. Whiting and colleagues[63] studied 45 horses during a refeeding period of 50 days following seizure caused by chronic starvation. Despite a careful diet of 10 days of free-choice hay before the addition of supplementary barley corn silage, 20% of the horses died. An association between initial BCS and survival was identified with those horses of BCS 1 out of 9 or less having a decreased chance of survival. Horses died at a mean of 7.9 days (range 1–19 days) after feeding. When a horse loses more than 50% of BW, the prognosis for survival is reportedly poor.[63]

Witham and Stull[64] (1998) studied 3 potential diets for feeding of horses with acute and chronic starvation: alfalfa hay, oat hay, and a combined oat hay and commercial ration, each fed for a 10-day period with equal calorie/energy provision. Horses fed the commercial ration (18.3% starch as fed) showed significantly higher postprandial concentrations of serum glucose and insulin than those on forage-only diets and a reduction in magnesium and phosphorus, potentially indicating refeeding syndrome. The diet of oat hay (<3% starch as fed) had a less dramatic impact on serum insulin level but serum phosphorus and magnesium levels remained low. Alfalfa hay (<3% starch as fed) proved the most successful diet, with minimal impact on serum insulin, and although phosphorus level remained low, an improvement was seen in serum magnesium level. Alfalfa is also high in dietary crude protein, which may be of benefit. Oil can be added to safely increase energy/calorie intake; however, this does not add to the magnesium or phosphorus intake and may prove unpalatable. Although alfalfa hay is difficult to come by in some areas, good-quality grass hay can be successfully used with a vitamin and mineral balancer.[21,34] Feeding should start at no more than 50% of the predicted digestible energy requirement (**Boxes 3 and 4**) given in multiple, small feeds to allow for decreased gastric volume and delayed gastric emptying, which may be seen in starved horses.[21,65]

Box 3
Refeeding protocol for use in cases of chronic starvation

Days 1 to 3
  Feed ≤ 50% of the calculated maintenance DE requirements per day (based on predicted weight of horse in moderate condition).
  Alfalfa hay (low glycemic index, rich in crude protein and minerals) or good-quality grass hay with a low-calorie forage balancer to supplement protein, vitamin, and mineral intake (must include thiamine, magnesium, phosphorus, and potassium).
  Forage analysis recommended. Avoid forages with NSC content greater than 10% DM basis. Molasses-free alfalfa pellets/products also suitable if low NSC content
  Divide ration into 6 small feeds per day.
  Monitor serum phosphorus, potassium, and magnesium.[4] If finances do not allow, a more conservative approach to refeeding should be taken to avoid metabolic instability.
  Inclusion of bran (0.1–0.5 kg/d/500-kg horse) has been used to supplement phosphorus.[4]

Days 4 to 5
  Gradually increase to 75% DE requirements.
  Divide ration into 6 small feeds per day.

Days 6 to 10
  Gradually increase to 100% DE requirements.
  Divide ration into 3 to 4 feeds per day.

Days 11 to 120
  Continue at 100% DE requirements gradually increasing quantity to 125% DE if consumed.
  Grain should not be introduced until BCS is moderate.
  Manage expectations; full rehabilitation may take 6 months.
  Gentle exercise (eg, hand walking) to promote development of muscle, limit deposition of adipose tissue, and promote well-being is recommended.[4]

Abbreviations: DE, digestible energy; DM, dry matter; NSC, nonstructural carbohydrate.

Adapted from Johns I. Veterinary management of starved and neglected horses. *In Practice.* 2014;36(3):144-152; with permission.

Box 4
Approaches for stimulating appetite in horses

Dietary
  Provide a variety of feeds in small amounts
  Discard uneaten feed and provide fresh
  Offer highly palatable feeds
    Molassed or unmolassed sugar beet pulp
    Molassed or unmolassed alfalfa products
    Add flavorings (garlic, ginger, fenugreek, banana, cherry)
  Add honey or molasses
  Sweet feed
    Pelleted senior feeds
    Soaked pelleted feeds
    Fiber-rich, low-sugar, and low-starch mash products
    Soaked mashes (eg, bran), warmed in winter
  Hand grazing and walking
  Fresh cut grass (green chop)
  Coarse fibrous feeds
  Appetite-stimulant supplements

Behavioral
  Thoroughly clean all feed containers
  Improve access to feed (elevate)
  Turnout on grass if possible
  Provide companion animals
  Feed with other animals present (competition): may have negative effects

Medical
  Provide analgesia if discomfort present
  Treat for gastric ulcers or provide prophylaxis (omeprazole)
  Administer appetite stimulants
    Antihistamines
    Cyproheptadine
    Benzodiazepines (controversial, short acting)
    Oral B vitamins (anecdotal)
    Anabolic steroids (controversial)

Additional nursing care includes establishing a warm environment to reduce calorie expenditure. This warm environment is preferable to heavy rugs that will burden a weak horse. If possible, hand walking and access to companions improve demeanor and appetite. Use of a sling may be necessary. Furthermore, wounds over bony prominences, which occur in horses that are recumbent for prolonged periods of time, should be treated and padded as needed.

Feeding for Failing Dentition

Horses with poor dentition benefit from access to pasture because fresh grass is soft and easy to masticate and digest. Pasture lengths more than 6 cm are helpful to aid prehension if incisors are poor; however, mature grass may become coarse.[34] If pasture restriction is required because of concurrent issues such as equine metabolic syndrome, PPID, or obesity, softer hays and haylage with a high leaf to stem ratio and appropriate nonstructural carbohydrate (NSC) content (<10% dry matter basis) can be useful.[66] Soaking hay may assist by softening stalky hay and further reducing the NSC content (see Megan Shepherd and colleagues' article, "Nutritional Considerations When Dealing with an Obese Adult Equine," in this issue). If diastemata are present, chopped fiber can contribute to interdental feed packing and should be avoided.[67]

As dental compromise progresses, grass cubes, grass pellets, or high-fiber commercial pellets (crude fiber levels 15%–25%) can be introduced to maintain BW. Sugar beet pulp (molassed or unmolassed [if the individual has concurrent insulin dysregulation] varieties are available and must always be fed soaked) and alfalfa cubes/pellets are additional sources of fiber. Furthermore, alfalfa products boost intake of amino acids and encourage appetite. Most dentally challenged horses still enjoy having forage, especially pasture, available, despite quidding, because the chewing action prevents boredom, may decrease the risk of gastric ulceration, and allows the horse to continue to share a field with more able companions.[58] If a horse experiences long-stem or short-stem forage choke or impaction colic, then soaked pelleted forage or soaked high-fiber commercial feeds may be safer, ideally divided into 4 to 5 feeds/d to mimic trickle feeding, especially because consumption of processed feeds may be more rapid than long-stem forage. Frequent feeding is often impractical for owners, and most horses do well on 3 feeds/d if pasture is available and the horse is allowed sufficient time to finish the meal or given a free-choice approach. A treat ball filled with a pelleted feed may also help extend eating time, if the horse can tolerate pellets without choking. Compounded senior horse rations can be used for part or all of the ration and many provide a good source of crude protein (12%–16%) and lysine to help maintain muscle mass.

Once dental compromise is advanced, high-fiber pellets can be soaked or a high-fiber mash provided to make up 100% of the ration. Specialist nutritional advice can be helpful at this stage. Some senior horse mashes are designed with low sugar and starch levels suitable for horses at risk of laminitis. Soaking feeds increases the volume of the meal, which may limit calorie intake per meal, requiring more frequent feeding. Soaked rations should be freshly made up to avoid refusal of stale feeds and warmed on cold days to encourage appetite, particularly if periodontal disease is present. Oils such as linseed/flaxseed, corn, vegetable (soybean), and canola are calorie dense and a good option for dentally challenged horses. Oils should be introduced slowly to avoid colic and palatability issues but can be increased up to 250 to 500 mL/500-kg horse per day.[58] Supplementary vitamin E should be given, when feeding supplemental oil, to reduce lipoperoxidation at 1.5 IU/mL oil.[68] Alternatively, stabilized calcium-supplemented rice bran and processed flaxseed are naturally high in oils and may suit the fussy eater.[59] For horses with equine metabolic syndrome (EMS) and PPID, it is advisable to check the nutritional content of any supplementary products such as rice bran because there may be wide individual variation in NSC content.

Nutritional Support for Gastrointestinal Disease

The approach to nutritional management of horses with gastrointestinal disorders depends on the type of condition present. Although several key points are addressed here, please see Myriam Hesta and Marcio Costa's article, "How Can Nutrition Help with Gastrointestinal Tract-Based Issues," in this issue for additional information. For horses with gastric ulceration, improving pasture access, reducing the amount of NSCs in the diet, providing multiple small meals, and increasing forage intake may all be of benefit in reducing the incidence and severity of the condition.[69] The addition of alfalfa to the forage, up to 25% of the daily intake, can be helpful by providing additional buffering capacity to the gastric contents.[35,70] Horses with cyathostomiasis or other colonic inflammatory disorders require a diet that achieves mechanical and functional rest for the colon.[71] Immature cool-season grasses and good-quality pelleted complete feeds are easily digested, low in bulk, and low in insoluble fibers, and should be fed little and often. Adequate provision of protein is essential at 1 g/kg BW/d as a minimum.[71] Most complete pelleted feeds provide this level; however, soybean meal, sugar beet pulp, and commercial balancers can be used as additional sources of protein along with small amounts of alfalfa. Oils such as corn, canola, vegetable (soybean), or flaxseed (250–500 mL/500-kg horse/d) are potential means to provide extra energy while resting the colon, although they may be less effective in animals with extensive disease. Supplementary vitamin E should be given to reduce lipoperoxidation at 1 to 2 IU/kg BW once daily.[72]

Nutritional Management of Hepatic Disease/Insufficiency

In the absence of clinical or clinicopathologic signs of hepatic insufficiency, major changes to the diet of a horse with compensated liver disease are thought to be unnecessary once dietary hepatotoxins have been ruled out.[73] Nutritional management is most useful in cases of hepatic insufficiency with or without hepatic encephalopathy (HE), although much of the information is sourced from human literature. Metabolic issues likely to be faced during hepatic insufficiency include decreased glycogen storage, decreased gluconeogenesis, insulin dysregulation, and catabolism of body proteins and fat stores.[73] Forages such as less mature (higher quality) grass, grass hay, or haylage should be available with frequent small feedings of supplementary concentrates to help regulate blood glucose levels.[61] To prevent catabolism of endogenous protein sources, dietary protein should not be restricted; however, avoidance of excessive protein levels is prudent if HE is present (**Box 5**). Until recently, use of protein sources with a high ratio of branched chain amino acids (BCAAs) to aromatic amino acids (AAAs) were recommended in the prevention of HE, such as legume hays, sorghum, wheat bran, and corn.[62] The benefit of this has become less clear following studies in humans to suggest that vegetable-based proteins, which tend to have lower BCAA to AAA ratios, seem more beneficial for patients with HE than animal-based proteins, some of which have higher BCAA to AAA ratios.[74] Oral administration of lactulose reduces the production and absorption of intestinal ammonia from dietary protein by causing mild hindgut acidosis.[63] Lactulose is readily taken by even anorexic horses and is suitable for long-term administration. Reducing dietary intake of iron may be of benefit in limiting the hepatic injury associated with chronic iron exposure.[51,75] The antioxidant effect of vitamin E (1–2 IU/kg BW/d) has been shown in some studies to attenuate hepatic inflammation and fibrosis in humans and may slow progression of hepatic disease.[76]

In anorexic horses it is better to feed what the horse will voluntarily consume. There are several approaches that can be used to encourage feed intake (see **Box 3**). Warming feed can improve consumption, as can the addition of flavorings such as ginger and garlic. In a palatability trial of equine concentrate feeds, feeds flavored with fenugreek, banana, and cherry were consumed more quickly than feed with the more traditional flavors such as peppermint and carrot.[77] Horses voluntarily consume sufficient dried garlic to cause Heinz body anemia if given access; however, dietary levels of 15 mg/kg dried garlic are considered safe for long-term consumption.[78,79]

Nutritional Management of Chronic Renal Disease

The primary objective when feeding horses with chronic kidney disease is to improve body condition, if possible, and to maintain condition for as long as possible.[80] It is important to ensure unlimited access to fresh water, because of impaired urinary concentrating ability and the resulting increase in water requirements. Dietary management relies on the provision of a low-protein diet, ideally based on as much pasture access as possible.[80] Fresh grass also has the benefit of having high concentrations of

---

Box 5
Feeding for hepatic disease/insufficiency

Compensated hepatic disease
  Nutritional requirements as per a healthy horse
  Consider vitamin E supplementation
  Screen current rations (forage/feedstuffs) for presence of dietary hepatotoxins, including:
  • Excessive iron/copper: use of multiple supplements
  • Dietary mycotoxins such as aflatoxins and fumonisins

Hepatic insufficiency
  Provide sufficient energy and protein to avoid endogenous catabolism and gluconeogenesis
  Grazing (10–14 h) or full turnout depending on body condition/pasture; if photosensitization present, consider turnout overnight
  Grass hay or haylage when grazing limited/stabled
  Avoid short/intense periods of grazing; may cause hindgut disturbance and promote ammoniagenesis
  Concentrate/complementary feeds (4–6 small meals per day or mix with forage for trickle effect)
    Commercial pellets/mix (DE range 8–10 MJ/kg, crude protein 8%–10%) suggested at 0.5 to 1 kg/100 kg BW/d
    Or home-prepared sources of fiber and starch, such as molassed sugar beet pulp, alfalfa cubes, micronized maize, milo (sorghum)
  Avoid exceeding 1 g/kg BW of starch per single meal; may cause hindgut disturbance/ increase risk of gastric ulceration and so forth
  Vegetable oil supplementation
    0.1 to 0.5 mL/kg BW; provision of dietary energy and essential fatty acids; introduce gradually to avoid palatability issues
  Supplementation of fat soluble vitamins A, E, D, K, and zinc (further reading, Durham[73] 2013)
  Additional vitamin E provision essential when using supplementary oils

Hepatic Encephalopathy - HE
  Basic feeding as above
  Avoid excessive use of high-protein-content feedstuffs such as leguminous hay, alfalfa, sugar beet, linseed, soya
  Oral administration lactulose 0.3 mL/kg every 6 to 24 h

Adapted from Durham AE. Nutrition for hepatic insufficiency. In: Geor RJ, Harris P, Coenen M, eds. *Equine Applied and Clinical Nutrition.* Elsevier; 2013:592-596; with permission.

---

natural antioxidants. When pasture is not available, then it is preferable to use grass hay, because legume hays have higher calcium and protein content.[52] Concentrate feeding may be required, especially in horses with poor appetites, and these should be highly palatable and easily digestible. Oats are often used, because they are very palatable and have a high energy content. In affected animals with reduced appetite, other possibilities may include pelleted senior feeds, which are often higher in fat and energy content, but may not be as low in phosphorus, calcium, or protein as would be ideal. The provision of adequate dietary protein is recommended, and 1.0 to 1.5 g/kg BW/d is a reasonable goal.[80] The adequacy of dietary protein intake can be assessed indirectly by monitoring the blood urea nitrogen/Cr ratio, with values greater than 15 (mg/dL) or 0.075 (µmol/L:mmol/L) suggesting excessive protein intake, whereas values less than 10 (mg/dL) or 0.05 (µmol/L:mmol/L) may indicate inadequate protein intake.[80] Oils (vegetable/soybean, corn, canola, linseed/flaxseed) can be a useful source of energy, and may be provided in the form of a high-fat senior pelleted feed or the direct addition of oil to the feed. Oils high in linoleic acid (corn, soybean) may be less desirable, because diets high in linoleic acid have been shown to be detrimental in dogs with kidney disease.[81] Because the provision of omega-3 polyunsaturated fatty acids has been shown to be beneficial in chronic kidney disease in other species,[81] it seems reasonable to consider including products high in omega-3s when supplementing equine patients as well.[80]

SUMMARY

Management of underweight horses requires detailed evaluation of the individual's nutritional needs and the composition of the diet provided. It also requires thorough assessment for underlying disease that may be contributing to, or responsible for, the weight loss observed. Dietary changes should be carefully implemented, especially in starved horses, in order to avoid secondary complications such as refeeding syndrome.

DISCLOSURES

N. Jarvis and H. McKenzie have no commercial or financial conflicts of interest and no active external funding relevant to this article.

REFERENCES

1. Tamzali Y. Chronic weight loss syndrome in the horse: a 60 case retrospective study. Equine Vet Educ 2006;18(6):289–96.
2. McFarlane D. Diagnostic testing for equine endocrine diseases: confirmation versus confusion. Vet Clin North Am Equine Pract 2019;35(2):327–38.
3. Costello J, Firshman AM, Brown JC, et al. Response to thyrotropin-releasing hormone (TRH) in a horse with hyperthyroidism associated with a functional thyroid adenoma. Can Vet J 2019;60(11):1189–93.
4. Argo CM. Feeding thin and starved horses. In: Geor RJ, Harris P, Coenen M, editors. Equine applied and clinical nutrition. Edinburgh: Elsevier; 2013.
5. Stratton-Phelps M. Nutritional management of the hospitalised horse. In: Corley KT, Stephen JO, editors. The equine hospital manual. Oxford (United Kingdom): Blackwell Publishing; 2008. p. 261–311.
6. Mohammed HO, Divers TJ, Summers BA, et al. Vitamin E deficiency and risk of equine motor neuron disease. Acta Vet Scand 2007;49:17.
7. Green P, Tong JM. The role of the veterinary surgeon in equine welfare cases. Equine Vet Educ 2004;16(1):46–56.
8. du Toit N, Burden FA, Dixon PM. Clinical dental examinations of 357 donkeys in the UK. Part 2: epidemiological studies on the potential relationships between different dental disorders, and between dental disease and systemic disorders. Equine Vet J 2009;41(4):395–400.
9. Nicholls VM, Townsend N. Dental disease in aged horses and its management. Vet Clin North Am Equine Pract 2016;32(2):215–27.
10. Ireland JL, Clegg PD, McGowan CM, et al. Disease prevalence in geriatric horses in the United Kingdom: veterinary clinical assessment of 200 cases. Equine Vet J 2012;44(1):101–6.
11. Chinkangsadarn T, Wilson GJ, Greer RM, et al. An abattoir survey of equine dental abnormalities in Queensland, Australia. Aust Vet J 2015;93(6):189–94.
12. Brown SL, Arkins S, Shaw DJ, et al. Occlusal angles of cheek teeth in normal horses and horses with dental disease. Vet Rec 2008;162(25):807–10.
13. Ralston SL, Foster DL, Divers T, et al. Effect of dental correction on feed digestibility in horses. Equine Vet J 2001;33(4):390–3.

14. Tremaine H, Casey M. A modern approach to equine dentistry. 1. Oral examination. In Pract 2012;34:2–10.
15. Di Filippo PA, Vieira V, Rondon DA, et al. Effect of dental correction on fecal fiber length in horses. J Equine Vet Sci 2018;64:77–80.
16. Ireland JL, Clegg PD, McGowan CM, et al. A cross-sectional study of geriatric horses in the United Kingdom. Part 1: Demographics and management practices. Equine Vet J 2011;43(1):30–6.
17. Bonin SJ, Clayton HM, Lanovaz JL, et al. Comparison of mandibular motion in horse chewing hay and pellets. Equine Vet J 2007;39:258–62.
18. Rahmani V, Hayrinen L, Kareinen I, et al. History, clinical findings and outcome of horses with radiographical signs of equine odontoclastic tooth resorption and hypercementosis. Vet Rec 2019;185(23):730.
19. Staszyk C, Bienert A, Kreutzer R, et al. Equine odontoclastic tooth resorption and hypercementosis. Vet J 2008;178:371–9.
20. Love S, Murphy D, Mellor D. Pathogenicity of cyathostome infection. Vet Parasitol 1999;85(2–3):113–21, discussion 121–12, 215-125.
21. Johns I. Veterinary management of starved and neglected horses. Practice 2014; 36(3):144–52.
22. McFarlane D, Hale GM, Johnson EM, et al. Fecal egg counts after anthelmintic administration to aged horses and horses with pituitary pars intermedia dysfunction. J Am Vet Med Assoc 2010;236(3):330–4.
23. Steinbach T, Bauer C, Sasse H, et al. Small strongyle infection: consequences of larvicidal treatment of horses with fenbendazole and moxidectin. Vet Parasitol 2006;139(1–3):115–31.
24. Oliver-Espinosa O. Diagnostics and treatments in chronic diarrhea and weight loss in horses. Vet Clin North Am Equine Pract 2018;34(1):69–80.
25. Lester HE, Matthews JB. Faecal worm egg count analysis for targeting anthelmintic treatment in horses: points to consider. Equine Vet J 2014;46(2):139–45.
26. Peregrine AS, McEwen B, Bienzle D, et al. Larval cyathostominosis in horses in Ontario: an emerging disease? Can Vet J 2006;47(1):80–2.
27. Kaspar A, Pfister K, Nielsen MK, et al. Detection of Strongylus vulgaris in equine faecal samples by real-time PCR and larval culture - method comparison and occurrence assessment. BMC Vet Res 2017;13(1):19.
28. Steuer AE, Loynachan AT, Nielsen MK. Evaluation of the mucosal inflammatory responses to equine cyathostomins in response to anthelmintic treatment. Vet Immunol Immunopathol 2018;199:1–7.
29. Giles SL, Nicol CJ, Harris PA, et al. Dominance rank is associated with body condition in outdoor-living domestic horses (Equus caballus). Appl Anim Behav Sci 2015;166:71–9.
30. Ingólfsdóttir HB, Sigurjónsdóttir H. The benefits of high rank in the wintertime—a study of the Icelandic horse. Appl Anim Behav Sci 2008;114(3–4):485–91.
31. Cymbaluk NF, Christison GI. Environmental effects on thermoregulation and nutrition of horses. Vet Clin North Am Equine Pract 1990;6(2):355–72.
32. Cymbaluk NF. Thermoregulation of horses in cold, winter weather: a review. Livest Prod Sci 1994;40:65–71.
33. Siciliano PD. Nutrition and feeding of the geriatric horse. Vet Clin North Am Equine Pract 2002;18(3):491–508.
34. Argo CM. Nutritional management of the older horse. Vet Clin North Am Equine Pract 2016;32(2):343–54.

35. Sykes BW, Hewetson M, Hepburn RJ, et al. European college of equine internal medicine consensus statement–equine gastric ulcer syndrome in adult horses. J Vet Intern Med 2015;29(5):1288–99.

36. Pedersen SK, Cribb AE, Read EK, et al. Phenylbutazone induces equine glandular gastric disease without decreasing prostaglandin E2 concentrations. J Vet Pharmacol Ther 2018;41(2):239–45.

37. Hough ME, Steel CM, Bolton JR, et al. Ulceration and stricture of the right dorsal colon after phenylbutazone administration in four horses. Aust Vet J 1999;77(12): 785–8.

38. Karcher LF, Dill SG, Anderson WI, et al. Right dorsal colitis. J Vet Intern Med 1990; 4(5):247–53.

39. Boshuizen B, Ploeg M, Dewulf J, et al. Inflammatory bowel disease (IBD) in horses: a retrospective study exploring the value of different diagnostic approaches. BMC Vet Res 2018;14(1):21.

40. Barr BS. Infiltrative intestinal disease. Vet Clin North Am Equine Pract 2006; 22(1):e1–7.

41. East LM, Savage CJ, Traub-Dargatz JL. Weight loss in the horse: a focus on abdominal neoplasia. Equine Vet Educ 1999;11(4):174–8.

42. Smith MR, Stevens KB, Durham AE, et al. Equine hepatic disease: the effect of patient- and case-specific variables on risk and prognosis. Equine Vet J 2003; 35(6):549–52.

43. Durham AE, Smith KC, Newton JR. An evaluation of diagnostic data in comparison to the results of liver biopsies in mature horses. Equine Vet J 2003;35(6): 554–9.

44. Johns IC. In horses with liver disease, does histological evaluation of biopsies provide better prognostic information than results of blood tests. Equine Vet Educ 2019;31:163–5.

45. Dunkel B, Jones SA, Pinilla MJ, et al. Serum bile acid concentrations, histopathological features, and short-, and long-term survival in horses with hepatic disease. J Vet Intern Med 2015;29(2):644–50.

46. Durham AE, Newton JR, Smith KC, et al. Retrospective analysis of historical, clinical, ultrasonographic, serum biochemical and haematological data in prognostic evaluation of equine liver disease. Equine Vet J 2003;35(6):542–7.

47. Durham AE. A clinical approach to liver disease in the horse. BEVA Veterinary Management of the Geriatric Horse. Buck (United Kingdom): Princes Risborough; 2016.

48. Caloni F, Cortinovis C. Effects of fusariotoxins in the equine species. Vet J 2010; 186(2):157–61.

49. Durham A. A study into the association of dietary mycotoxins with liver disease in horses. J Vet Intern Med 2018;32:867–78.

50. Caloni F, Cortinovis C. Toxicological effects of aflatoxins in horses. Vet J 2011; 188(3):270–3.

51. Theelen MJP, Beukens M, Grinwis GCM, et al. Chronic iron overload causing haemochromatosis and hepatopathy in 21 horses and 1 donkey. Equine Vet J 2019; 51:304–9.

52. Schott HC 2nd. Chronic renal failure in horses. Vet Clin North Am Equine Pract 2007;23(3):593–612, vi.

53. McLeland S. Diseases of the equine urinary system. Vet Clin North Am Equine Pract 2015;31(2):377–87.

54. Brosnahan MM, Paradis MR. Demographic and clinical characteristics of geriatric horses: 467 cases (1989-1999). J Am Vet Med Assoc 2003;223(1):93–8.

55. Ashley FH, Waterman-Pearson AE, Whay HR. Behavioural assessment of pain in horses and donkeys: application to clinical practice and future studies. Equine Vet J 2005;37:565–75.
56. Moses VS, Bertone AL. Nonsteroidal anti-inflammatory drugs. Vet Clin North Am Equine Pract 2002;18(1):21–37, v.
57. Skerritt GC, McLelland J. Mammalian locomotion. In: Skerritt GC, McLelland J, editors. Functional anatomy of the limbs of domestic animals. Bristol (United Kingdom): John Wright & Sons; 1984. p. 224–35.
58. Jarvis NG. Nutrition of the aged horse. Vet Clin North Am Equine Pract 2009; 25(1):155–166, viii.
59. Jarvis N, Paradis MR, Harris P. Nutrition considerations for the aged horse. Equine Vet Educ 2019;31(2):102–10.
60. Sanders RE, Schumacher J, Brama PAJ, et al. Mandibular condylectomy in a standing horse for treatment for osteoarthritis of the temporomandibular joint. Equine Vet Educ 2014;26:624–8.
61. Henneke DR, Potter GD, Kreider JL, et al. Relationship between condition score, physical measurements and body fat percentage in mares. Equine Vet J 1983; 15(4):371–2.
62. Stull C. Nutrition for rehabilitating the starved horse. J Equine Vet Sci 2003;23: 456–7.
63. Whiting TL, Salmon RH, Wruck GC. Chronically starved horses: predicting survival, economic, and ethical considerations. Can Vet J 2005;46(4):320–4.
64. Witham CL, Stull CL. Metabolic responses of chronically starved horses to refeeding with three isoenergetic diets. J Am Vet Med Assoc 1998;212(5):691–6.
65. Kronfeld DS. Starvation and malnutrition of horses: recognition and treatment. J Equine Vet Sci 1993;13:289–303.
66. Harris P, Dunnett C. Nutritional tips for veterinarians. Equine Vet Educ 2018;30: 486–96.
67. Miles AEW, Grigson C. Colyer's variation and diseases of the teeth of animals (revised edition). Cambridge (United Kingdom): CambridgeUniversity Press; 1990.
68. Warren LK, Vineyard KR. Fat and fatty acids. In: Geor RJ, Harris P, Coenen M, editors. Equine applied and clinical nutrition. New York (NY): Elsevier; 2013. p. 136–55.
69. Galinelli N, Wambacq W, Broeckx BJG, et al. High intake of sugars and starch, low number of meals and low roughage intake are associated with Equine Gastric Ulcer Syndrome in a Belgian cohort. J Anim Physiol Anim Nutr (Berl) 2019. https:// doi.org/10.1111/jpn.13215.
70. Zavoshti FR, Andrews FM. Therapeutics for equine gastric ulcer syndrome. Vet Clin North Am Equine Pract 2017;33(1):141–62.
71. Bozorgmanesh R, Magdesian KG. Nutritional considerations for horses with colitis. Part 1: Nutrients and enteral nutrition. Equine Vet Educ 2018;30(10):564–8.
72. Finno CJ, Valberg SJ. A comparative review of vitamin E and associated equine disorders. J Vet Intern Med 2012;26(6):1251–66.
73. Durham AE. Nutrition for hepatic insufficiency. In: Geor RJ, Harris P, Coenen M, editors. Equine applied and clinical nutrition. Edinburgh: Elsevier; 2013. p. 592–6.
74. Campion D, Giovo I, Ponzo P, et al. Dietary approach and gut microbiota modulation for chronic hepatic encephalopathy in cirrhosis. World J Hepatol 2019; 11(6):489–512.
75. Casteel SW. Metal toxicosis in horses. Vet Clin North Am Equine Pract 2001;17(3): 517–27.

76. Nagashimada M, Ota T. Role of vitamin E in nonalcoholic fatty liver disease. IUBMB Life 2019;71(4):516–22.

77. Goodwin D, Davidson HPB, Harris P. Selection and acceptance of flavours in concentrate diets for stabled horses. Appl Anim Behav Sci 2005;95:223–32.

78. Riviere JE, Boothe DM, Czarnecki-Maulden GL, et al. Safety of dietary supplements for horses, dogs and cats (animal nutrition series). Washington, DC: National Research Council; 2009.

79. Pearson W, Boermans HJ, Bettger WJ, et al. Association of maximum voluntary dietary intake of freeze-dried garlic with Heinz body anemia in horses. Am J Vet Res 2005;66(3):457–65.

80. Schott HC. Urinary tract disease. In: Geor RJ, Harris P, Coenen M, editors. Equine applied and clinical nutrition. Edinburgh, Elsevier; 2013.

81. Brown SA, Brown CA, Crowell WA, et al. Beneficial effects of chronic administration of dietary omega-3 polyunsaturated fatty acids in dogs with renal insufficiency. J Lab Clin Med 1998;131(5):447–55.

Nutritional Considerations When Dealing with an Obese Adult Equine

Megan Shepherd, DVM, PhD, DACVN[a],[*],
Patricia Harris, MA, PhD, VetMB, MRCVS, DipECVCN[b],
Krishona L. Martinson, PhD[c]

KEYWORDS

- Body condition score (BCS) • Morphometrics • Ideal body weight
- Weight loss resistance • Metabolic • Ration

KEY POINTS

- Equine obesity adversely affects health.
- Maximizing feeding duration (i.e. chewing time) helps support gastrointestinal health and prevent the development of unwanted behaviors.
- Forage will often need to be complemented with an equine-specific amino acid-vitamin-mineral product to ensure appropriate macro and micronutrient intake.
- Monitoring is critical to prescribed weight loss success. If there is apparent weight loss resistance, then explore owner compliance, as there may be barriers to implementing the prescribed plan. If the equine is not losing weight, also consider possible increases in structured exercise to increase energy expenditure.
- Feeding less than 1.25% BW in dry matter per day is generally not recommended. However, for severely weight loss–resistant equines, especially ponies, reducing to 1% of current BW in dry matter may be needed, but only under veterinary supervision.

INTRODUCTION: WHY EQUINE OBESITY MATTERS

Obesity can be generally defined as the accumulation of an excessive quantity of adipose tissue that may impair health.[1] Obesity arises when there is an imbalance between energy intake and energy expenditure. Equine obesity can adversely affect health by increasing the risk of insulin dysregulation (ID)[2–4] and laminitis,[5–7] reducing

[a] Nutrition, Department of Large Animal Clinical Sciences, Virginia-Maryland College of Veterinary Medicine, Phase II Duck Pond Drive, Virginia Tech Mail Code 0442, Blacksburg, VA 24061, USA; [b] WALTHAM Petcare Science Institute, Waltham-on-the-Wolds, Melton Mowbray, Leics LE14 4RT, England; [c] Department of Animal Science, University of Minnesota, 1364 Eckles Avenue, St Paul, MN 55108, USA
* Corresponding author.
E-mail address: meshephe@vt.edu

Vet Clin Equine 37 (2021) 111–137
https://doi.org/10.1016/j.cveq.2020.12.004
0749-0739/21/© 2021 Elsevier Inc. All rights reserved.
vetequine.theclinics.com

heat tolerance[8] and reproductive efficiency.[9] In addition, as observed in other species, obesity may be proinflammatory[10–12] and/or increase the risk of orthopedic disease.[13] In addition, obese equines are less likely to make full recoveries from laminitis,[14] are more likely to develop myocardial hypertrophy,[15] and may be more likely to develop post–abdominal surgery complications.[16,17] Furthermore, foals from obese mares may have a higher risk of developmental orthopedic disease and insulin dysregulation (see Morgane Robles and colleagues' article, "Nutrition of Broodmares," in this issue).[18]

The prevalence of being overweight or obese varies around the world (**Table 1**), but is present in roughly 30% of the equine population of industrialized countries. Furthermore, the incidence appears to vary by breed-type[19–23] and season.[24] Ponies and some horse breeds (e.g., warmbloods, Andalusians, Icelandic) appear to be more prone to obesity, perhaps due to being more metabolically efficient.[23,25–29]

Despite the relatively high prevalence and numerous comorbidities, obesity is still a relatively underappreciated welfare issue in equines.[30,31] Laminitis is perhaps the most concerning of the comorbidities.[32,33] In addition to obesity, laminitis risk is influenced by diet[32,34–41] and may be associated with changes in the gut microbiome/microbiota.[32] Although an association between obesity and gut/fecal microbes has been established in other species,[42–45] the role of gut microbes in naturally occurring obese equines, versus diet-induced obese equines,[25] is unclear. Forage digestibility does not yet appear to generally differ between overweight and lean equids[46,47]; however, the gut microbiota[48] and serum acetate (a significant energy source for equines)[47,49] appear to differ between lean and overweight equines. Ponies and horses appear to have differences in their gut microbiota, which may be tied to metabolic

Table 1
Prevalence of overweight/obese equines by location and breed type

Location and Reference	Total Number	Breed Type	% Overweight/Obese[a]
US locations			
United States[54]	1215	Horses and ponies	21
Minnesota[20]	629	Horses and ponies	38
Virginia[55]	300	Horses	32
Minnesota, Alabama, and Kentucky[22]	314	Saddle-type horses	36
Minnesota[22]	89	Warmbloods	2
Minnesota[21]	138	Draft horses	42
Oklahoma[22]	261	Adult miniature horses	30
Non-US locations			
Australia[23]	229	Horses and ponies	23
North Somerset, England[24]	97	Horses and pones	27 (winter) 35 (summer)
Great Britain[19]	792	Horses and ponies	31
United Kingdom[56]	331	Horses and ponies	28
United Kingdom[51]	158	Horses	18
Glasgow, Scotland[57]	319	Horses	45
Saskatoon, Canada[58]	290	Horses	28

[a] As defined by the authors: typically reported as a body condition score of at least 6 on a 9-poinit scale or converted to a 9-point scale.

differences.[25] Furthermore, gut microbes may be associated with an equine's body weight loss rate.[46] This is not perhaps surprising, as gut microbes help equines extract a significant amount of energy (>50% of daily energy requirements) from high fiber, forage-based diets through fermentation (see Patricia Harris and Megan Shepherd's article, "What Would Be Good for All Veterinarians to Know About Equine Nutrition," in this issue).[29,50] More research is needed to further elucidate the link between gut microbes, obesity, and metabolic changes (see Myriam Hesta and Marcio Costa's article, "How Can Nutrition Help with Gastrointestinal Tract-Based Issues," in this issue).

The best way to manage equine obesity is to prevent it. Adipose tissue has lower energy requirements than more metabolically active tissue (eg, muscle). Therefore, strategic negative energy balance is needed for a successful weight loss program. There are several potential challenges to implementation, including the subjective nature of assigning a body condition score (BCS), lack of owner recognition of obesity, and the difficulties in making necessary management changes.[20–23,30,51] Veterinarians should avoid obesity shaming terminology (eg, fat, chunky) and judgment toward the owner, as these may negatively influence success.[52,53]

This article focuses on the nutritional management of equine obesity. However, other factors, such as overall health, activity level, and exercise also should be considered. For equines with chronic conditions that may predispose them to unintended weight loss (eg, chronic kidney disease), prescribed weight loss should be pursued with caution or not pursued at all, depending on the prognosis.

DIAGNOSING OBESITY

Methods for estimating body fat include deuterium oxide, BCS, cresty neck scores (CNS), ultrasound, morphometric measurements, and ideal body weight (BW) equations. Deuterium oxide is considered a gold standard and represents both internal (eg, visceral) and external (eg, subcutaneous) fat deposits; however, this method is not currently practical due to cost and methodology.[59,60] Tools to diagnose obesity also may be used to monitor the success of a weight loss plan. See also Myriam Hesta and Megan Shepherd's article, "How to Perform a Nutritional Assessment in a First Line/General Practice, in this issue regarding patient assessment.

BCS is the most common and practical method for diagnosing obesity.[60–62] In the United States and United Kingdom, equine obesity is commonly diagnosed using a 9-point subjective BCS.[62] The original Henneke BCS system was based on body fat percentage, calculated by rump fat thickness (see limitations of ultrasound later in this article), in quarter horse broodmares.[62] However, Dugdale and colleagues[63] and Fowler and colleagues[60] compared BCS to body fat percentage, calculated from deuterium oxide, in 77 adult horses and ponies and 15 thoroughbreds, respectively. Both determined that BCS was positively correlated with body fat percentage; however, the ability to predict body fat percentage declined with increasing BCS.[60,63] Assigning a BCS score involves a subjective assessment of subcutaneous fat mass on a 9-point scale with 1 indicating emaciation and a score of 9 indicating obesity.[60,62,63] Overweight (ie, fleshy, fat) is characterized by a BCS of ≥ 6[56] and obesity as ≥ 7[20,23,55,58] of 9, depending on the opinion of the authors, or a body fat mass of more than 20%.[63] Furthermore, few investigators differentiate the use of "overweight" and "obese" terminology in publications.[24,57]

CNS is used to assess neck crest adiposity and can be complementary to BCS.[64,65] Assigning a CNS score involves a subjective assessment of fat mass over the nuchal ligament on a 5-point scale, with 0 indicating no crest/fat over the nuchal ligament and

5 indicating that the crest droops to one side. Both BCS and CNS may correlate with metabolic parameters such as insulin, glucose, leptin, and triglycerides, although this varies by study.[64,66] However, the subjective nature of BCS and CNS opens the door to evaluator bias and does not directly account for internal fat.[63,67]

Ultrasound assessment of subcutaneous fat is, technically, an objective means to diagnose obesity.[60,68,69] Sites previously assessed for fat thickness in the horse include ribs, shoulder, lumbar, and rump, with the latter used most commonly.[60,62,69] Westervelt and colleagues[68] reported that ultrasound rump fat was useful for predicting total body fat, as determined by postmortem fat extraction, in horses and ponies. Fowler and colleagues[60] reported that ultrasound subcutaneous neck fat correlated better with deuterium oxide total body fat than shoulder, rib, rump or tailhead fat in nonobese thoroughbreds, which may not represent other breeds or obese horses. Subcutaneous fat thickness does not capture internal fat. Furthermore, changes in rump and rib fat thickness have been inversely associated with BW change (ie, thicker with BW loss) during weight loss protocols in the winter, possibly due to redistribution of fat in response to adverse environmental conditions.[70] In addition, ultrasound evaluation of rump fat thickness is sensitive to probe placement, position, and/or pressure.[47] Thus, this objective means to diagnose obesity does not seem practical outside of a research setting.

Morphometric measurements are a relatively practical means for objectively diagnosing obesity.[20–22,55,60,71] Body mass index (BMI) is calculated as BW (kg) divided by squared height (meters2) and in some studies has correlated positively with body condition score.[16,55,71] However, BMI does not correlate with percent body fat in the horse.[72] Fowler and colleagues[60] reported that heart girth-to-BW ratio correlated with total body fat via deuterium oxide and was superior to subcutaneous ultrasound thickness. Both crest height or neck circumference-to-height ratio were suitable morphometrics for assessment of CNS, and these morphometrics may be used to compliment BCS assessment. Furthermore, Potter and colleagues[72] developed a new body condition index based on morphometric parameters compared with body fat, as measured by deuterium oxide.

DESIGNING A GENERAL WEIGHT LOSS PLAN

Energy restriction, while meeting essential nutrient requirements and managing satiety, is key to a successful weight loss plan. Establishing a program to promote weight loss may simply require changing the amount/type of feed, restricting grazing, and/or increasing the exercise load. Voluntary dry matter (DM) intake (DMI) in equines varies widely (1.5%–5.5% weight[73]); therefore, simply cutting out energy-dense feeds, while providing ad libitum amounts of forage, may not provide adequate energy restriction for some. Consequently, restricting and monitoring the amount of forage provided and consumed is often required. Designing a detailed weight loss plan that addresses the nuances of each individual and available resources will improve the success of the plan. As with any equine, the ration must include fresh and palatable water, available at all times (see also Patricia Harris and Megan Shepherd's article, "What Would Be Good for All Veterinarians to Know About Equine Nutrition," in this issue).

WHAT TO FEED
Forage

Maximizing calories coming from forage is important to help promote satiety, support gastrointestinal health, and support normal foraging behavior.[74–76] Insoluble fiber in forages (eg, cellulose) is slowly fermented by gut microbes, supports a neutral hindgut pH and the symbiotic gut microbiota, and promotes overall gut health.[77] Furthermore, every effort should be made to maximize long-stem grass forage in the diet (see

Patricia Harris and Megan Shepherd's article, "What Would Be Good for All Veterinarians to Know About Equine Nutrition," in this issue).

A forage with low to average caloric density is ideal, as it allows for a better balance between energy restriction and maintenance of satiety.[78] More mature forage is higher in neutral detergent fiber (NDF) and acid detergent fiber (ADF), which represent the structural fibers in the cell wall.[79,80] Neutral detergent fiber content is negatively correlated with intake of both hay[80] and pasture.[81] Acid detergent fiber content is a negative indicator of forage digestibility (total tract, including fermentation), although this does not appear to be absolute.[82,83] Generally, forage with an NDF of less than 65% and ADF less than 45% is considered acceptable for healthy, adult horses. Unfortunately, preserved forages (eg, hay) may be sold without a nutrient analysis in most countries. Therefore, consumers often have to purchase forage based on availability and physical assessment. Visually, mature hay typically has a low leaf-to-stem ratio (eg, is more stemmy) and has more seed heads (in grasses) or flowers (in legumes). Furthermore, the burden usually falls on the consumer to conduct a forage nutrient analysis. See Nerida Richards and collegaues' article, "Nutritional and Non-Nutritional Aspects of Forage," in this issue regarding forages and analysis. Forage should be of good hygiene (eg, free from mold and dust) and stored in an area shielded from rain/moisture (see Patricia Harris and Megan Shepherd's article, "What Would Be Good for All Veterinarians to Know About Equine Nutrition," in this issue).

Availability of forage type varies by region and is available in different forms (**Box 1**).[77,84–87] Through the northern hemisphere, cool-season grasses (eg, orchardgrass, timothy, fescue), warm-season grasses (eg, Bermuda grass, teff; **Box 2**),[80,81,88–90] and legumes (eg, alfalfa; **Box 3**)[78,79] are available. Ideally, legumes should be avoided, as they

---

Box 1
Forage type

Forage type of classification refers to taxonomy and key characteristics of each. Note that the stage of plant maturity often has a greater impact on nutrient content and quality than forage type. Forage is generally available in a variety of forms, including fresh/pasture, hay, haylage, or silage. Furthermore, commercially available pelleted, cubed, or chopped hays are available. See Patricia Harris and Megan Shepherd's article, "What Would Be Good for All Veterinarians to Know About Equine Nutrition," in this issue for more information about forage type and hygiene. See also Myriam Hesta and Megan Shepherd's article, "How to Perform a Nutritional Assessment in a First Line/General Practice, in this issue regarding forage assessment, and Nerida Richards and colleagues' article, "Nutritional and Non-Nutritional Aspects of Forage," in this issue regarding forage-based deficiencies and toxicities.

Silage may be lower in WSC than hay or haylage, as the fermentation process uses these components. The energy density of haylage and silage varies, but is generally more energy dense than hay.[35] Generally, the weather is agreeable for hay making in the United States; therefore, feeding grass or alfalfa haylage or silage to horses is not common.

For the obese equine, commercial forage would ideally be manufactured from grass hays. Commercially available forage is helpful when hay availability is low. Furthermore, pelleted and cubed forage may be used in the face of poor dentition (see Nicola Jarvis and Harold C. McKenzie's article, "Nutritional Considerations When Dealing with an Underweight Adult or Senior Horse," in this issue), as they require less mastication and take up water when soaked. In ruminants, having long-stem forage (ie, bailed hay) is superior for rumen function and health versus forage that is ground or chopped below. However, the role of forage length on gastrointestinal function is less understood in the horse. However, less time is spent chewing pelleted forage, as compared with long-stem forage. Therefore, long-stem forage should be fed when possible to reduce the risk of gastric ulcers and to better mimic the horse's natural foraging behavior.

> **Box 2**
> **Warm-season grass**
>
> Teff has a lower equine digestible energy, NSC, and crude protein, and higher amounts of NDF, on a DM basis, compared with alfalfa and cool-season grasses. The calcium-to-phosphorus ratio and nitrate-nitrogen content of Teff should be examined before initiating grazing (see Nerida Richards and colleagues' article, "Nutritional and Non-Nutritional Aspects of Forage," in this issue).

are generally more energy dense than grasses.[78,81] Warm-season grass hays, like Bermudagrass, tend to be lower in digestible energy (DE), nonstructural carbohydrates (NSC), and crude protein, and higher in NDF.[80,81,89,90] Generally, straw may be used to replace a small portion (<50%, preferably no more than 30%) of grass hay.[74,91] For donkeys, straw may make up 100% of forage. Straw is higher in NDF and ADF, thus helps to maximize satiety during calorie restriction.[92] However, poor quality or hygienic straw, or if straw makes up most of the forage, can lead to rapid weight loss. The risk of equine gastric ulcer syndrome increases when straw is the main forage[76] (see Myriam Hesta and Marcio Costa's article, "How Can Nutrition Help with Gastrointestinal Tract-Based Issues," in this issue). Straw should be shaken to remove excess seed heads due to potential for oral trauma from the awns. Slowly introducing straw over the course of 10 to 14 days may help reduce the risk of colic secondary to impaction.[93] Ideally, the introduction of straw to the diet would be done under the guidance of an equine nutritionist and/or veterinarian. Water consumption may increase when fed straw.

Ration Balancers

The diet/ration should meet all essential nutrient goals, as established by the National Research Council (NRC; https://nrc88.nas.edu/nrh/)[73] or other recognized guidelines (see Patricia Harris and Megan Shepherd's article, "What Would Be Good for All Veterinarians to Know About Equine Nutrition," in this issue). The goal is to reduce fat mass while minimizing any loss of lean tissue (eg, muscle). Meeting, or exceeding, protein requirements is important for the maintenance of lean muscle mass, which in turn positively influences basal metabolic rate (**Box 5**). The ability for the forage alone to meet the protein needs depends on forage quality (see Patricia Harris and Megan Shepherd's article, "What Would Be Good for All Veterinarians to Know About Equine Nutrition"; and Kristine L. Urschel and Erica C. McKenzie's article, "Nutritional Influences on Skeletal Muscle and Muscular Disease," in this issue) (**Box 5**). Supplemental protein (or amino acids) may be needed to complement the forage, particularly in the United Kingdom and Europe and especially when feeding restricted intakes. In addition, protein and micronutrient (ie, vitamins and mineral)

> **Box 3**
> **Alfalfa**
>
> Alfalfa hay is commonly fed to equines, but is not a good choice for the overweight equine due to the higher energy density. If alfalfa hay is the only option, selecting a more mature (eg, flowering) alfalfa is one method of reducing the energy density. In one study, alfalfa in the bud stage (less mature) had an average 2.45 Mcal/kg DE, whereas flowering alfalfa (more mature) had less, at 2.14 Mcal/kg DE. Reducing DM target to 1.25% of current body weight, dividing the hay into small meals and feeding frequently, and/or using a slow feed hay net will likely be necessary to limit time spent without forage availability.

provision should match the equine's life stage (eg, adult maintenance, work, growth), regardless of the degree of forage or calorie restriction needed to achieve weight loss.

Forage needs to be complemented with a mineral-vitamin source to provide the micronutrients that the forage lacks. Common essential nutrients that are often not met by forage alone include sodium, chloride, copper, zinc, selenium, and vitamin E.[78] Others (eg, calcium) may be deficient when limit-feeding forage. Sodium chloride requirements may easily be met by providing free choice access to a white or trace mineral (≥95% sodium chloride) block, preferably near a fresh water source. However, anecdotal reports claim that some horses are reluctant to lick or consume minerals from a block, especially during cold weather. Trace mineral requirements may be met by adding an equine-specific granular or block vitamin-mineral supplement. Note, a micromineral supplement that works well in one area (eg, selenium poor soil) may not complement the forage well from another area (eg, selenium-rich soil; see also Nerida Richards and colleagues' article, "Nutritional and Non-Nutritional Aspects of Forage," in this issue). Vitamin E is low in processed forage (eg, hay); therefore, vitamin E supplementation (eg, equine-specific vitamin-mineral supplement) is needed when feeding primarily processed forage. Although granular or block vitamin-mineral products may generally be fed ad libitum near a water source, precise monitoring of intake is challenging. For equines with higher sodium and chloride requirements (eg, working, sweating), loose salt may be needed and fed at a precise daily amount.

Equine-specific balancer pellets (ie, ration balancers) are highly fortified commercial products that may be used in place of a granular or block vitamin-mineral source. Balancer pellets often contain 30% crude protein on an as-fed basis, as compared with approximately 16% crude protein as a maximum in most commercial feeds, and are meant to be fed in specified (not ad libitum) small quantities (eg, 0.5–1.0 kg per day for a 500-kg equine). Thus, ration balancers can be fed in a single daily meal or, for obese or laminitis-prone equines, may be divided into multiple meals. Balancer pellets are a good option to provide vitamins and minerals in equines consuming a primarily forage diet because (1) it gives the caregiver something to feed, which is often an important factor in the human-animal-bond, and (2) they are generally readily consumed and thus easier to monitor intake. Follow manufacturer's feeding instructions, or work with an equine nutritionist, to refine the appropriate balancer and required feeding rate to best complement the forage feed and needs of the individual horse.

When feeding to promote weight loss, using energy-dense feeds (eg, grains, commercial sweet feeds, commercial senior feeds, and brans with 2.6–3.3 Mcal/kg as fed) can lead to a dramatic reduction in total daily DM when trying to reduce overall calorie intake. This in turn increases the risk of gastrointestinal, metabolic, and behavioral complications, as mentioned later in this article. Therefore, feeding lower caloric or less energy-dense feeds is preferred. Commercially available "lite" or "weight control" (ie formulated to be fed without additional forage) are generally lower in calories than many other commercial feeds and may be used when forage is not available; however, these feeds may be more energy dense than many grass forages, thus professionals should consider the total DM and energy intake per day. Furthermore, consider the level of fortification and whether an additional vitamin-mineral source is needed or not, especially if such feeds are not being fed at the manufacturer's recommended levels.

How Much to Feed

Feeding based on a DM target is a practical option and the only option when a nutrient analysis for the forage or feedstuff does not exist. Target DM intake also may be based on ideal weight (see Estimating target body weight, later in this article); however, using current weight may be more practical in that it reduces the number of calculations. Regardless of how a weight loss plan is developed, the ultimate goal is for the equine to lose weight.

How much to feed based on current body weight

Estimating current body weight. The most accurate way to measure an equine's BW is by using a calibrated scale. The most practical way to estimate an equine's BW is by using a BW tape calibrated for equines; however, estimated BW will vary by BW tape used and user. There are 2 ways to orient the BW tape. One is to place the tape around the heart girth, behind the elbow, perpendicular to the ground and over the highest point of the withers. Another way is to place the tape around the heart girth, behind the elbow, but not perpendicular to the ground, as the top of the BW tape is placed just behind (vs over) the withers. BW (kg) also may be estimated using a measuring tape and the following calculation ((girth circumference cm^2 × body length cm)/11,877), with body length measured from the point of the shoulder to the tuber ischi.[55] Additional calculations are available for miniature horses,[94] ponies,[95] yearlings,[96] and weaning.[97,98] Furthermore, the following equation was formulated for estimating German warmblood BW (kg) = (−1160 + 2.594 × wither height in cm) + (1.336 × heart girth in cm) + (1.538 × body circumference in cm) + (6.226 × cannon bone circumference in cm) + (1.487 × neck circumference in cm) + (13.63 × BCS point), with BCS on a 9-point scale.[61] Mobile applications are available to automatically calculate BW from morphometric data (eg, height, girth circumference, neck circumference, and body length) and breed type.[20–22,99]

How much to feed. For the equid that simply needs a controlled diet (eg, an equine that consumes ≥3% of weight in daily DM or that is fed too much of an energy-dense feed), limiting total daily DM to 2% of current weight per day (**Box 4**), preferably of a low to moderate energy-dense forage, may result in adequate weight loss.[73,74] For some equines, limiting forage to 1.25% to 1.5% of current weight in DM per day may be needed; however, the authors recommend working with an equine nutritionist before feeding below 1.5% current weight. Note, some equines are quite metabolically efficient (weight loss resistant) or have reduced energy expenditure (eg, voluntary or prescribed due to laminitis or orthopedic disease), thus, for some cases, further restriction is needed (not <1% current weight on DM basis) and only with veterinary monitoring.[74,100] Each reduction in daily DM requires more intensive monitoring due to limited gut fill and increased time between meals, which can increase the risk of gastrointestinal, metabolic, and behavioral complications.[92,100–105] The primary potential metabolic complication is hyperlipidemia; donkeys and pregnant/lactating mares are at higher risk.[106,107] Hyperlipidemia occurs secondary to negative energy balance and is a sign of too rapid weight loss for that individual. Behavioral abnormalities that may occur when forage is limited include cribbing, wood chewing, ingesting wood shavings/bedding, and coprophagy.[92,108–110] Although dry feeds (eg, hay, commercial pelleted, or textured feed) never have zero moisture, they should have limited moisture. Hay should have at least 85% DM (ie, no more than 15% moisture) and preferably closer to 90%.[77] Therefore, the as-fed amount is generally 1 kg, for every 10 kg, greater than the amount on a DM basis, for example, if the daily DM target is 9 kg, then 10 kg of hay would be needed to account for the weight of the moisture in the hay (and 5 kg if the target is 4.5 kg DM). However, exact amounts should be tailored to the equine's weight.

How much to feed based on estimated target body weight

Estimating target body weight. Target BW may be estimated based on equations that include morphometrics (eg, girth circumference, neck circumference, height, and body length) and breed type.[20–22] Inclusion of morphometrics not influenced by

---

Box 4
Feeding based on dry matter target

Example case: warmblood gelding with a body weight of 635 kg, BCS 7/9, unremarkable topline, body length = 170 cm and wither height = 167 cm

A dry matter (DM) target of 2% may be calculated based on current body weight or estimated target body weight.

Daily DM target, calculated from current body weight:
• 635 kg × 0.02 = 12.7 kg DM

Daily DM target, calculated from estimated target body weight (kg), based on BCS (see the section, Estimating target body weight):
• 635 kg – 34 kg = 601 kg
• 601 kg × 0.02 = 12.0 kg DM

Daily DM target, calculated from estimated target body weight (kg), based on morphometrics (see the section, Estimating target body weight):
• Target body weight (kg) = (4.92 × body length in cm) + (4.64 × height in cm) – 1016 = (4.92 × 170 cm) + (4.64 × 167 cm) – 1016 = 595 kg
• 595 kg × 0.02 = 11.9 kg DM

Daily hay target, on an as-fed (AF) basis (ie, the weight you would feed the gelding each day), if grass hay has 90% dry matter:
• 12.7 kg BM/0.9 = 14.1 kg AF
• 12.0 kg/0.9 = 13.3 kg AF
• 11.9 kg/0.9 = 13.2 kg AF

Initial recommendations should be adjusted every 2 to 4 weeks as needed to meet weight loss target. Feeding less than 1.25% BW in dry matter per day is generally not recommended. However, for severely weight loss–resistant equines reducing to 1% of current BW in dry matter may be needed, only under veterinary supervision.

Checking protein intake

NRC average adult maintenance daily protein requirement for 635 kg adult equine = 800 g

Average crude protein (CP) content of US grass hay = 11% on a DM basis
• 11 g CP per 100 g DM
• 110g CP per kg DM

If feeding 2.0% of current body weight per day in DM, the protein provision is calculated as follows:
• 635 kg × 0.02 = 12.7 kg DM × 110g CP/kg DM = 1397g CP

Therefore, in this scenario, if feeding 2.0% current body weight in DM of an average quality US grass hay, the gelding's CP requirement is met.

---

adiposity (eg, height and body length), along with breed type, improve the accuracy of the estimated target BW. Furthermore, mobile applications are available to automatically calculate estimated ideal BW.[20–22,99]

Target BW also may be estimated based on current and target BCS.[62] For most equines, a target BCS of 5/9 is a good starting point. However, for equines with orthopedic disease, a target BCS of 4/9 may be ideal, to reduce stress and strain on joints. Conversely, for equines with chronic disease that may lead to uncontrolled BW loss (eg, kidney, liver disease) or equines prone to BW loss over the winter, a target BCS of 6/9 may be ideal. The general BW per 1 point within the 9 point BCS score in horses was reported to be 16 to 20 kg.[111] However, breed-specific BW per 9-point BCS score have been documented and ranges from 3.0% to 6.8% of BW (**Table 2**).[20–22] See example case (see **Box 4**) in this article. Limitations of using BCS to estimate ideal

Table 2
Body weight (BW) needed to change 1 body condition score (BCS) arranged by breed type

Equine-Type and Reference	BW (kg) Associated with a Change in 1 BCS (9-Point Scale)	BW (%) Associated with a Change in 1 BCS (9-Point Scale)
Arabians[20]	34	3.0–3.5
Ponies[20]	29	3.0–3.5
Stock horses (eg, American quarter horse, American paint)[20]	28	3.0–3.5
Draft horses[21]	39	2.8–6.8
Warmbloods[21]	17	2.8–6.8
Miniature horses[22]	8	2.8–6.8
Saddle-type (eg, American saddlebred, Morgan)[20,22]	15	2.8–6.8
Thoroughbreds[20,22]	26	2.8–6.8

BW are (1) BCS does not account for changes to internal (eg, abdominal/visceral) fat, and (2) equines at their target BCS may still have excess internal fat.[67] Regardless of the limitations, estimating ideal BW based on BCS is included here because BCS is the most common and practical, although subjective, means for diagnosing obesity.

How much to feed. If calculating the daily DM target based on estimated target weight, start with 2% of target weight (see **Box 4**). The authors encourage veterinarians to work with an equine nutritionist if daily DM needs to be restricted to less than 1.5% of estimated target weight.[100]

How to Feed

Restricted forage should be divided into at least 2 daily meals; more meals is ideal to limit time without forage access to ≤5 hours, at least during daylight hours (ie, giving the last meal as late as possible during the day).[101,102]

Making the Forage Last

Hay nets/grills can slow the rate of intake and extend meal time, which is particularly important when limiting daily DM.[112–117] The smaller the opening, the slower the rate of intake. In one study, hay nets with medium (4.4 cm) and small (3.2 cm) openings reduced DMI rate (kg/h) by 27% and 40% (1.1 kg/h and 0.9 kg/h), respectively, as compared with DMI rate without a hay net (1.5 kg/h).[113] This reduction resulted in doubling of time spent feeding (5.0 and 6.5 hours, respectively, vs 3.0 hours).[113] Some equines do appear capable of adjusting to hay nets over time.[117,118] Conversely, using a very small hole, or layering multiple small hole nets, is not recommended.[118] Furthermore, hay nets should be checked for wear and replaced as needed.[117] Using a slow-feed/small-medium opening hay nets is encouraged, especially when limiting daily DM to less than 1.5% of weight.[77,117]

Food toys may be used to slow consumption and provide environmental enrichment.[116] Some food toys work best with pelleted feeds, such as pelleted grass hay. When using food toys, the pelleted grass hay should be included in the daily DM goal. Equines may get frustrated when food toys are empty[119]; therefore, if used, remove food toys once emptied.

Monitoring

Regular monitoring is critical for determining if the initially prescribed weight loss plan is successful. The frequency of monitoring (eg, every week, every other week, monthly) should be individually tailored. If there are concerns of rapid weight loss (eg, initial plan was too restrictive or presence of illness), then weekly rechecks may be needed. Once a healthy weight loss trend has been established, monthly rechecks are likely appropriate.

Generally, the goal is for the overweight equine to lose 0.5% to 1.0% of weight per week.[70,74,100,108,120] This typically correlates to loosing 0.5/9 to 1/9 BCS points per month.[74,100,120] However, equines can lose significant weight without losing BCS, perhaps due to internal fat dynamics.[112,121] Furthermore, most caregivers do not have easy access to a calibrated scale and thus use equine-calibrated weight tapes or weight equations (see , previously in this article). Although weight tapes are generally good for monitoring trends, they only account for changes in heart girth circumference. Other morphometrics, like measuring rump width[121] and belly girth circumference at the widest point of the belly, may be helpful to track.[24,108,122]

If weight loss is too slow or has not occurred, review compliance regarding exactly what is fed, how much is being fed, and activity (eg, maybe the caregivers were compliant, but activity has reduced due to season or injury). If after 4 to 6 weeks there has been limited change in weight, BCS, or morphometrics, despite adherence to the plan, then DMI needs to be reduced. If daily DMI is already at 1.25% of current weight, then efforts should be made to secure a lower calorie forage and continue to monitor and check with an equine nutritionist (see previously in this article regarding exceptions). If the caregiver has not been compliant, investigate the cause and help the caregiver establish a management plan that is sustainable.

Achieving a healthy BCS is half the battle, as maintaining a healthy weight will require continued diligence. Once target BCS is achieved, the caloric goal should be adjusted to maintain healthy weight. Therefore, routine assessment (eg, monthly) of weight and BCS should continue until weight has stabilized (ie, stable over several months) to ensure that the diet/ration is appropriate. Physical activity and environmental factors (eg, air temperature) influence energy expenditure; therefore, the diet/ration may need regular adjustment. Caregivers should not expect to ever return to free choice forage feeding, and continue modifications including the use of a slow feeder (eg, small-medium opening hay net), selecting mature/relatively low-calorie forage, or, when on pasture, using a grazing muzzle. Aside from monitoring the success of the weight loss plan, the equine should be monitored for gastrointestinal, metabolic, and behavioral complications. Furthermore, the diet/ration should continue to include ad libitum access to fresh water and meet all essential nutrient requirements.

Special Considerations

The preceding guidelines may not be a good fit for every equine and/or may not be practical for every caregiver. Therefore, this section includes guidelines for nuances that may impact the success of the prescribed weight loss plan.

How Much to Feed Based on Digestible Energy

Designing a weight loss plan based on an energy/calorie goal is a more precise way to establish an effective weight loss plan, as energy requirements vary by individual and energy density varies across forage sources. However, a forage nutrient analysis is needed, as the DE content of forage cannot be accurately predicted based on physical parameters.

If forage analysis is available, using the NRC (https://nrc88.nas.edu/nrh/) low adult maintenance calculation of 33.3 kcal/kg of current weight is a place to start (**Box 5**).[73] After setting or updating the daily energy goal and designing a plan, it is best to check the daily DM provision. Ideally, the daily DM is initially 1.5% to 2.0% of current weight. If the forage is too energy dense, such that daily DM provision is less than 1.25% of current weight, then a lower calorie forage should be obtained or an equine nutritionist should be consulted. For overweight equines that are active (ie, overweight performance equine), this level of energy restriction may be too restrictive. Conversely, should the initial weight loss plan not be successful (see "Monitoring" section), and the caregiver has been compliant, then further reduce energy by 10% to 20%.

Using the Current Diet and Diet History to Refine the Plan

The current diet provides context, and assessment of the current diet allows the weight loss diet to be more specifically tailored to the individual. A diet history should be collected to get a general perspective of where the calories are coming from and how the individual is being fed. It is helpful to inquire about the type and form of forage fed (eg, pasture type access, long-stem hay, cubed, pelleted), and if and what type of complementary feed/concentrate is fed (eg, textured feed, bran). The structure of questions used to collect a diet history will influence the level of detail given.[123] Evaluating the current diet is generally time-consuming and a detailed analysis is not practical for all practitioners. Ideally, practitioners should be properly compensated for time spent managing the obese equine, including time spent evaluating the current diet, but this is often challenging. Therefore, the weight loss plan may be initiated "from scratch" and modified as needed. See Myriam Hesta and Megan Shepherd's article, "How to Perform a Nutritional Assessment in a First Line/General Practice, in this issue regarding how to conduct a nutritional assessment.

Donkeys

Like equids, the incidence of obesity in donkeys is significant, with 26% and 34% reported in the United Kingdom and Europe,[124,125] although less in areas where donkeys are more commonly used for work.[126] Like obese horses and ponies, obese donkeys are more likely to have lower insulin sensitivity[127] and may have higher blood insulin concentrations[127,128] than lean donkeys.

Box 5
Feeding based on digestible energy target

Example case: warmblood gelding with a body weight of 635 kg, BCS 7/9 and unremarkable topline

Daily digestible energy target = 33.3 kcal/kg body weight:
- 635 kg × 33.3 kcal/kg = 21,146 kcal = 21.2 Mcal
  Daily hay provision, in dry matter, if the hay has 2.06 Mcal/lb DM:
- 21.2 Mcal/2.06 Mcal/lb DM = 10.3 kg DM
  Check DM, as a percentage of body weight:
- 10.3 kg DM/635 kg = 1.6% body weight, which is ok to start at because daily dry matter is 1.5% to 2.0% body weight

Daily hay provision, as fed, if the hay has 90% dry matter:
- 10.3 kg DM/0.9 = 11.4 kg AF

Like other equids, obesity in donkeys is diagnosed using a donkey-specific subjective 9-point BCS system.[129] Donkeys are considered obese when BCS exceeds 6 of 9.[127] In addition, a 5-point BCS donkey-specific system has been developed by the Donkey Sanctuary.[124,130] A subjective 5-point neck score and an objective neck circumference-to-height ratio has also been developed, as donkeys typically deposit more fat in the neck than horses and ponies.[128] Subcutaneous fat measured by ultrasound seems to correlate well with BCS.[131] The use of objective means to measure body fat (eg, deuterium oxide) has not yet been used. Current weight may be estimated using the following calculations[128,129]:

- kg weight for a donkey with a BCS of $\geq 7/9$ = ([heart girth circumference$_{cm}^{2.575}$] × [height$_{cm}^{0.240}$])/3968
- kg weight for a donkey with a BCS of $\leq 6/9$ = ([heart girth circumference$_{cm}^{2.12}$] × [height$_{cm}^{0.688}$])/3801

BMI has been used in donkeys (weight$_{kg}$/height $_m^2$), though not universally.[128]

Donkeys are physiologically more efficient in that they have higher fiber digestion (total-tract) and relatively lower energy expenditure, compared with horses.[132,133] Paired with often a sedentary companion animal lifestyle (compared with donkeys in regular work[126,129]), it is no surprise that obesity is a major problem. Straw or high NDF, lower calorie forage (eg, NDF $\geq 70\%$ DM) may be needed to promote healthy weight loss while minimizing time between meals and maximizing forage intake.[130] Straw may provide most of the forage intake.[134] Regardless, of the forage fed, the forage should be complemented with an equine-specific vitamin-mineral source. Methods to slow intake should be considered, as for other equines.

Seniors

Age is not a disease; however, there are age-associated conditions that are relevant to the topic of obesity, such as potential of increased risk of colic, pituitary pars intermedius dysfunction (PPID), dental disease, and orthopedic disease.[120,135–139] Propensity for inflammation increases with age and increased "inflamm-aging" is associated with obesity.[140,141]

Equids with PPID are at risk of insulin dysregulation (discussed in detail later in this article) and laminitis.[134] PPID may lead to loss of lean muscle mass,[142] thus a diet that modestly exceeds protein requirements[73] may be ideal (see Kristine L. Urschel and Erica C. McKenzie's article, "Nutritional Influences on Skeletal Muscle and Muscular Disease," in this issue). Equids with PPID may be polydipsic,[134] so extra care should be taken to ensure easy access to fresh water.

For the overweight senior equines, including donkeys,[124,143] unable to effectively masticate long-stem forage, consider replacing the long-stem forage with soaked processed low-starch and sugar forage or forage alternatives. Forage is generally available in a variety of forms, including commercially available pelleted, cubed, or chopped hays. Grass hay-based processed forage (eg, chopped, cubed, pelleted) is often preferred over alfalfa-based and commercial senior feeds due the lower calorie content. Similar to when feeding long-stem forage, processed forage should be complimented with a vitamin-mineral product.

Activity and Athletes

Promoting voluntary activity can help increase energy expenditure and thus limit the need for more severe calorie and DM restriction. Furthermore, instituting a structured exercise plan, when appropriate, may help limit muscle loss during a prescribed weight loss plan. Muscle mass positively influences basal metabolic rate; therefore, preserving muscle mass is advantageous when mobilizing fat mass during a prescribed weight loss plan.[70] Regular (5 days a week) 25-minute low-intensity exercise (15-minute trot with warm up and down) may improve insulin sensitivity.[74,144] See Kristine L. Urschel and Erica C. McKenzie's article, "Nutritional Influences on Skeletal Muscle and Muscular Disease," in this issue regarding nutrition and muscle.

Characterization of an equine as an athlete is relatively subjective, although the NRC does provide guidance regarding categories of work.[73] The NRC energy requirements for work may overestimate the needs for the overweight athlete. Regardless, the ration should still meet all essential nutrient requirements, which are higher for the athlete than the adult equine at maintenance.[73] If overweight or obese, even if in regular work, the potential to have insulin dysregulation (see the next section) needs to be considered when designing the ration. See Kristine L. Urschel and Erica C. McKenzie's article, "Nutritional Influences on Skeletal Muscle and Muscular Disease," in this issue regarding nutrition and muscle.

Equines with Insulin Dysregulation

Presence or absence of hyperinsulinemia alone is not the most precise way to determine if an equine has insulin dysregulation.[145] Dynamic tests needed to diagnose insulin dysregulation may not be practical for on-farm use, although oral sugar tests are commonly conducted.[145–147] Regardless, limiting dietary NSC can complement the weight loss plan by limiting metabolic complications that may be associated with the current obese state.

Nonstructural Carbohydrates

Nonstructural carbohydrates include sugars, starch, and fructan. Grains (eg, barley, oats) and grain-based concentrates tend to have higher NSC concentration (37%–67% DM), especially in the form of starch, compared with forages (typically 6%–20% DM).[148] Limiting dietary NSC, including avoiding sweet treats, is indicated in equines with insulin dysregulation and/or laminitis.[147,149] Effective weight loss may resolve concurrent hyperinsulinemia, if present.[144]

Sugars and fructan are analytically represented as water-soluble carbohydrates (WSC). The role of fructans on insulin dynamics is not yet clear, as the monosaccharide subunits are linked by beta-glycosidic bonds, which are not degraded by mammalian enzymes.[150] Fructans are rapidly fermented by microbes in the equine cecum and large colon.[151,152] However, fructans may be fermented before the large intestine and influence insulinemic and glycemic responses to a forage meal.[41,153,154] Furthermore, fructan ingestion influences hindgut microbes[32,155,156] and a type of fructan (inulin) has been used to induce laminitis.[36,37,41] Although specific forage fructan (eg, phlein, higher degree of polymerization than inulin) has not been directly linked to changes in hindgut microbes or laminitis in vivo, changes in hindgut microbes have been demonstrated in vitro.[157]

Grass WSC content varies within the forage species, day, and across the growing season.[81,158–160] For example, the warm-season grass teff is lower in WSC and associated with lower peak insulin response in the fall compared with cool-season grasses.[81,161] Generally, grass WSC can be reduced if cut or consumed (1) at a more mature state, (2) when not stressed (eg, cold, drought), or (3) during the early morning (provided temperatures are above freezing).

Generally, in senior and obese equines, feeds and forage with greater than 10% to 12% NSC[147,149] on a DM basis are discouraged, as they may increase the risk of insulin dysregulation and laminitis.[40,162] Without a forage analysis, the NSC content cannot be inferred. However, efforts to limit NSC intake should be implemented.

Instituting a weight loss plan by limit-feeding forage may result in less total daily NSC intake, especially if forage was previously fed ad libitum and/or higher NSC forages were fed.

Reducing Hay Nonstructural Carbohydrates by Soaking and Steaming

Should the obese equine have insulin dysregulation, a low NSC (ideally <10% DM)[147] forage is considered ideal. However, when forage options are limited, soaking reduces NSC, specifically WSC, and may reduce postprandial insulin.[79,86,163–166] The amount of WSC lost may be influenced by water temperature, soak duration, and hay density (solid flake or shaken lose).[86,165–167] In one study, soaking hay for 16 hours reduced WSC on average 28% in 8°celcius water (winter) and 46% in 16°celcius water (summer); although the reduction was less than 10% for some hays.[165,166] In another study, soaking hay for 12 hours reduced WSC on average 71% in 22°celcius water (cold).[79] Furthermore, soaking hay for 12 hours reduced WSC 43%.[86] It can be hard to come up with a single practical guideline for soaking hay given the unpredictable variation across and within studies.[165] Martinson and colleagues[79,167] suggest limiting soaking to 60 minutes. Rendle and colleagues[74] suggest soaking hay up to 6 hours in cold water or 1 hour in warm water, based on prior work.[163,165,166,168] However, along with WSC loss, DM and other nutrient losses occur.[79,86,165] To account for a DM loss, the daily hay target has been recommended to be increased by 20% when hay is soaked (eg, 1.8% vs 1.5% of weight in presoak DM).[74] Minerals, such as potassium and phosphorus, are also reduced during soaking.[167] Therefore, as previously stated, the forage should be complemented with equine-specific vitamin and mineral sources. Soaking also increases the microbial content of hay, if not fed immediately, and the water used to soak hay should be discarded carefully.[169] Although steaming can be used to reduce mold counts, it is not a reliable way to reduce components of NSC.[170] Although steaming after soaking may be used to reduce microbial counts,[169,171] it is not normally practical.

Total WSC will be lower in silage than hay made from the same field, as microbes use WSC as energy substrate.[86,87,172] Haylage WSC can, however, still be high depending on the initial content, as preservation is primarily through exclusion of air rather than fermentation. See Patricia Harris and Megan Shepherd's article, "What Would Be Good for All Veterinarians to Know About Equine Nutrition"; and Nerida Richards and colleagues' article, "Nutritional and Non-Nutritional Aspects of Forage," in this issue for more information about forage and WSC. Grass haylage, and sometimes silage, is commonly fed to performance and maintenance horses outside of the United States.[77,87,173–175] However, the weather is generally more suitable for hay making in the United States, therefore, silage and haylage are less commonly fed to horses.

Pasture Access for the Obese Equine: Slowing Fresh Forage Consumption with Grazing Muzzles

Insulin dysregulation and laminitis have been associated with pasture consumption.[7,176,177] Furthermore, equines prefer short grass,[178] which may concentrate NSC in cool-season grasses. Pasture management influences forage NSC and thereby potentially insulin regulation.[179] Stressed (eg, overgrazed or drought) or unfertile soil can increase the accumulation of NSC.

Feeding hay, versus pasture, allows for more precise and controlled feeding, as pasture intake is a major factor for obesity.[24] However, fresh forage from pasture may be the most practical option in certain environments (eg, if there is no dry lot or forage-free outdoor housing). Ponies can ingest nearly 5% of their weight in DM per day,[122,180] and horses grazing for 15 hours a day can consume between 1.4% and

2.5% of their weight depending on the time of year and forage availability.[181] Furthermore, ponies can ingest 1% of their weight in DM if grazing is limited to 3 hours,[182,183] and horses have been shown to accelerate pasture DM intake rates, especially when grazing is restricted to ≤9 hours each day.[184] Therefore, time-restricted grazing is not an effective means to limit pasture forage intake.[184] However, eliminating pasture forage access may not always be practical or desirable. Furthermore, keeping an equine stalled reduces voluntary exercise and thus energy expenditure.

Grazing muzzles do reduce pasture forage intake, although reported reductions vary between 30% and 80%.[180,183,185] Grazing muzzles can enable equines to have some access to pasture, where they can expend more energy than confined in a dry lot and fed hay.[186] Grazing muzzles are not welcome by all caregivers, and potential issues mentioned include rubbing, altered social interactions, and increased wearing of the teeth; however, the consequences of not limiting pasture intake are much greater (eg, laminitis and obesity). Furthermore, wearing grazing muzzles for 24 hours a day resulted in no observed impact on various physiologic stress measures in miniature horses.[182,187] The author (PH) does not routinely recommend 24-hour use, and suggests muzzles should be used as one part of a weight management program. Ponies can be particularly adept at removing muzzles. Muzzles come in a variety of shapes, and care should be taken to properly fit and ensure full adaptation before leaving the equine unattended. Check muzzles daily for wear and adjust as needed.[188] Weekly evaluation of weight and BCS should be taken to determine the individual equine's grazing efficacy while wearing the muzzle.[183] Muzzles should be worn the entire time the equine is on pasture, as compensatory intake can occur in animals left on pasture once the grazing muzzle has been removed.[180,183,189] Muzzles that prevent water access should be avoided.

Supplements

Levothyroxine sodium may help promote weight loss and insulin sensitivity,[190] although more research is needed.[74] Levothyroxine should not be prescribed in the obese equine without implementation of a diet plan. A variety of nutraceuticals and supplements are marketed for managing the equine with insulin dysregulation (eg, chromium, magnesium).[191] To date, the published evidence of their success in managing obesity or insulin dysregulation is weak to absent.[120,147,192] Furthermore, some nutraceuticals and supplements that have been studied have not been compared with a control or placebo.[193] Therefore, nutraceuticals claiming to improve insulin regulation should be viewed and used with caution[194] (see Ruth Bishop and David A. Dzanis article', "Staying on the Right Side of the Regulatory Authorities"; and Ingrid Vervuert and Meri Stratton-Phelps' article, "The Safety and Efficacy in Horses of Certain Nutraceuticals that Claim to Have Health Benefits," in this issue).

SUMMARY

Obesity is a relatively underappreciated, but widespread (up to 30% or even more in some populations), welfare issue in equines with serious health implications and should be prevented; if not prevented, it should be corrected. Strategic calorie restriction is often needed to promote healthy weight loss. However, DM provision should be maximized by feeding low energy-dense feeds (eg, low-quality to moderate-quality forage). Feeding management strategies should be used as needed to limit time between meals to less than 5 hours, at least during daylight hours. Monitoring is essential for determining if the initial weight loss plan is successful. Furthermore, especially for equines at low DM intake (<1.5% body weight per day), monitoring for gastrointestinal issues, hypertriglyceridemia, and abnormal behavior is important. Finally, when in doubt, consult with an equine nutritionist, preferably one who is experienced and up-to-date with their CPD.

REFERENCES

1. Anon. Obesity and overweight. Available at: https://www.who.int/news-room/fact-sheets/detail/obesity-and-overweight. Accessed October 12, 2020.
2. Hoffman RM, Boston RC, Stefanovski D, et al. Obesity and diet affect glucose dynamics and insulin sensitivity in thoroughbred geldings. J Anim Sci 2003; 81:2333–42.
3. Frank N, Elliott S, Brandt L, et al. Physical characteristics, blood hormone concentrations, and plasma lipid concentrations in obese horses with insulin resistance. J Am Vet Med Assoc 2006;228:1383–90.
4. Vick M, Adams A, Murphy B, et al. Relationships among inflammatory cytokines, obesity, and insulin sensitivity in the horse. J Anim Sci 2007;85:1144–55.
5. Coleman MC, Belknap JK, Eades SC, et al. Case-control study of risk factors for pasture-and endocrinopathy-associated laminitis in North American horses. J Am Vet Med Assoc 2018;253:470–8.
6. Treiber K, Kronfeld D, Geor R. Insulin resistance in equids: possible role in laminitis. J Nutr 2006;136:2094S–8S.
7. Carter R, Treiber K, Geor R, et al. Prediction of incipient pasture-associated laminitis from hyperinsulinaemia, hyperleptinaemia and generalised and localised obesity in a cohort of ponies. Equine Vet J 2009;41:171–8.
8. Sillence M, Noble G, McGowan C. Fast food and fat fillies: the ills of western civilisation. Vet J 2006;172:396–7.
9. Vick M, Sessions D, Murphy B, et al. Obesity is associated with altered metabolic and reproductive activity in the mare: effects of metformin on insulin sensitivity and reproductive cyclicity. Reprod Fertil Dev 2006;18:609–17.
10. Suagee JK, Corl BA, Geor RJ. A potential role for pro-inflammatory cytokines in the development of insulin resistance in horses. Animals (Basel) 2012;2:243–60.
11. Bruynsteen L, Erkens T, Peelman LJ, et al. Expression of inflammation-related genes is associated with adipose tissue location in horses. BMC Vet Res 2013;9:240.
12. Burns TA, Geor RJ, Mudge MC, et al. Proinflammatory cytokine and chemokine gene expression profiles in subcutaneous and visceral adipose tissue depots of insulin-resistant and insulin-sensitive light breed horses. J Vet Intern Med 2010; 24:932–9.
13. Kealy RD, Lawler DF, Ballam JM, et al. Effects of diet restriction on life span and age-related changes in dogs. J Am Vet Med Assoc 2002;220:1315–20.
14. Menzies-Gow NJ, Stevens K, Barr A, et al. Severity and outcome of equine pasture-associated laminitis managed in first opinion practice in the UK. Vet Rec 2010;167:364–9.
15. Heliczer N, Gerber V, Bruckmaier R, et al. Cardiovascular findings in ponies with equine metabolic syndrome. J Am Vet Med Assoc 2017;250:1027–35.
16. Hill JA, Tyma JF, Hayes GM, et al. Higher body mass index may increase the risk for the development of incisional complications in horses following emergency ventral midline celiotomy. Equine Vet J 2020;52(6):799–804.
17. Packer MJ, German AJ, Hunter L, et al. Adipose tissue-derived adiponectin expression is significantly associated with increased post operative mortality in horses undergoing emergency abdominal surgery. Equine Vet J Suppl 2011;(39):26–33.

18. Robles M, Nouveau E, Gautier C, et al. Maternal obesity increases insulin resistance, low-grade inflammation and osteochondrosis lesions in foals and yearlings until 18 months of age. PLoS One 2018;13:e0190309.

19. Robin CA, Ireland JL, Wylie CE, et al. Prevalence of and risk factors for equine obesity in Great Britain based on owner-reported body condition scores. Equine Vet J 2015;47:196–201.

20. Martinson KL, Coleman RC, Rendahl AK, et al. Estimation of body weight and development of a body weight score for adult equids using morphometric measurements. J Anim Sci 2014;92:2230–8.

21. Catalano DN, Coleman RJ, Hathaway MR, et al. Estimation of actual and ideal bodyweight using morphometric measurements and owner guessed bodyweight of adult draft and warmblood horses. J Equine Vet Sci 2016;39:38–43.

22. Catalano DN, Coleman RJ, Hathaway MR, et al. Estimation of actual and ideal bodyweight using morphometric measurements of miniature, saddle-type, and thoroughbred horses. J Equine Vet Sci 2019;78:117–22.

23. Potter SJ, Bamford NJ, Harris PA, et al. Prevalence of obesity and owners' perceptions of body condition in pleasure horses and ponies in south-eastern Australia. Aust Vet J 2016;94:427–32.

24. Giles SL, Rands SA, Nicol CJ, et al. Obesity prevalence and associated risk factors in outdoor living domestic horses and ponies. PeerJ 2014;2:e299. Available at: https://www.ncbi.nlm.nih.gov/pmc/articles/PMC3970797/. Accessed May 29, 2020.

25. Langner K, Blaue D, Schedlbauer C, et al. Changes in the faecal microbiota of horses and ponies during a two-year body weight gain programme. PLoS One 2020;15:e0230015.

26. Bamford NJ, Potter SJ, Harris PA, et al. Breed differences in insulin sensitivity and insulinemic responses to oral glucose in horses and ponies of moderate body condition score. Domest Anim Endocrinol 2014;47:101–7.

27. Schedlbauer C, Blaue D, Gericke M, et al. Impact of body weight gain on hepatic metabolism and hepatic inflammatory cytokines in comparison of Shetland pony geldings and warmblood horse geldings. PeerJ 2019;7:e7069.

28. Ragnarsson S, Jansson A. Comparison of grass haylage digestibility and metabolic plasma profile in Icelandic and standardbred horses. J Anim Physiol Anim Nutr 2011;95:273–9.

29. Vermorel M, Vernet J, Martin-Rosset W. Digestive and energy utilisation of two diets by ponies and horses. Livest Prod Sci 1997;51:13–9.

30. Owers R, Chubbock S. Fight the fat! Equine Vet J 2013;45:5.

31. Anon. The rise in equine obesity. Available at: https://veterinary-practice.com/article/the-rise-in-equine-obesity. Accessed May 12, 2020.

32. Milinovich G, Trott D, Burrell P, et al. Changes in equine hindgut bacterial populations during oligofructose-induced laminitis. Environ Microbiol 2006;8:885–98.

33. Steelman SM, Chowdhary BP, Dowd S, et al. Pyrosequencing of 16S rRNA genes in fecal samples reveals high diversity of hindgut microflora in horses and potential links to chronic laminitis. BMC Vet Res 2012;8:231.

34. Garner H, Coffman J, Hahn A, et al. Equine laminitis of alimentary origin: an experimental model. Am J Vet Res 1975;36:441–4.

35. Bailey S, Rycroft A, Elliott J. Production of amines in equine cecal contents in an in vitro model of carbohydrate overload. J Anim Sci 2002;80:2656–62.

36. van Eps A, Pollitt C. Equine laminitis induced with oligofructose. Equine Vet J 2006;38:203–8.

37. Kalck KA, Frank N, Elliott SB, et al. Effects of low-dose oligofructose treatment administered via nasogastric intubation on induction of laminitis and associated alterations in glucose and insulin dynamics in horses. Am J Vet Res 2009;70:624–32.
38. Baskerville CL, Chockalingham S, Harris PA, et al. The effect of insulin on equine lamellar basal epithelial cells mediated by the insulin-like growth factor-1 receptor. PeerJ 2018;6:e5945.
39. Asplin K, Sillence M, Pollitt C, et al. Induction of laminitis by prolonged hyperinsulinaemia in clinically normal ponies. Vet J 2007;174:530–5.
40. Treiber K, Hess T, Kronfeld D, et al. Dietary energy sources affect insulin sensitivity and Beta-cell responsiveness of trained Arabian geldings during endurance exercise. J Anim Physiol Anim Nutr 2005;89:427–33.
41. Bailey S, Menzies-Gow N, Harris P, et al. Effect of dietary fructans and dexamethasone administration on the insulin response of ponies predisposed to laminitis. J Am Vet Med Assoc 2007;231:1365–73.
42. Ley R, Backhed F, Turnbaugh P, et al. Obesity alters gut microbial ecology. Proc Natl Acad Sci U S A 2005;102:11070–5.
43. Guo X, Xia X, Tang R, et al. Real-time PCR quantification of the predominant bacterial divisions in the distal gut of Meishan and Landrace pigs. Anaerobe 2008;14:224–8.
44. Turnbaugh P, Gordon J. The core gut microbiome, energy balance and obesity. J Physiol 2009;587:4153–8.
45. Handl S, Heilmann RM, German A, et al. Fecal microbiota and fecal calprotectin and S100A12 concentrations in lean and obese dogs. Journal of Veterinary Internal Medicine 2012;24.
46. Morrison PK, Newbold CJ, Jones E, et al. The equine gastrointestinal microbiome: impacts of age and obesity. Front Microbiol 2018;9:3017.
47. Shepherd ML, Ponder MA, Burk AO, et al. Fibre digestibility, abundance of faecal bacteria and plasma acetate concentrations in overweight adult mares. J Nutr Sci 2014;3:e10.
48. Biddle AS, Tomb J-F, Fan Z. Microbiome and blood analyte differences point to community and metabolic signatures in lean and obese horses. Front Vet Sci 2018;5:225.
49. Morrison PK, Newbold CJ, Jones E, et al. The equine gastrointestinal microbiome: impacts of weight-loss. BMC Vet Res 2020;16:78.
50. McNeil N. The contribution of the large intestine to energy supplies in man. Am J Clin Nutr 1984;39:338–42.
51. Stephenson HM, Green MJ, Freeman SL. Prevalence of obesity in a population of horses in the UK. Vet Rec 2011;168:131.
52. Ravary A, Baldwin MW, Bartz JA. Shaping the body politic: mass media fat-shaming affects implicit anti-fat attitudes. Pers Soc Psychol Bull 2019;45:1580–9.
53. Vogel L. Fat shaming is making people sicker and heavier. CMAJ 2019;191:E649.
54. Brooks SA, Makvandi-Nejad S, Chu E, et al. Morphological variation in the horse: defining complex traits of body size and shape. Anim Genet 2010;41(Suppl 2):159–65.
55. Thatcher CD, Pleasant RS, Geor RJ, et al. Prevalence of overconditioning in mature horses in southwest Virginia during the summer. J Vet Intern Med 2012;26:1413–8.

56. Harker I, Harris P, Barfoot C. The body condition score of leisure horses competing at an unaffiliated championship in the UK. J Equine Vet Sci 2011; 31:253–4.
57. Wyse CA, Mcnie KA, Tannahil VJ, et al. Prevalence of obesity in riding horses in Scotland. Vet Rec 2008;162:590–1.
58. Kosolofski HR, Gow SP, Robinson KA. Prevalence of obesity in the equine population of Saskatoon and surrounding area. Can Vet J 2017;58:967–70.
59. Dugdale AH, Curtis GC, Milne E, et al. Assessment of body fat in the pony: part II. Validation of the deuterium oxide dilution technique for the measurement of body fat. Equine Vet J 2011;43:562–70.
60. Fowler AL, Pyles MB, Bill VT, et al. Relationships between measurements of body fat in thoroughbred horses. J Equine Vet Sci 2020;85:102873.
61. Kienzle E, Schramme SC. Body condition scoring and prediction of body weight in adult warm blooded horses. Pferdeheilkunde 2004;20:517–24.
62. Henneke DR, Potter GD, Kreider JL, et al. Relationship between condition score, physical measurements and body-fat percentage in mares. Equine Vet J 1983; 15:371–2.
63. Dugdale AH, Grove-White D, Curtis GC, et al. Body condition scoring as a predictor of body fat in horses and ponies. Vet J 2012;194(2):173–8. Available at: http://www.ncbi.nlm.nih.gov/pubmed/22578691.
64. Carter R, Geor R, Staniar W, et al. Apparent adiposity assessed by standardised scoring systems and morphometric measurements in horses and ponies. Vet J 2009;179:204–10.
65. Giles SL, Nicol CJ, Rands SA, et al. Assessing the seasonal prevalence and risk factors for nuchal crest adiposity in domestic horses and ponies using the Cresty Neck Score. BMC Vet Res 2015;11:13.
66. Anon. EQUIFAT: A novel scoring system for the semi-quantitative evaluation of regional adipose tissues in Equidae. Available at: https://journals.plos.org/plosone/article?id=10.1371/journal.pone.0173753. Accessed April 1, 2020.
67. Siegers EW, de Ruijter-Villani M, van Doorn DA, et al. Ultrasonographic measurements of localized fat accumulation in Shetland pony mares fed a normal v. a high energy diet for 2 years. Animal 2018;12:1602–10.
68. Westervelt R, Stouffer J, Hintz H, et al. Estimating fatness in horses and ponies. J Anim Sci 1976;43(4):781–5.
69. Staub C, Venturi E, Cirot M, et al. Ultrasonographic measures of body fatness and their relationship with plasma levels and adipose tissue expression of four adipokines in Welsh pony mares. Domest Anim Endocrinol 2019;69:75–83.
70. Argo CM, Curtis GC, Grove-White D, et al. Weight loss resistance: a further consideration for the nutritional management of obese Equidae. Vet J 2012; 194:179–88.
71. Donaldson M, McFarlane D, Jorgensen A, et al. Correlation between plasma alpha-melanocyte-stimulating hormone concentration and body mass index in healthy horses. Am J Vet Res 2004;65:1469–73.
72. Potter SJ, Harris PA, Bailey SR. 63 Derivation of a new body condition index to estimate body fat percentage from morphometric measurements: comparison with body condition score. J Equine Vet Sci 2015;35:410–1.
73. NRC. Nutrient requirements of horses. 6th edition. Washington, DC: The National Academies Press; 2007.
74. Rendle D, McGregor Argo C, Bowen M, et al. Equine obesity: current perspectives. UK-Vet Equine 2018;2:1–19.

75. Stanley SO, Cant JP, Osborne VR. A pilot study to determine whether a tongue-activated liquid dispenser would mitigate abnormal behavior in pasture-restricted horses. J Equine Vet Sci 2015;35:973–6.

76. Luthersson N, Nielsen KH, Harris P, et al. Risk factors associated with equine gastric ulceration syndrome (EGUS) in 201 horses in Denmark. Equine Vet J 2009;41:625–30.

77. Harris PA, Ellis AD, Fradinho MJ, et al. Review: Feeding conserved forage to horses: recent advances and recommendations. Animal 2017;11:958–67.

78. Anon. Common feed profiles | Equianalytical. Available at: https://equi-analytical.com/common-feed-profiles/. Accessed December 11, 2019.

79. Martinson K, Jung H, Hathaway M, et al. The effect of soaking on carbohydrate removal and dry matter loss in orchardgrass and alfalfa hays. J Of Equine Vet Sci 2012;32:332–8.

80. Staniar WB, Bussard JR, Repard NM, et al. Voluntary intake and digestibility of teff hay fed to horses. J Anim Sci 2010;88:3296–303.

81. DeBoer ML, Hathaway MR, Kuhle KJ, et al. Glucose and insulin response of horses grazing alfalfa, perennial cool-season grass, and teff across seasons. J Equine Vet Sci 2018;68:33–8.

82. Harbers LH, McNally LK, Smith WH. Digestibility of three grass hays by the horse and scanning electron microscopy of undigested leaf remnants. J Anim Sci 1981;53:1671–7.

83. Van Soest P, Robertson J, Lewis B. Methods for dietary fiber, neutral detergent fiber, and nonstarch polysaccharides in relation to animal nutrition. J Dairy Sci 1991;74:3583–97.

84. Harris P, Sillence M, Inglis R, et al. Effect of short (< 2CM) lucerne chaff addition on the intake rate and glycaemic response of a sweet feed. Pferdeheilkunde 2005;21:87–8.

85. Robison CI, Nielsen BD, LeCompte RA, et al. Chopping hay before feeding does not influence fecal particle size, blood variables, or water intake in 3-year-old Arabians. J Equine Vet Sci 2017;54:118–22.

86. Müller CE, Nostell K, Bröjer J. Methods for reduction of water soluble carbohydrate content in grass forages for horses. Livestock Sci 2016;186:46–52.

87. Müller CE, Udén P. Preference of horses for grass conserved as hay, haylage or silage. Anim Feed Sci Technology 2007;132:66–78.

88. DeBoer ML, Martinson KL, Kuhle KJ, et al. Plasma amino acid concentrations of horses grazing alfalfa, cool-season perennial grasses, and teff. J Equine Vet Sci 2019;72:72–8.

89. Hansen TL, Chizek EL, Zugay OK, et al. Digestibility and retention time of coastal bermudagrass (cynodon dactylon) hay by horses. Animals (Basel) 2019;9:1148.

90. DeBoer ML, Sheaffer CC, Grev AM, et al. Yield, nutritive value, and preference of annual warm-season grasses grazed by horses. Agron J 2017;109:2136–48.

91. Dosi MCM, Kirton R, Hallsworth S, et al. Inducing weight loss in native ponies: is straw a viable alternative to hay? Vet Rec 2020;187(8):e60.

92. McGreevy PD, Cripps PJ, French NP, et al. Management factors associated with stereotypic and redirected behaviour in the thoroughbred horse. Equine Vet J 1995;27:86–91.

93. Curtis L, Burford JH, England GCW, et al. Risk factors for acute abdominal pain (colic) in the adult horse: a scoping review of risk factors, and a systematic review of the effect of management-related changes. PLoS One 2019;14: e0219307.

94. Bruce AM, Wagner E, Tyler P. Weight estimation in miniature horses and Shetland ponies. J Anim Sci 2010;93:204.

95. Owen KM, Wagner EL, Dowler LE, et al. Estimation of body weight in ponies. J Anim Sci 2008;86:431.

96. Wilson KR, Jackson SP, Abney CS, et al. Body weight estimation methods as influenced by condition score, balance, and exercise status in horses. Proceedings 19th Equine Nutrition and Physiology Symposium Tucson, AZ, May 31-June 3, 2005:57–62.

97. Wilson KR, Gibbs PG, Potter GS, et al. Comparison of different body weight estimation methods to actual weight of horses. In Proceedings 18th Equine Nutrition and Physiology Symposium. East Lancing, MI: 2003. p, 238–42.

98. Staniar WB, Kronfeld DS, Hoffman RM, et al. Weight prediction from linear measures of growing thoroughbreds. Equine Vet J 2004;36:149–54.

99. Anon. Horse apps. Available at: https://extension.umn.edu/horse/horse-apps. Accessed May 27, 2020.

100. Kienzle E, Fritz J. Nutritional laminitis-preventive measures for the obese horse. Tierarztl Prax Ausg G Grosstiere Nutztiere 2013;41:257–64.

101. Bass L, Swain E, Santos H, et al. Effects of feeding frequency using a commercial automated feeding device on gastric ulceration in exercised quarter horses. J Equine Vet Sci 2018;64:96–100.

102. Luthersson N, Nielsen KH, Harris P, et al. The prevalence and anatomical distribution of equine gastric ulceration syndrome (EGUS) in 201 horses in Denmark. Equine Vet J 2009;41:619–24.

103. Coenen M. [The occurrence of feed-induced stomach ulcers in horses]. Schweiz Arch Tierheilkd 1990;132:121–6.

104. Murray MJ, Eichorn ES. Effects of intermittent feed deprivation, intermittent feed deprivation with ranitidine administration, and stall confinement with ad libitum access to hay on gastric ulceration in horses. Am J Vet Res 1996;57:1599–603.

105. Ralston SL, Baile CA. Factors in the control of feed intake of horses and ponies. Neurosci Biobehav Rev 1983;7:465–70.

106. Reid SW, Mohammed HO. Survival analysis approach to risk factors associated with hyperlipemia in donkeys. J Am Vet Med Assoc 1996;209:1449–52.

107. Watson TD, Murphy D, Love S. Equine hyperlipaemia in the United Kingdom: clinical features and blood biochemistry of 18 cases. Vet Rec 1992;131:48–51.

108. Bruynsteen L, Moons CPH, Janssens GPJ, et al. Level of energy restriction alters body condition score and morphometric profile in obese Shetland ponies. Vet J 2015;206:61–6.

109. Cooper JJ, Albentosa MJ. Behavioural adaptation in the domestic horse: potential role of apparently abnormal responses including stereotypic behaviour. Livestock Prod Sci 2005;92:177–82.

110. Curtis GC, Barfoot CF, Dugdale AHA, et al. Voluntary ingestion of wood shavings by obese horses under dietary restriction. Br J Nutr 2011;106(Suppl 1):S178–82.

111. G Heusner. Ad libitum feeding of mature horses to achieve rapid weight gain. In: 13th Equine Nutr. Phys. Symp. Gainesville, FL, January 21-23, 1993;86.

112. Glunk EC, Hathaway MR, Grev AM, et al. The effect of a limit-fed diet and slow-feed hay nets on morphometric measurements and postprandial metabolite and hormone patterns in adult horses. J Anim Sci 2015;93:4144–52.

113. Glunk EC, Hathaway MR, Weber WJ, et al. The effect of hay net design on rate of forage consumption when feeding adult horses. J Equine Vet Sci 2014;34:986–91.

114. Aristizabal F, Nieto J, Yamout S, et al. The effect of a hay grid feeder on feed consumption and measurement of the gastric pH using an intragastric electrode device in horses: a preliminary report. Equine Vet J 2014;46:484–7.

115. Martinson K, Wilson J, Cleary K, et al. Round-bale feeder design affects hay waste and economics during horse feeding. J Anim Sci 2012;90:1047–55.

116. Rochais C, Henry S, Hausberger M. "Hay-bags" and "slow feeders": Testing their impact on horse behaviour and welfare. Appl Anim Behav Sci 2018; 198:52–9.

117. Ellis AD, Fell M, Luck K, et al. Effect of forage presentation on feed intake behaviour in stabled horses. Appl Anim Behav Sci 2015;165:88–94.

118. Ellis AD, Redgate S, Zinchenko S, et al. The effect of presenting forage in multi-layered haynets and at multiple sites on night time budgets of stabled horses. Appl Anim Behav Sci 2015;171:108–16.

119. Goodwin D, Davidson HPB, Harris P. A note on behaviour of stabled horses with foraging devices in mangers and buckets. Appl Anim Behav Sci 2007;105: 238–43.

120. McGowan CM, Dugdale AH, Pinchbeck GL, et al. Dietary restriction in combination with a nutraceutical supplement for the management of equine metabolic syndrome in horses. Vet J 2013;196:153–9.

121. Dugdale AH, Curtis GC, Cripps P, et al. Effect of dietary restriction on body condition, composition and welfare of overweight and obese pony mares. Equine Vet J 2010;42:600–10.

122. Dugdale AH, Curtis GC, Cripps PJ, et al. Effects of season and body condition on appetite, body mass and body composition in ad libitum fed pony mares. Vet J 2011;190:329–37.

123. MacMartin C, Wheat HC, Coe JB, et al. Effect of question design on dietary information solicited during veterinarian-client interactions in companion animal practice in Ontario, Canada. J Am Vet Med Assoc 2015;246:1203–14.

124. Morrow LD, Smith KC, Piercy RJ, et al. Retrospective analysis of post-mortem findings in 1,444 aged donkeys. J Comp Pathol 2011;144:145–56.

125. Dai F, Dalla Costa E, Murray LMA, et al. Welfare conditions of donkeys in Europe: initial outcomes from on-farm assessment. Animals 2016;6:5.

126. Pritchard JC, Lindberg AC, Main DCJ, et al. Assessment of the welfare of working horses, mules and donkeys, using health and behaviour parameters. Prev Vet Med 2005;69:265–83.

127. Pritchard A, Nielsen B, McLean A, et al. Insulin resistance as a result of body condition categorized as thin, moderate, and obese in domesticated U.S. Donkeys (Equus asinus). J Equine Vet Sci 2019;77:31–5.

128. Mendoza FJ, Estepa JC, Gonzalez-De Cara CA, et al. Energy-related parameters and their association with age, gender, and morphometric measurements in healthy donkeys. Vet J 2015;204:201–7.

129. Pearson RA, Owassat M. A guide to live weight estimation and body condition scoring of donkeys. July 2000. 14 pp. Centre for Tropical Veterinary Medicine, University of Edinburgh, UK and Institut Agronomique et Veterinaire, Hassan II, Rabat, Morocco. ISBN: 0-907146-11-2. 2000. Available at: https://agris.fao.org/agris-search/search.do?recordID=GB2012111895. Accessed June 29, 2020.

130. Burden F. Practical feeding and condition scoring for donkeys and mules. Equine Vet Education 2012;24:589–96.

131. Quaresma M, Payan-Carreira R, Silva SR. Relationship between ultrasound measurements of body fat reserves and body condition score in female donkeys. Vet J 2013;197:329–34.

132. Pearson RA, Archibald RF, Muirhead RH. The effect of forage quality and level of feeding on digestibility and gastrointestinal transit time of oat straw and alfalfa given to ponies and donkeys. Br J Nutr 2001;85:599–606.

133. Carretero-Roque L, Colunga B, Smith DG, et al. Digestible energy requirements of Mexican donkeys fed oat straw and maize stover. Trop Anim Health Prod 2005;37(Suppl 1):123–42.

134. Horn R, Bamford NJ, Afonso T, et al. Factors associated with survival, laminitis and insulin dysregulation in horses diagnosed with equine pituitary pars intermedia dysfunction. Equine Vet J 2019;51:440–5.

135. Brosnahan M, Paradis M. Demographic and clinical characteristics of geriatric horses: 467 cases (1989-1999). J Am Vet Med Assoc 2003;223:93–8.

136. Miller MA, Moore GE, Bertin FR, et al. What's new in old horses? Postmortem diagnoses in mature and aged equids. Vet Pathol 2016;53:390–8.

137. McFarlane D. Pathophysiology and clinical features of pituitary pars intermedia dysfunction. Equine Vet Education 2014;26:592–8.

138. McFarlane D. Equine pituitary pars intermedia dysfunction. Vet Clin North Am Equine Pract 2011;27:93–113.

139. Ralston SL, Breuer LH. Field evaluation of a feed formulated for geriatric horses. J Equine Vet Sci 1996;16:334–8.

140. Siard-Altman MH, Harris PA, Moffett-Krotky AD, et al. Relationships of inflamm-aging with circulating nutrient levels, body composition, age, and pituitary pars intermedia dysfunction in a senior horse population. Vet Immunol Immunopathol 2020;221:110013.

141. Adams AA, Katepalli MP, Kohler K, et al. Effect of body condition, body weight and adiposity on inflammatory cytokine responses in old horses. Vet Immunol Immunopathol 2009;127:286–94.

142. Mastro LM, Adams AA, Urschel KL. Whole-body phenylalanine kinetics and skeletal muscle protein signaling in horses with pituitary pars intermedia dysfunction. Am J Vet Res 2014;75:658–67.

143. du Toit N, Burden FA, Dixon PM. Clinical dental examinations of 357 donkeys in the UK. Part 1: Prevalence of dental disorders. Equine Vet J 2009;41:390–4.

144. Bamford NJ, Potter SJ, Baskerville CL, et al. Influence of dietary restriction and low-intensity exercise on weight loss and insulin sensitivity in obese equids. J Vet Intern Med 2019;33:280–6.

145. Bertin FR, de Laat MA. The diagnosis of equine insulin dysregulation. Equine Vet J 2017;49:570–6.

146. Frank N, Bailey S, Durham A, et al. Recommendations for the Diagnosis and Treatment of Equine Metabolic Syndrome (EMS). Equine Endocrinology Group. Available at: HYPERLINK "https://nam03.safelinks.protection.outlook.com/?url=https%3A%2F%2Fsites.tufts.edu%2Fequineendogroup%2Ffiles%2F2016%2F11%2F2016-11-2-EMS-EEG-Final.pdf&data=04%7C01%7CJ.Surendrakumar%40elsevier.com%7Cbcdd085ac66643759dd408d8da822fdc%7C9274ee3f94254109a27f9fb15c10675d%7C0%7C0%7C637499600164773109%7CUnknown%7CTWFpbGZsb3d8eyJWIjoiMC4wLjAwMDAiLCJQIjoiV2luMzIiLCJBTiI6Ik1haWwiLCJXVCI6Mn0%3D%7C1000&sdata=9%2B9PYNyygrgk1s8zrulaB6GgX2vxYt1VUmNxXw3I0HU%3D&reserved=0" https://sites.tufts.edu/equineendogroup/files/2016/11/2016-11-2-EMS-EEG-Final.pdf.

147. Durham AE, Frank N, McGowan CM, et al. ECEIM consensus statement on equine metabolic syndrome. J Vet Intern Med 2019;33:335–49.
148. Equi-Analytical L. Grass Hay Accumulated crop years: 05/01/2000 through 04/30/2016. 2016. Available at: https://equi-analytical.com/common-feed-profiles/.
149. Frank N, Geor R, Bailey S, et al. Equine metabolic syndrome. J Vet Intern Med 2010;24:467–75.
150. Longland A, Byrd B. Pasture nonstructural carbohydrates and equine laminitis. J Nutr 2006;136:2099S–102S.
151. Niness K. Inulin and oligofructose: what are they? J Nutr 1999;129:1402S–6S.
152. James S, Muir J, Curtis S, et al. Dietary fibre: a roughage guide. Intern Med J 2003;33:291–6.
153. Coenen M, Mösseler A, Vervuert I. Fermentative gases in breath indicate that inulin and starch start to be degraded by microbial fermentation in the stomach and small intestine of the horse in contrast to pectin and cellulose. J Nutr 2006; 136:2108S–10S.
154. Borer KE, Bailey SR, Menzies-Gow NJ, et al. Effect of feeding glucose, fructose, and inulin on blood glucose and insulin concentrations in normal ponies and those predisposed to laminitis. J Anim Sci 2012;90(9):3003–11. Available at: http://www.ncbi.nlm.nih.gov/pubmed/22585777.
155. Crawford C, Sepulveda MF, Elliott J, et al. Dietary fructan carbohydrate increases amine production in the equine large intestine: implications for pasture-associated laminitis. J Anim Sci 2007;85:2949–58.
156. Newbold CJ, Macías B, Crawford C, et al. Changes in the bacterial populations in the equine hindgut following the addition of inulin to the diet. 2009. Available at: https://pure.aber.ac.uk/portal/en/publications/changes-in-the-bacterial-populations-in-the-equine-hindgut-following-the-addition-of-inulin-to-the-diet(c0166ace-1b9e-4b18-bcce-622de37bd6d0).html. Accessed May 15, 2020.
157. Ince JC, Longland AC, Moore-Colyer MJS, et al. In vitro degradation of grass fructan by equid gastrointestinal digesta. Grass Forage Sci 2014;69:514–23.
158. Kagan IA, Kirch BH, Thatcher CD, et al. Seasonal and diurnal variation in simple sugar and fructan composition of orchardgrass pasture and hay in the piedmont region of the United States. J Equine Vet Sci 2011;31:488–97.
159. Kagan IA, Goodman JP, Seman DH, et al. Effects of harvest date, sampling time, and cultivar on total phenolic concentrations, water-soluble carbohydrate concentrations, and phenolic profiles of selected cool-season grasses in Central Kentucky. J Equine Vet Sci 2019;79:86–93.
160. Williams CA, Kenny LB, Burk AO. Effects of grazing system, season, and forage carbohydrates on glucose and insulin dynamics of the grazing horse. J Anim Sci 2019;97:2541–54.
161. DeBoer ML, Hathaway MR, Weber PSD, et al. Glucose and insulin response of aged horses grazing alfalfa, perennial cool-season grass, and teff during the spring and late fall. J Equine Vet Sci 2019;72:108–11.
162. Treiber K, Boston R, Kronfeld D, et al. Insulin resistance and compensation in thoroughbred weanlings adapted to high-glycemic meals. J Anim Sci 2005; 83:2357–64.
163. Argo CM, Dugdale AHA, McGowan CM. Considerations for the use of restricted, soaked grass hay diets to promote weight loss in the management of equine metabolic syndrome and obesity. Vet J 2015;206:170–7.
164. Carslake HB, Argo CMcG, Pinchbeck GL, et al. Insulinaemic and glycaemic responses to three forages in ponies. Vet J 2018;235:83–9.

165. Longland AC, Barfoot C, Harris PA. Effects of soaking on the water-soluble carbohydrate and crude protein content of hay. Vet Rec 2011;168:618.

166. Longland AC, Barfoot C, Harris PA. Effect of period, water temperature and agitation on loss of water-soluble carbohydrates and protein from grass hay: implications for equine feeding management. Vet Rec 2014;174:68.

167. Martinson KL, Hathaway M, Jung H, et al. The effect of soaking on protein and mineral loss in orchardgrass and alfalfa hay. J Equine Vet Sci 2012;32:776–82.

168. Mack SJ, Dugdale AH, Argo CM, et al. Impact of water-soaking on the nutrient composition of UK hays. Vet Rec 2014;174:452.

169. Moore-Colyer MJS, Lumbis K, Longland A, et al. The effect of five different wetting treatments on the nutrient content and microbial concentration in hay for horses. PLoS One 2014;9:e114079.

170. Earing JE, Hathaway MR, Sheaffer CC, et al. Effect of hay steaming on forage nutritive values and dry matter intake by horses. J Anim Sci 2013;91:5813–20.

171. Moore-Colyer MJS, Taylor JLE, James R. The effect of steaming and soaking on the respirable particle, bacteria, mould, and nutrient content in hay for horses. J Equine Vet Sci 2016;39:62–8.

172. Anon. Feed Composition Library | Dairy One. Available at: https://dairyone.com/services/forage-laboratory-services/feed-composition-library/. Accessed May 29, 2020.

173. Ringmark S, Roepstorff L, Essén-Gustavsson B, et al. Growth, training response and health in standardbred yearlings fed a forage-only diet. Animal 2013;7:746–53.

174. Müller CE, Hultén C, Gröndahl G. Assessment of hygienic quality of haylage fed to healthy horses. Grass Forage Sci 2011;66:453–63.

175. Lindåse S, Müller C, Nostell K, et al. Evaluation of glucose and insulin response to haylage diets with different content of nonstructural carbohydrates in 2 breeds of horses. Domest Anim Endocrinol 2018;64:49–58.

176. USDA. Lameness and laminitis in US horses. Fort Collins (CO): Center for Epidemiology and Animal Health, National Animal Health Monitoring System; 2000.

177. Treiber K, Kronfeld D, Hess T, et al. Evaluation of genetic and metabolic predispositions and nutritional risk factors for pasture-associated laminitis in ponies. J Am Vet Med Assoc 2006;228:1538–45.

178. Fleurance G, Duncan P, Mallevaud B. Daily intake and the selection of feeding sites by horses in heterogeneous wet grasslands. Anim Res 2001;50:149–56.

179. Fitzgerald DM, Pollitt CC, Walsh DM, et al. The effect of different grazing conditions on the insulin and incretin response to the oral glucose test in ponies. BMC Vet Res 2019;15:345.

180. Longland AC, Barfoot C, Harris PA. The effect of wearing a grazing muzzle vs not wearing a grazing muzzle on pasture dry matter intake by ponies. J Equine Vet Sci 2011;31:282–3.

181. Dowler LE, Siciliano PD, Pratt-Phillips SE, et al. Determination of pasture dry matter intake rates in different seasons and their application in grazing management. J Equine Vet Sci 2012;32:85–92.

182. Davis K, Iwaniuk M, Dennis R, et al. Effects of grazing muzzles on voluntary exercise and physiological stress in a miniature horse herd. J Equine Vet Sci 2019;76:101.

183. Longland AC, Barfoot C, Harris PA. Effects of grazing muzzles on intakes of dry matter and water-soluble carbohydrates by ponies grazing spring, summer, and

autumn swards, as well as autumn swards of different heights. J Equine Vet Sci 2016;40:26–33.

184. Glunk EC, Pratt-Phillips SE, Siciliano PD. Effect of restricted pasture access on pasture dry matter intake rate, dietary energy intake, and fecal pH in horses. J Equine Vet Sci 2013;33:421–6.

185. Glunk EC, Sheaffer CC, Hathaway MR, et al. Interaction of grazing muzzle use and grass species on forage intake of horses. J Equine Vet Sci 2014;34:930–3.

186. SHINGU Y, Kawai M, INABA H, et al. Voluntary intake and behavior of Hokkaido native horses and light half-bred horses in woodland pasture. J Equine Sci 2000;11:69–73.

187. Davis KM, Iwaniuk ME, Dennis RL, et al. Effects of grazing muzzles on behavior and physiological stress of individually housed grazing miniature horses. Appl Anim Behav Sci 2020;231:105067.

188. National Equine Welfare Council (NEWC). NEWC grazing muzzle guidance. 2015. Available at: http://www.newc.co.uk/wp-content/uploads/2015/09/NEWC-Grazing-Muzzle-download-007_FINAL-1-sm.pdf. Accessed June 29, 2020.

189. Pollard D, Wylie CE, Verheyen KLP, et al. Identification of modifiable factors associated with owner-reported equine laminitis in Britain using a web-based cohort study approach. BMC Vet Res 2019;15:59.

190. Frank N, Elliott SB, Boston RC. Effects of long-term oral administration of levothyroxine sodium on glucose dynamics in healthy adult horses. Am J Vet Res 2008;69:76–81.

191. Marycz K (University of E and LS, Moll E (Mutyhle EDG (Germany)), Grzesiak J (University of E and LS. Influence of functional nutrients on insulin resistance in horses with equine metabolic syndrome. *Pakistan Veterinary Journal (Pakistan)*. 2016. Available at: http://agris.fao.org/agris-search/search.do?recordID= PK2016000477. Accessed February 24, 2020.

192. Chameroy KA, Frank N, Elliott SB, et al. Effects of a supplement containing chromium and magnesium on morphometric measurements, resting glucose, insulin concentrations and insulin sensitivity in laminitic obese horses. Equine Vet J 2011;43:494–9.

193. Manfredi JM, Stapley ED, Nadeau JA, et al. Investigation of the effects of a dietary supplement on insulin and adipokine concentrations in equine metabolic syndrome/insulin dysregulation. J Equine Vet Sci 2020;88:102930.

194. Tinworth KD, Harris PA, Sillence MN, et al. Potential treatments for insulin resistance in the horse: a comparative multi-species review. Vet J 2010;186:282–91.

Nutritional Influences on Skeletal Muscle and Muscular Disease

Kristine L. Urschel, BSc, PhD[a], Erica C. McKenzie, BSc, BVMS, PhD[b],*

KEYWORDS

- Skeletal muscle • Growth • Exercise • Muscle disorders

KEY POINTS

- Proper nutritional management is necessary for the growth and maintenance of muscle mass, to support muscle contraction, to promote muscle recovery following exercise, and in the management and prevention of muscular disorders.
- Key nutrients needed to support muscle include protein, carbohydrates, fat, vitamin E, and selenium.
- Additional research is indicated to optimize muscle health and performance across the lifespan of the horse.

INTRODUCTION

In an athletic species such as the horse, the development and maintenance of muscle mass is of the utmost importance. Regardless of whether the horse is an elite athlete or sedentary, nutrition plays an essential role in skeletal muscle health. In addition to ensuring that adequate amounts of protein and energy are provided in the ration to support the growth and maintenance of skeletal muscle, adequate selenium and vitamin E are also critical for muscle health. In addition, several heritable muscular disorders can be managed primarily through nutritional interventions.

In mature horses, muscle accounts for 40% to 55% of body weight (BW).[1] The moisture and protein content of muscle range from 68% to 77% and 19% to 22% wet weight, respectively, varying by muscle type, horse age, and breed. Other major components of skeletal muscle include fat (generally <5%), glycogen (1%–2%), and minerals (~1%).[2–5] The content of the essential amino acids, relative to lysine content, is very consistent across muscle groups, as shown in **Table 1**. The mineral composition of skeletal muscle is provided in **Table 2**.

[a] Department of Animal and Food Sciences, University of Kentucky, 612 W.P. Garrigus Building, Lexington, KY 40546, USA; [b] Department of Clinical Sciences, Carlson College of Veterinary Medicine, Oregon State University, 227 Magruder Hall, 700 Southwest 30th Street, Corvallis, OR 97331, USA
* Corresponding author.
E-mail address: klurschel@uky.edu

Vet Clin Equine 37 (2021) 139–175
https://doi.org/10.1016/j.cveq.2020.12.005
0749-0739/21/© 2020 Elsevier Inc. All rights reserved.

Table 1
Essential amino acid composition of equine skeletal muscle

	Badiani et al,[4] 1997	Seong et al,[5] 2016
Histidine	57	43–56
Isoleucine	58	46–48
Leucine	97	95–96
Lysine	100	100
Methionine	31	26–30
Phenylalanine	52	46–49
Threonine	54	52
Valine	61	49–52

Amino acid composition is expressed as a percentage of the lysine content, calculated by [amino acid content (g/100 g) ÷ lysine content (g/100 g)] × 100. Data were obtained from studies examining the composition of horse meat. Depending on the cut of meat, lysine content varied from 1.57 to 1.92 g/100 g. Seong and colleagues[5] reported the individual compositions of 10 different muscle groups (cuts of meat), whereas Badiani and colleagues [4] reported only the composition of the upper hindlimb muscles.

Data from Badiani A, Nanni N, Gatta PP, Tolomelli B, Manfredini M. Nutrient profile of horsemeat. *J Food Compos Anal.* 1997;10:254-269; and Seong PN, Park KM, Kang GH, et al. The Differences in Chemical Composition, Physical Quality Traits and Nutritional Values of Horse Meat as Affected by Various Retail Cut Types. *Asian-Australas J Anim Sci.* 2016;29:89-99.

AN OVERVIEW OF MUSCLE FIBER STRUCTURE AND PHYSIOLOGY
The Muscle Fiber

The plasma membrane of each individual muscle fiber is known as the sarcolemma, and it has a series of invaginations projecting toward the center of the muscle fiber, known as the transverse tubules (T tubules). Notable structures within the muscle

Table 2
Mineral composition of equine skeletal muscle

Mineral	Muscle Content
Calcium (g)	0.04
Phosphorus (g)	3.1
Magnesium (mg)	250
Sodium (mg)	369
Potassium (mg)	3841
Chloride (mg)	560
Sulfur (mg)	2250
Iron (mg)	204
Copper (mg)	21.6
Zinc (mg)	115
Manganese (mg)	2.5
Selenium (mg)	0.27

Values for calcium, phosphorus, magnesium, sodium, chloride and sulfur are per kilogram muscle wet weight and values for iron, copper, zinc, manganese and selenium are per kilogram muscle dry weight.

Data from Coenen M. Macro and trace elements in equine nutrition. In: Geor RJ, Harris PA, M. C, eds. *Equine Applied and Clinical Nutrition: Health, Welfare and Performance.* New York: Saunders Elsevier; 2013:190-228.

fibers include multiple nuclei, abundant chains of myofibrils, and the sarcoplasmic reticulum. The multiple nuclei result from the fusion of muscle stem cells to form the individual muscle fiber. The myofibrils run parallel to the length of the muscle fiber, give the muscle its contractile properties, and are formed through the specific arrangement of 2 myofilaments: the thick and thin filaments. The thick filament is composed of myosin and the thin filament contains actin, troponin, and tropomyosin. The interaction between the thick and the thin filaments forms a repeating unit known as the sarcomere. Each myofibril is surrounded by a structure known as the sarcoplasmic reticulum, which associates with the T tubules of the sarcolemma. Figures showing the structural features of muscle fibers can be found elsewhere, including a review article by Frontera and Ochala.[6]

Muscle Fiber Types

Muscle fibers are not uniform between muscles or even within an individual muscle. Based on the isoform of the myosin heavy chain protein, 3 distinct muscle fiber types have been identified in the skeletal muscle of horses: types I, IIA, and IIX.[7] Before the late 1990s, IIX fibers were classified as IIB fibers based on myosin ATPase histochemical staining.[8] However, molecular techniques showed that horses do not express the IIB myosin heavy chain isoform that has been reported in smaller mammals such as rats.[7] Each muscle fiber type has unique structural, contractile, and metabolic properties.[9] In general, type I fibers hydrolyze ATP more slowly and are termed slow twitch fibers. They show a more oxidative phenotype, with a smaller diameter, plentiful blood supply, more fat stores, a greater mitochondrial density, and a greater activity of oxidative enzymes. In contrast, type II fibers hydrolyze ATP more rapidly and are termed fast twitch fibers, meaning they form cross-bridges more rapidly and are able to generate more force during contraction. They have a more prominent sarcoplasmic reticulum, greater glycogen stores, greater glycolytic capacity, and a larger diameter compared with type I fibers. Functionally, type IIX fibers have a larger cross-sectional area and contract more rapidly than IIA fibers and generally have a lower oxidative capacity. However, in trained horses, the type IIX fibers may have an oxidative capacity that approaches levels seen in the type I and IIA fibers.[10]

Muscle fiber formation occurs before birth, with postnatal muscle growth occurring exclusively through hypertrophy. To the best of the authors' knowledge, the effects of maternal nutrition on fetal muscle fiber development has not been studied in horses. However, in other species, it is well documented that poor maternal nutrition, through either overfeeding or underfeeding, can result in effects on muscle fiber numbers and size at birth and can lead to differences in body composition that last throughout the animal's life.[11,12] For example, lambs from ewes overfed or underfed during gestation had larger muscle fibers at birth; however, by 3 months of age, both groups of lambs had smaller muscle fibers with a higher fat content compared with lambs from control-fed ewes.[12] The effects of maternal nutrition on muscle fiber numbers and growth merits additional research in horses because of the importance of skeletal muscle for subsequent athletic performance.

Muscle fiber type composition varies by muscle type, depth, and horse breed. Front limb muscles have more type I fibers and fewer type IIX fibers than the propulsive hind end muscles.[13] Type I fibers increase in frequency and type IIX fibers decrease in frequency with progressing gluteus medius muscle depth.[7,8] At the same depth of the gluteus medius muscle, Thoroughbreds had fewer type I fibers than Arabians,[14] reflective of the greater speed or endurance capabilities of the Thoroughbreds and Arabians, respectively. Similarly, the gluteus medius muscles of Thoroughbred and

Standardbred foals have greater maximum oxidative capacity, compared with Quarter horse foals of the same age.[15]

Satellite Cells

Muscle stem cells, known as satellite cells, are involved in postnatal muscle growth and repair by fusing with existing muscle fibers, contributing nuclei, mitochondria, and other organelles needed to support muscle growth and function. Although there is limited research on the nutritional factors influencing satellite cell function in horses, it is well accepted in other livestock species that an adequate plane of nutrition is necessary for optimal stem cell growth.[16] Incubating equine satellite cells with β-hydroxy-β-methylbutyrate (HMB), a metabolite of the amino acid leucine, altered the expression of genes related to many important functions, including differentiation, proliferation, inflammatory response, protein synthesis, and cellular energy use.[17] Satellite cells harvested from horses that received tributryn, a glycerol molecule with 3 butyrate molecules attached, for 30 days showed increased satellite cell activation relative to untreated horses.[18] The proposed mechanism of action of the tributyrin was that butyrate acts as a histone deacetylase inhibitor, which was then able to influence cellular gene expression. However, although both HMB and tributyrin contain butyrate moieties and both influence satellite cell function, these molecules are not metabolically related and, to the best of the authors' knowledge, do not interconvert.

Muscle Contraction

Figures outlining the processes of skeletal muscle contraction can be found in most veterinary physiology textbooks and in review articles of skeletal muscle physiology.[6] Acetylcholine is released from the motor neuron and binds to receptors on the muscle fiber's sarcolemma, causing sodium to flow into the cell, depolarizing the muscle fiber. Voltage-gated calcium channels on the T tubules and the sarcoplasmic reticulum open and calcium flows into the muscle sarcoplasm from the sarcoplasmic reticulum. When calcium binds to troponin on the thin filament there is a conformational change, exposing myosin-binding sites on actin. Meanwhile, myosin on the thick filament binds and hydrolyzes the cellular energy currency ATP to ADP, and the actin and myosin bind to form a cross-bridge. Once the cross-bridge forms, myosin undergoes a conformational change, pulling the thin filament over the thick filament, resulting in a shortened sarcomere, and ultimately muscle contraction. From a nutritional standpoint, muscle contraction requires appropriate intracellular and extracellular concentrations of 3 key ions, sodium, potassium, and calcium, and adequate energy substrate, particularly glucose or fatty acids, to make ATP. In addition, because the myofibrils are proteins, protein is a critical nutrient for muscle structure and function.

REGULATION OF MUSCLE PROTEIN SYNTHESIS

Muscle protein content is determined by the balance between rates of muscle protein synthesis and degradation: if synthesis exceeds degradation, protein will be accreted and muscle mass will increase. Muscle protein synthesis is the main factor that regulates muscle mass in humans.[19,20] In mammals, the activation of muscle protein synthesis is regulated by the mammalian target of rapamycin (mTOR) signaling pathway (**Fig. 1**).[19] Insulin, amino acids, and exercise independently activate different upstream signaling pathways, which then converge to activate the mTOR protein. Once activated, mTOR is then able to activate other proteins, ultimately allowing the assembly of the cellular machinery and the initiation of protein synthesis. In horses, feeding results in an increase in mTOR signaling, likely caused by the increase in both circulating

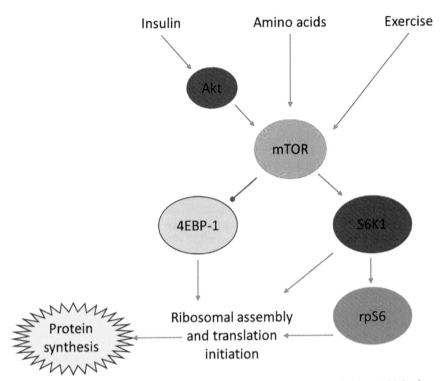

Fig. 1. The mTOR signaling pathway that regulates muscle protein synthesis. mTOR is phosphorylated and activated by several independent types of anabolic stimuli, including amino acids, glucose, and exercise. Once activated, mTOR phosphorylates several downstream targets, including 4E-BP1, S6K1, and rpS6, resulting in ribosomal assembly, translation initiation, and ultimately protein synthesis. Green arrows indicate that the protein or process is activated and the red arrow indicates that the protein is inhibited by phosphorylation.

insulin and amino acids.[21,22] The activation of mTOR signaling was more responsive to feeding, the same amount and type of protein in a test meal feeding protocol (1.2 g/kg BW), in yearlings than in older horses.[22] This finding is in agreement with the greater rates of average daily gain in yearlings. A recent study showed that mTOR signaling can be maximized with the intake of a meal of a commercial complementary feed containing 0.25 g protein/kg BW.[23] This finding is in agreement with data in young men where the rate of muscle protein synthesis, measured using stable isotopes, is maximized when ~0.25 g/kg BW of a high-quality protein, such as whey, is provided in a single meal.[24] In humans, soy protein is less effective at stimulating muscle protein synthesis than whey, skim milk, and beef, possibly because of lower levels of the essential amino acids in plant-based proteins.[20] The effect of protein source on the activation of muscle protein synthesis in horses has not been studied. However, because of differences in protein digestibility between forage and grain sources,[25,26] it is expected that a greater amount of forage protein would be needed to elicit the same degree of signaling than a primarily cereal grain or oilseed protein source.

In other species, the branched chain amino acid (BCAA) leucine seems to be particularly effective at activating mTOR signaling and increasing muscle protein synthesis.[27,28] The addition of leucine to a meal containing suboptimal levels of protein increases muscle protein synthesis to levels comparable with higher levels of protein intake.[28,29] The effects of leucine supplementation of muscle mTOR signaling have not been studied in horses in vivo; however, in vitro, muscle satellite cells showed increased downstream mTOR signaling when a physiologic concentration of leucine was provided in the culture medium.[30]

In humans, resistance exercise results in an increase in muscle protein synthesis, continuing even 48 hours after the bout of exercise.[31] However, exercise has also been shown to increase muscle protein breakdown.[31] In order to achieve a net accretion of muscle protein, feeding must occur in proximity to exercise in order to increase plasma insulin concentrations to a level that suppresses muscle protein degradation. There is a synergistic effect of exercise and protein feeding on rates of muscle protein synthesis,[32] with the greatest benefits occurring when feeding occurs within about an hour of exercise in humans. From dose-response studies in young adults, the consumption of a protein drink containing ∼0.25 g/kg BW of whey or egg protein following a single heavy-load bout of leg resistance exercise supported maximal rates of postexercise muscle protein synthesis.[24,33] There is also evidence that smaller amounts of protein can support similar increased rates of muscle protein synthesis, provided the protein is enriched with leucine to a level of ∼0.04 g/kg BW (the amount provided in 0.25 g/kg BW of whey protein).[34] In humans, plasma insulin concentrations of ∼15 to 30 mU/L are needed to suppress muscle protein breakdown.[35] In horses, the consumption of 0.25 g/kg BW protein from a commercial feed, the amount of protein needed to maximize mTOR signaling, resulted in plasma insulin concentrations of ∼20 mU/L.[23] However, whether this insulinemic response was sufficient to suppress muscle protein breakdown in healthy horses is currently unknown.

In conclusion, because there is limited research regarding muscle mTOR signaling in horses, and to the authors' knowledge no direct measurements of equine muscle protein synthesis using isotopes, the impact of nutrition on equine skeletal muscle protein synthesis must be largely extrapolated from humans. It is important to acknowledge that there may be limitations associated with relying on such data to understand the nutritional regulation of equine muscle mass because of differences in typical rations, digestive anatomy and physiology, and in muscle fiber type proportions. There is clearly a need for additional equine-specific research to elucidate optimal dietary strategies for the development and maintenance of skeletal muscle in horses.

PRIMARY FUEL SOURCES AND METABOLISM

Muscle contraction requires energy (ATP) and, as exercise intensity increases, so do ATP needs. ATP must be made by each individual cell from dietary energy sources. Skeletal muscle is able to make ATP using both aerobic and anaerobic pathways[36]: glucose can be metabolized both aerobically and anaerobically, whereas fatty acids (eg, acetate, linoleic acid) can only be metabolized aerobically.

Anaerobic Energy Production

Muscle cells obtain glucose from either the blood or from glycogen stores in the liver and muscle. Glycolysis is a series of enzymatic steps occurring in the cell's cytosol and converts glucose to 2 pyruvate molecules, resulting in a net yield of 2 ATP. In the absence of adequate oxygen, this pyruvate is converted to lactic acid. The conversion of glucose to lactic acid is the major anaerobic pathway of ATP synthesis in muscle cells; however, there are 2 additional pathways that can also generate ATP anaerobically. First, the enzyme creatine kinase (CK) can transfer a high-energy phosphate group from creatine phosphate to ADP, forming creatine and ATP. Second, in the adenosine deaminase pathway, 2 ADP molecules are used to generate an ATP and an AMP.[37] The AMP is then further metabolized, resulting in an increase in blood concentrations of ammonia, uric acid, and allantoin, and a net loss of purine nucleotides from the muscle.[38] Both of these pathways are able to generate ATP rapidly; however, the overall contribution of these pathways to total energy production is much lower than for anaerobic glycolysis.

Aerobic Energy Production

If a cell has an adequate supply of oxygen, the pyruvate formed through glycolysis is transported to the cell's mitochondria and converted to acetyl coenzyme A, which is then metabolized through the Krebs (citric acid) cycle, resulting in the production of CO_2 and a small amount of ATP. The Krebs cycle is also coupled to 2 other processes: the electron transport chain and oxidative phosphorylation, which results in the bulk of the aerobic ATP production and is the portion of the pathway that consumes oxygen. Compared with glycolysis, aerobic glucose metabolism is slower but yields more ATP per glucose ($\sim$36 ATP compared with 2 with glycolysis). Fatty acids, volatile fatty acids, and amino acids are also metabolized to intermediates that can enter the Krebs cycle and therefore can be used to make ATP aerobically. A comprehensive figure of the metabolic pathways responsible for ATP formation in the muscle of horses can be found in a review article by Votion and colleagues.[36]

Energy Metabolism at Rest

As summarized by Harris,[39] a 450-kg horse is estimated to have 40,000 g of adipose triacylglyceride, 1400 to 2800 g of muscle triacylglyceride, 3150 to 4095 g of muscle glycogen, and 90 to 220 g of liver glycogen, all of which can be used to make ATP. At rest, aerobic ATP synthesis predominates. Circulating acetate and glucose can account for up to 32% and 78%, respectively, of the hindlimb aerobic ATP synthesis in resting horses receiving an all-forage diet.[40] When cereal grains are incorporated into the diet, the contributions that glucose and acetate make to the oxidative metabolism in the hindlimb increase and decrease, respectively.[40]

Energy Metabolism During Exercise

During low-intensity exercise, aerobic glucose and fatty acid metabolism can support the muscle's energy demands, but more intense exercise requires the anaerobic metabolism of glucose. Muscle stores of creatine phosphate ($\sim$60 mmol/kg dry weight [DW]) and ATP (20–25 mmol/kg DW) are far lower than muscle stores of glycogen (>500 mmol/kg DW), so creatine phosphate and ATP are only able to sustain the first several seconds of exercise.[41,42] In intense exercise lasting more than a few seconds, muscle glycogen is the major energy substrate.[43] Strenuous treadmill exercise and prolonged endurance exercise can deplete muscle glycogen stores by as much as 50% to 75%.[44,45] However, less intense or shorter-duration exercise, such as a 1.6-km (1-mile) Thoroughbred race or a 70-minute moderate-intensity treadmill test, resulted in muscle glycogen depletion of $\sim$20% to 30%.[46,47]

There is an inverse relationship between exercise intensity and the amount of ATP that can be made by aerobic pathways, which in turn influences substrate use. At 30% of maximal oxygen uptake (Vo_{2max}), glucose, glycogen, and lipids supported $\sim$10%, 30%, and 60%, respectively, of the energy expenditure, whereas, at 60% Vo_{2max}, these values were $\sim$5%, 70%, and 25%, respectively.[48] The mobilization of adipose triacylglycerides and glycogen stores is triggered by exercise-induced hormonal changes, specifically increases in circulating epinephrine, cortisol, and glucagon concentrations, and a decrease in circulating insulin concentrations.[49] The anaerobic adenosine deaminase pathway of ATP production is most important during high-intensity exercise[50]; however, even submaximal exercise can lead to some degree AMP deamination.[38]

Modifying Dietary Fat and Carbohydrate Provision

Although horses lack a gallbladder and so cannot store bile, they still have the ability to digest and absorb fat.[51] Horses adapted to high-fat diets, up to ~25% to 30% of the digestible energy content, have an increased capacity to oxidize fatty acids during low-intensity to moderate-intensity exercise, as shown by a lower respiratory exchange ratio,[52,53] reduced glucose use,[52,54] and increased activity of enzymes involved in the oxidative energy pathways,[53] compared with horses receiving lower-fat diets. In these studies, most of the exercise consisted of walking (~1.5 m/s) and trotting (4 m/s) on a treadmill, with the duration of exercise ranging from 40 minutes to more than 2 hours.[52–54] An important caveat is that, in those studies where fat supplementation was shown to have beneficial effects, horses were adapted to these rations for a minimum of 5 to 10 weeks.[52,53]

Thoroughbred horses in training receiving a diet with 12% of digestible energy as fat had higher resting muscle glycogen concentrations and faster run times than horses receiving a control diet, although glycogen use during exercise was not influenced by fat supplementation.[47] More recently, Pagan and colleagues[55] reported that, following 3 consecutive days of incremental exercise tests that resulted in an ~33% depletion in muscle glycogen stores, horses receiving a low-nonstructural-carbohydrate (NSC) (12.3%), high-fat (14.3%) concentrate replenished less glycogen over 72 hours (63% repletion) than those receiving concentrates that were moderate (46.5% NSC; 7.8% fat) or high (65.2% NSC; 4.8% fat) in NSC, who restored 94% of their glycogen stores in the 72 hours postexercise. However, more work is needed to confirm these findings. Some practical considerations associated with high-fat feeding include ensuring that horses are gradually adapted to the increased fat/oil intake over 2 to 3 weeks to prevent digestive upset and ensuring that the remainder of the diet is properly balanced to provide adequate vitamins (especially vitamin E), minerals, and protein. Carbohydrate provision before or during exercise can also modify energy metabolism during exercise. If carbohydrates were administered either intravenously during exercise or as a grain meal fed shortly before exercise, there was an increase in the portion of energy needs met by blood glucose metabolism and a reduction in lipid oxidation, although this did not spare muscle glycogen use.[56,57]

Amino Acids as a Muscle Fuel

Although amino acids can be metabolized aerobically and could potentially be used to provide ATP during exercise, it is not thought that this occurs to any large extent, except possibly during prolonged endurance exercise.[58,59] BCAAs (leucine, isoleucine, and valine) have been suggested as a potential energy source during prolonged low-intensity exercise. Skeletal muscle is the only tissue that contains the entire enzymatic pathway for BCAA oxidative metabolism, and decreases in the blood concentrations of these amino acids have been reported during endurance exercise.[59,60] The provision of 25 g of an amino acid mixture, containing primarily the BCAAs, to Quarter horses 30 minutes before and immediately following a treadmill conditioning session resulted in lower plasma lactate concentrations and lower heart rate, suggesting improved aerobic work capacity.[61] However, the supplementation of either 18 g of BCAA 1 hour before exercise[62] or 30 g of BCAA both 30 minutes before and immediately following exercise[63] to Standardbred horses in training did not alter any plasma markers of energy metabolism. Amino acids likely play a more pivotal role in muscle recovery following exercise than they do as an energy substrate during exercise.

Muscle Glycogen Repletion

Following moderate or intense exercise, it can take 48 to 72 hours to replenish muscle glycogen concentrations in horses,[64,65] even when a ration with high NSCs (NSC; 51% of dry matter [DM], ~2.3 g NSC/kg BW/meal) is fed for 72 hours following the glycogen-depleting exercise.[65] In humans, a similar degree of depletion can be restored within 24 hours with high levels of NSC intake (6.6–9 g/kg BW).[66] In the early postexercise period, muscle glycogen synthesis rates in humans are ~40 mmol/kg DW/h) following oral NSC intake (5 g/kg BW).[67] In horses, such high levels of NSC intake are not feasible because of health concerns, including colic and laminitis (discussed in Patricia Harris and Megan Shepherd's article, "What Would Be Good for All Veterinarians to Know About Equine Nutrition"; Myriam Hesta and Marcio Costa's article, "How Can Nutrition Help with Gastrointestinal Tract-Based Issues," elsewhere in this issue). Therefore, postexercise glycogen synthesis has only been studied in response to lower levels of NSC intake, ranging from ~1 to 2.5 g/kg BW per meal or through dosing.[65,68,69] Providing 1 g/kg BW glucose as a multiple gavage at 0, 2, and 4 hours postexercise resulted in a glycogen synthesis rate of 9 mmol/kg DW/h in the 6-hour period following exercise, which was not different than the 7 mmol/kg DW/h that resulted if no additional carbohydrate was provided.[69] Similarly, when a 1-g/kg BW glucose gavage at 0, 2, and 4 hours postexercise was combined with 0.1-g/kg BW leucine at 0 and 2 hours, differences in muscle glycogen content in the 24 hours following exercise were not seen, compared with water administration alone.[70] Even with what would be considered an aggressive postexercise NSC feeding protocol (~2.5 g NSC/kg BW/meal), in the first 24 hours following exercise cessation, muscle glycogen concentrations were not different compared with lower NSC treatments.[65,68] Furthermore, only modest benefits to high NSC intake were seen in the period 48 to 72 hours following exercise.[65] Whole-body insulin sensitivity does not increase following a bout of exercise in horses[71]; therefore, horses may require a greater increase in postexercise plasma insulin concentrations to support glycogen synthesis. Although not practical outside of a research setting, the intravenous infusion of glucose (3 g/kg BW over 6 hours), beginning 15 minutes after exercise, more than doubled serum insulin concentrations to those provoked by a similar amount of glucose given orally, and resulted in higher rates of glycogen synthesis (21 mmol/kg DW/h) in the 6 hours postexercise period.[69] The slow rate of glycogen repletion is particularly a concern in disciplines that involve multiple bouts of glycogen-depleting exercise within a short time frame, such as 3-day eventing, because exercising with depleted muscle glycogen stores has been associated with impaired anaerobic metabolism.[44]

As reviewed by Waller and Lindinger,[72] oral carbohydrate provision is limited in its ability to promote glycogen repletion postexercise in horses, and therefore other nutritional strategies have been investigated. It was proposed that the provision of an acetate could spare the oxidation of glucose by muscles in the postexercise recovery period. Compared with no supplementation, an acetate (1.6 g/kg BW) and glucose (0.67 g/kg BW) solution resulted in a greater rate of glycogen repletion (22 vs 6.8 mmol/kg DW/h) in the first 4 hours following exercise, although no differences in muscle glycogen concentration between treatments were evident after 24 hours.[73] More practical for either horse owners or clinicians, the provision of a commercial hypotonic rehydration electrolyte solution, designed to replace 8 L of sweat loss, following glycogen-depleting exercise increased the rate of glycogen repletion (15 vs 5.7 mmol/kg DW/h) in the first 4 hours following exercise compared with an untreated group, and these differences were sustained after 24 hours.[46] Although some strategies have been successful in increasing glycogen synthesis rates relative to a control treatment, the rates were still only one-third to one-half the rates reported in human muscle following consumption of large amounts of carbohydrates.[67] Because large intakes of NSC should be discouraged in horses, because of the concerns outlined in Patricia Harris and Megan Shepherd's article, "What Would Be Good for All Veterinarians to Know About Equine Nutrition"; Myriam Hesta and Marcio Costa's article, "How Can Nutrition Help with Gastrointestinal Tract-Based Issues," elsewhere in this issue, it is important to continue to work to identify alternative strategies to promote more rapid glycogen repletion.

PROTEIN AND ENERGY FOR MUSCLE GROWTH AND MAINTENANCE

In French draft breeds, muscle increased from 36% to 46% of BW by 12 months of age.[74] Similarly, in neonatal Thoroughbreds, muscle represented 36% of BW, compared with 53% in mature Thoroughbreds.[1] The rapid rate of muscle accretion early in life is reflected in the dietary protein requirements. In a horse estimated to reach 500 kg at maturity, crude protein (CP) requirements at 1, 6, and 12 months of age are 8.0, 3.1, and 2.6 g/kg BW/d, respectively (**Table 3**).[75] Protein synthesis is an energetically costly process and therefore it is also important to ensure that daily energy requirements are met in order to support optimal growth. Digestible energy requirements are also related to average daily gain at 97, 72, and 59 kcal/kg BW/d for horses 1, 6, and 12 months old (mature BW of 500 kg), respectively.[75]

Although recommendations exist for CP, horses require essential amino acids and enough amino nitrogen to make the nonessential amino acids. Lysine is well accepted as a limiting amino acid in growing horses,[76] and this is the only essential amino acid for which the National Research Council (NRC) has published recommendations.[75] Threonine[77] and methionine[78] have been suggested as potentially limiting amino acids in growing horses, although requirements have not been established. To estimate essential amino acid requirements, the NRC suggests using the profile of amino acids in a relevant protein source, such as skeletal muscle, and calculating requirements based on their ratio to lysine in that protein source.[79] For example, the NRC lysine requirement of a yearling is 112 mg/kg BW.[75] From **Table 1**, muscle threonine content is ~53% of lysine content and so the threonine requirement is estimated at 59 mg/kg BW. For rapidly growing horses, this is likely a reasonable approach to estimate amino acid requirements, but may be less appropriate in estimating amino acid requirements of mature horses, where the daily amino acid needs are primarily to replenish the horse's endogenous losses. For amino acids where there are high endogenous losses, this method could result in the underestimation of amino acid requirements. For example, in other species, threonine is contained in high amounts in intestinal mucin, resulting in high endogenous threonine losses.[80] It is also important to acknowledge that the lysine requirements provided in the NRC have not been empirically determined. Rather, they were extrapolated from the horse's CP requirement, or, in the case of lactating mares, they are based on the lysine output in the mare's milk.[75] If the current NRC lysine requirements do not accurately reflect the true requirements, this approach would inaccurately estimate the other amino acid requirements.

Although protein overfeeding is common in the equine industry[81] and helps to ensure that all amino acid requirements are adequately met, there are several potential consequences of such a strategy. As reviewed elsewhere, overfeeding protein results in increased nitrogenous waste excretion, which has both environmental and horse health implications because this nitrogen is volatized to ammonia.[81] Urinary nitrogen is excreted in the form of urea, which is energy requiring and heat producing and

Table 3
National Research Council dietary crude protein and lysine recommendations for horses across the lifespan (mature weight of 500 kg)

Class of Horse	Protein Requirement		Lysine Requirement	
	g/d	g/kg BW/d	g/d	mg/kg BW/d
Growing Horse				
2 mo	660	5.8	28	248
6 mo	676	3.1	29	134
12 mo	846	2.6	36	112
18 mo	799	2.0	34	88
2 y	770	1.8	33	77
Sedentary Horse				
Average	630	1.3	27	54
Pregnant Mare				
Early gestation (<5 mo)	630	1.3	27	54
Midgestation (7 mo)	729	1.4	31	60
Late gestation (11 mo)	893	1.6	38	67
Lactating Mare				
1 mo	1535	3.1	85	170
3 mo	1468	2.9	80	160
6 mo	1265	4.2	67	134
Exercising Horse				
Light (1–3 h/wk)	699	1.4	30	60
Moderate (3–5 h/wk)	768	1.5	33	66
Heavy (4–5 h/wk)	862	1.7	37	74
Very heavy (1 h/wk speed work; 6–12 h/wk slow work)	1004	2.0	43	86

All values were obtained from the 2007 Nutrient Requirements of Horses.
Data from National Research Council. Nutrient Requirements of Horses. Vol 6th. Washington DC: National Academies Press; 2007.

increases water output.[82,83] High protein intakes also resulted in increased plasma lactate concentrations both at rest[84] and following sprint exercise,[85] but did not result in a more rapid onset of fatigue in sprint exercise tests.[85] Therefore, there is a need to accurately determine amino acid requirements in horses, particularly in those with increased requirements because of growth, exercise, or lactation (discussed further in Morgane Robles and colleagues' article, "Nutrition of Broodmares," in this issue).

Depending on forage quality, energy tends to be a more limiting nutrient than protein, because generally, if a ration meets digestible energy requirements, then it will also meet protein requirements. The primary sites of digestion of the proteins found in forages and complementary feeds differ. Most forage protein cannot be accessed by enzymes until microbial cell wall digestion occurs and so it is digested microbially in the large intestine, whereas protein in cereal grains (oats, corn) and oilseeds (soybean meal) are digested primarily enzymatically in the small intestine, which is also the major site of amino acids absorption.[25,26] The capacity for the large intestine to absorb amino acids is still an area of active research. Early studies showed very limited ability for microbially derived amino acid to be absorbed by the horse.[86] However, more recently, amino acid transporters have been identified in the large intestine, and the large intestinal mucosa was able to absorb lysine in vitro.[87,88] Regardless, horses are able to obtain some amino acids from forage: horses consuming a variety of pasture types showed notable increases in plasma amino acid concentrations compared with fasting level after only 2 hours of grazing.[89] However, the amino acids found in complementary feeds are thought to be more digestible and more available to the horses. Horses consuming a ration including both hay and grain had a more rapid postprandial aminoacidemia and a significantly positive nitrogen balance compared with horses consuming only hay, despite both diets providing similar levels of amino acid intake.[90]

For adult horses at maintenance with low protein requirements, a grass forage with ~10% to 12% CP (as fed) should provide sufficient CP to meet requirements. A recent study showed that horses consuming alfalfa, cool season grass, and teff pastures at a daily intake level of 1.5% of BW (DM) consume sufficient lysine to meet requirements.[89] However, in cases where forage contains even less protein, it may not provide sufficient amounts of each of the essential amino acids. In these horses, a ration balancer, which is a concentrated source of protein, vitamins, and minerals, could be provided to meet protein requirements. Commercial ration balancers range in CP content from ~10% to 32%, and the specific ration balancer can be selected based on the protein content of the available forage. For example, a high-protein ration balancer (~30%–32% CP) typically complements a low-protein grass forage. For a higher-protein forage, such as alfalfa, it is unlikely that any additional amino acids are required and therefore a low-protein (~10%) ration balancer is a good choice to provide vitamins and minerals, while minimizing the overfeeding of protein. For growing, lactating, and exercising horses, protein and energy needs may not be met by a grass forage alone, necessitating an additional protein source such as alfalfa or a complementary feed. The best complementary feed to meet protein needs depends on how much additional energy and protein the horse requires beyond what can be provided by the forage available: if only a small amount of additional energy is required, then a small amount of a high-protein ration balancer could be fed. However, if the horse requires a substantial amount of additional energy, a lower-protein complementary feed (~12%–16% CP) may be a better option to account for higher levels of complementary feed intake while preventing excessive protein intake. Although some commercial concentrates have additional free amino acids added, typically comprising the potentially limiting amino acids (lysine, threonine, and/or methionine), this is not a universal practice because it increases the cost of feed production. Top dressing free amino acid products are available, although typically not very palatable. Furthermore, although free amino acid inclusion could be a way to ensure essential amino acids are provided in adequate quantities, while minimizing the total protein content, for this approach to be successful, better estimates of amino acid requirements are necessary.

MUSCLE IN AGED HORSES

As in other species, sarcopenia, a loss of muscle mass with age, has been reported in horses with and without pituitary pars intermedia dysfunction (PPID).[91,92] Anabolic resistance in human skeletal muscle with advanced age has been well documented.[93] A similar resistance is likely to be at least partially responsible for the loss of muscle mass in aged horses. In the 1 study that compared mTOR signaling in mature (8–14 years old) versus aged (>20 years old) horses, there was a reduction in activation of 1 of the downstream effectors of mTOR signaling.[94] Horses with PPID have a marked reduction in the cross-sectional area of both type IIA and IIX muscle fibers (ie, fast twitch)[95] compared with age-matched control horses, suggesting that PPID may reduce muscle protein synthesis. However, in studies that compared mTOR signaling in age-matched horses with and without PPID, there were no differences in mTOR signaling in response to either feeding or insulin infusion,[96,97] suggesting that the reported muscle loss in horses with PPID is not a result of a reduction in responsiveness of the muscle to anabolic stimuli.

MUSCLE ERGOGENIC SUPPLEMENTS

Ergogenic supplements are those that are given with the intention of improving stamina, performance, or recovery. Popular supplements that are marketed specifically for potential beneficial effects on skeletal muscle include amino acid supplements, HMB, and creatine.

Amino Acid Supplementation

In 3-year-old Thoroughbreds, intravenous administration of an amino acid (~0.22 g/kg BW/h) and glucose (~0.22 g/kg BW/h) mixture following exercise was more effective than amino acid infusion, glucose infusion, or saline infusion in supporting hindlimb protein synthesis.[98] Another study found that feeding a postexercise supplement (5 g/kg BW) containing electrolytes and amino acids resulted in greater mTOR signaling compared with a control supplement 4 to 48 hours postexercise.[99] Therefore, there are potentially benefits to feeding amino acids following exercise; however, more research is needed to optimize doses and to develop equine-specific postexercise feeding strategies.

In recent years, a new category of feed and supplements has entered the market, advertising benefits to a horse's so-called topline, the epaxial muscles. These products are high in protein and may even be enriched in leucine, and often present increased protein synthesis as a proposed mechanism of action. In some cases, recommendations are to provide the feed/supplement in conjunction with an exercise program, but this recommendation is not universal. Because this category of feeds/supplements is still new, there is an absence of research to support their efficacy. However, based on the available data from human nutrition, it seems that, unless the animal was previously fed an inadequate quantity or quality of protein, it is unlikely that these products would promote muscle growth and development in the absence of an accompanying tailored exercise regimen. Although some muscle scoring systems have been developed in recent years,[100] there is currently no system that is universally accepted to the same extent as the Henneke system for body condition scoring[101] to visually score a horse's skeletal muscle.

β-Hydroxy-β-methyl Butyrate

As reviewed elsewhere, there have been mixed reports on the benefits of the leucine metabolite HMB in humans during exercise training. Some studies report improvements in muscle mass, strength, and aerobic performance and decreased muscle damage, with other studies reporting no beneficial effects.[102] The typical dose of HMB administered in human studies is 3 g ($\sim$0.04 g/kg BW), resulting in plasma HMB concentrations of $\sim$400 μM.[102] It has been proposed that HMB seems to be most beneficial in previously untrained individuals undergoing strenuous exercise.[102] Supplementation seems to be particularly effective in elderly patients with sarcopenia, and has been shown to increase protein synthesis, lean body mass, and muscle strength in this group, even when individuals are sedentary.[102] Supplementation with HMB (15 g/d) in training and racing Thoroughbreds decreased serum CK activity, a marker of muscle damage, 30 minutes after a bout of exercise, compared with no exercise.[103] Satellite cells cultured in the presence of HMB (50–100 μM) had altered expression of genes related to protein turnover[17] and increased rates of protein synthesis.[104] Although HMB supplementation shows promise to improve muscle health and protein mass in horses, additional research is needed, particularly in exercising and aged horses.

Creatine

Creatine is a precursor to creatine phosphate, and in humans it may improve performance in disciplines that involve high intensity or strength.[105] However, the bioavailability of orally administered creatine is low in horses, presumably because, as herbivores, horses had no evolutionary need for intestinal transporters for a compound that is found almost exclusively in animal tissues.[106] Creatine supplementation in horses ($\sim$50–100 g/d by mouth) did not result in any improvements in exercise performance or muscle metabolism during aerobic or anaerobic exercise efforts.[106–108]

Carnitine

Carnitine is essential for the aerobic metabolism of fatty acids because it is a component of the membrane system that transports fatty acids from the cytosol into the mitochondria. In humans, there is evidence that carnitine supplementation increases Vo_{2max} and aids in postexercise muscle recovery.[109] In horses, it was recently proposed that muscle carnitine availability may limit fat oxidation during strenuous endurance exercise.[110] The effects of carnitine supplementation in horses have been mixed. One study found that 10 g/d of supplementation given either in feed or nasogastrically to lightly exercised horses resulted in a modest increase in plasma carnitine concentrations, but, when the same dose was given intravenously over 15 days, there was no increase in muscle carnitine content.[111] In another study, 10 g/d of carnitine supplementation in horses undergoing treadmill exercise training resulted in increased muscle carnitine concentrations, increased the proportion of type IIA muscle fibers, and increased muscle capillarity. However, these beneficial effects disappeared when exercise training ceased, even with the continued ingestion of carnitine.[112] An even greater level of carnitine supplementation ($\sim$50 g; 58% intravenously, 42% orally) to Warmbloods increased free carnitine extraction and the extraction of some acylcarnitines by the hindlimb muscles following low-intensity exercise, and the investigators suggested this may be beneficial in optimizing performance.[113]

In conclusion, amino acid supplementation seems to increase postexercise muscle protein synthesis in horses. There are insufficient data to support muscle-building effects of supplemental amino acids in the absence of exercise. At this time, there has not been extensive research focused on identifying supplements with ergogenic benefits in horses. However, there are some data both in vitro and in vivo to support the role of HMB in promoting the accretion of muscle mass. There is also evidence in vivo that carnitine supplementation may be beneficial for aerobic-type exercise. Additional research is warranted in this area in horses.

MUSCULAR DISORDERS INFLUENCED BY NUTRITION

Several muscular disorders of horses are instigated by or respond to nutrition. At present, the most well-recognized acquired muscular disorders arising from nutritional mismanagement relate to deficiencies of vitamin E and selenium. Several hereditary muscular disorders of horses are exacerbated or mitigated by nutritional factors. In conjunction with other management changes, nutritional manipulation can present a convenient, practical, and effective method of preventing or controlling these diseases.[114–116] Heritable muscular disorders for which nutrition plays an influential role in horses include several forms of exertional rhabdomyolysis, as well as hyperkalemic periodic paralysis (HYPP).

Exertional Rhabdomyolysis Disorders

Exertional rhabdomyolysis (ER), classically represented by the occurrence of stiffness, sweating, and reluctance to move during or after exercise, with myoglobinuria in severe cases, was linked decades ago to consumption of a high-starch rations during periods of rest in draft horses.[117,118] Although the management triggers associated with disease were correctly identified, the attribution of clinical signs to abnormally high systemic lactate concentrations has now been solidly disproved.[119–121] Several heritable muscular disorders with varying pathophysiologies are now recognized as the cause of ER in a wide range of light and heavy horse breeds.[115,118] An overview of heritable muscle disorders that can cause ER and that are potentially amenable to nutritional management are included in **Table 4**.

Type 1 Polysaccharide Storage Myopathy

At present, the most well-characterized ER disorder is type 1 polysaccharide storage myopathy (PSSM1; **Fig. 2**), which is an autosomal dominant glycogen storage disorder linked to a gain-of-function mutation in the glycogen synthase 1 gene (*GYS1*).[122] Affected individuals likely experience abnormal aerobic energy metabolism in skeletal muscle.[116,122] More than 20 light and heavy breeds have this disorder, but it has not been reported in Thoroughbreds, Fjords, Welsh ponies, or Clydesdales.[123,124] It is highly prevalent in Quarter horses, Percherons, and Belgian draft horses and can occur in crossbreeds.[115,124,125] Clinical signs vary and are not always exertion related. Many horses are asymptomatic.[115,126] In affected light breeds, the most common clinical presentation is typical signs of ER with concurrent increase of muscle enzyme activities, often after a period of rest.[127] Affected Warmbloods and draft horses less reliably show signs of rhabdomyolysis, and commonly show muscular weakness and atrophy.[128–132]

Horses homozygous for the *GYS1* mutation may be more clinically severe and potentially more resistant to management than heterozygotes.[126,132] Quarter horses that are concurrently heterozygous for a low-prevalence mutation in the ryanodine receptor 1 gene (*RYR1*), which is associated with ER and malignant hyperthermia, also

Table 4
Heritable muscular disorders of horses that can potentially be influenced by nutritional manipulation

Disorder	Commonly Affected Breeds	Gene and Affected Product	Signs	Diagnostic Techniques	Nutritional Manipulation
Type 1 PSSM	• Quarter horse • Paint • Appaloosa • Belgian • Percheron	• GYS1 • Muscle glycogen synthase	• Light breeds: ER • Drafts: weakness and atrophy	• Genetic testing • Submaximal exercise test • Muscle biopsy	• NSC ≤ 12% DM • ± Vegetable fat supplementation at 5%–10% DM depending on severity and caloric needs
Type 2 PSSM	• Warmbloods • Quarter horse	• Unknown	• Warmbloods: poor technical performance • Quarter horse: ER	• No scientifically validated genetic test available • CK, AST • Muscle biopsy	• NSC ≤ 20% DM • ± Vegetable fat supplementation at 5%–10% DM depending on severity and caloric needs ± amino acid or whey protein supplementation
RER	• Thoroughbred • Standardbred	• Unknown	• ER • Signs in training, not in racing	• No scientifically validated genetic test available • CK, AST	• NSC ≤ 20% DM • ± Fat supplementation up to 10% DM • Specifically formulated commercial feed product available
MFM	• Arabian • Warmblood	• Unknown	• ER in Arabs • Signs in training and racing	• No scientifically validated genetic test available • Muscle biopsy	• Anecdotal suggestions to reduce fat (oxidative load) • Whey protein supplement • Specifically formulated commercial feed product available
HYPP	• Quarter horse • Paint • Appaloosa • Pony of the Americas	• SCN4A • α-Subunit of the skeletal muscle sodium channel	• Tremors • Weakness • Cardiorespiratory signs	• Genetic testing	• Reduce potassium in ration to ≤1.5% using low-potassium hays, soaking hay, and supplemental feeds • Divided meals to limit potassium per meal • Careful selection of electrolyte products

Abbreviations: AST, aspartate aminotransferase, HYPP, hyperkalemic periodic paralysis; MFM, myofibrillar myopathy; PSSM, polysaccharide storage myopathy; RER, recurrent exertional rhabdomyolysis.

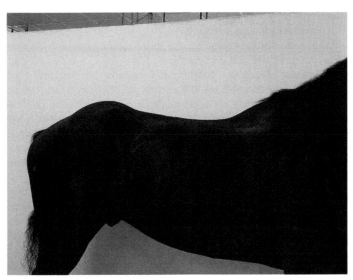

Fig. 2. A 6-year-old Percheron horse with generalized muscle atrophy attributed to underlying PSSM1. Atrophy of the epaxial and gluteal regions is particularly pronounced.

tend to have more severe clinical signs and greater resistance to management interventions.[132–134] Diagnosis of PSSM1 can be achieved via genetic testing through academic or commercial laboratories providing scientifically validated tests for the *GYS1* mutation. Concurrent submaximal exercise testing in light breeds helps to identify functional abnormalities associated with the mutation if serum CK level is inappropriately increased after a light exercise effort.[126] Histopathology assessment of semitendinosus or semimembranosus samples can be used in suspected horses with PSSM1 that lack the causative mutation.[123]

Nutritional management of PSSM1 has been extensively investigated and currently represents the most effective means of controlling signs of disease in affected horses.[116,135–137] High NSC intake in affected horses is suspected to contribute to abnormalities of oxidative substrate metabolism and muscle pain during exercise.[116,138,139] As a result, manipulation of the ration for these horses primarily involves reducing starch content by traditionally recommending a low NSC content for the ration, ranging from 4% to 12% DM.[115,135,139] A simple approach to adjusting the ration for a horse with PSSM1 is as follows:

- Determine digestible energy (DE) requirement according to NRC guidelines and other sources.[75,140] Serial monitoring of body condition should be performed over time to determine whether adjustments are required.[75] Some horses with PSSM are concurrently overweight at the time of diagnosis, and this must be accounted for when making ration adjustments (see Megan Shepherd and colleagues' article, "Nutritional Considerations When Dealing with an Obese Adult Equine," in this issue).
- Determine the desired NSC (approximated by water soluble carbohydrates (WSC) + starch) value based on clinical severity. Horses with severe signs are most likely to benefit from values less than or equal to 10% DM. Milder cases or non–Quarter horse breeds may tolerate rations with higher values, even exceeding 30%, particularly if they are fat supplemented, turned out, or regularly

exercised.[115,141,142] In mild cases, evaluating the ration and simply removing any high-NSC product may be adequate.

- Determine an appropriate forage for the ration base to achieve the desired NSC value. For horses with PSSM1, hay with less than 12% DM is desirable to minimize insulin responses.[143] Ideally, a chemical nutrient analysis would be conducted on forage to be fed. Hay can be soaked to reduce WSC values a small and unpredictable amount, although this may also reduce DE and other nutrients[144] (see Megan Shepherd and colleagues' article, "Nutritional Considerations When Dealing with an Obese Adult Equine," in this issue). If an appropriate forage or forage replacer cannot be identified, or forage cannot be fed for other reasons, commercial complete feed products low in starch and sugar can be used to substitute some or all forage.
- For additional supplementation to meet caloric demands, low-starch vegetable-based fat supplements can be included, such as vegetable oil (eg, corn, canola), low-starch calcium-balanced rice bran, or high–vegetable fat/oil commercial supplements. Such supplementation has been shown to provide positive effects during exercise in horses with PSSM1, in some cases even where horses continue to consume starch.[141] Enhancing dietary vegetable fat intake is encouraged for any clinically affected horse with PSSM1 if weight gain can be managed appropriately.[116,141,145]
- Ensure the ration meets vitamin and mineral needs, including vitamin E for horses without green pasture access, and selenium in regions of known deficiency.

Horses with PSSM1 may not show substantial clinical improvement or decline in muscle enzyme activity for several weeks after a ration change, likely reflecting time needed for alterations in relevant cellular processes.[139] Furthermore, provision of a structured daily or frequent exercise routine is critical to optimize clinical outcomes, and in some cases may be effective even in the absence of substantial dietary changes.[116,135,142,146] When appropriate recommendations are applied, it is expected that virtually all Quarter horses with PSSM1 will show reduced frequency of ER, and nearly two-thirds may cease to have any episodes.[135,147] It has not been verified whether similar success might be expected in other breeds with PSSM1.

Type 2 Polysaccharide Storage Myopathy

Horses that have muscular disease with clinical and histopathologic similarities to PSSM1 but that lack high muscle glycogen concentrations or the GYS1 mutation of PSSM1 are currently classified as having type 2 PSSM (PSSM2).[123,131] This disorder has been described in a range of Warmblood breeds, and in Quarter horses, Morgans, Thoroughbreds, Standardbreds, and Icelandic horses.[118,146,148] The cause and pathogenesis are not well characterized, although currently nearly 30% of Quarter horse PSSM cases, and up to 80% of Warmblood PSSM cases, are thought to reflect PSSM2.[118,123] Affected horses can present acutely with ER but more often present vague and chronic abnormalities such as reduced willingness to exercise, decreased technical performance, muscle soreness, and slow muscle atrophy, despite often normal muscle enzyme activities.[118,146,147] Diagnosis currently is challenging, and relies on muscle biopsy and ruling out other reasons for poor performance until a scientifically validated genetic test becomes available.[149,150]

Preliminary evidence suggests that horses with PSSM2 benefit from similar manipulations to their ration and exercise routine as horses with PSSM1.[146,147] The combination of exercise and dietary changes to optimize outcome is also critical; when only partial compliance is achieved, the probability of improvement in affected

Warmbloods is less than 30%.[146] In an owner survey, 80% of Warmbloods with PSSM2 showed improvement with management changes, although 40% remained affected to some degree with reluctance to perform appropriately during ridden activities.[147] Affected horses (~500 kg) should be fed a ration that provides for a range of DE from 16.4 to 24.6 Mcal/d (maintenance to moderate exercise) and less than 20% of daily DE from NSC, 15% to 20% of DE as fat (~330–440 g in a 20-MCal/84 MJ ration), and 697 to 836 g of protein per day.[147] Alternative recommendations for horses with PSSM2 have included 15% to 20% DE from NSC (~10%–12% DM), fat supplementation only if needed for body condition, and whey protein supplementation if muscle atrophy is evident.[115]

Recurrent Exertional Rhabdomyolysis

Approximately 5% to 10% of Thoroughbred and Standardbred racehorses have a heritable muscular disorder referred to as recurrent exertional rhabdomyolysis (RER).[151–153] Typically signs of muscle damage occur during training and not racing, with increases in muscle enzyme activities commonly accompanying signs of muscular discomfort during or after exercise.[152,153] There is strong evidence that RER relates to abnormalities of skeletal muscle calcium regulation. Thoroughbred horses with RER have a lower contracture threshold of intercostal muscle tissue in response to halothane and caffeine, which emulates a feature of malignant hyperthermia in other species.[154] In vitro application of dantrolene sodium, a drug used for a range of neuromuscular disorders, normalizes muscle contracture responses in RER horses.[151] Furthermore, rhabdomyolysis can be prevented in affected horses by oral administration of dantrolene before exercise.[155] It has proved challenging to identify the genetic profile of RER, suggesting complex inheritance.[151,156] The lack of a scientifically validated genetic test to confirm RER in horses complicates diagnosis, and muscle biopsy has limited utility because histopathologic abnormalities are nonspecific. Submaximal exercise testing has not proved reliable, although measurement of serum muscle enzyme activities around training exercise might help identify affected horses.[115]

Horses with RER can show a strong positive response to dietary manipulation within 1 week of reducing starch in the ration. The reason for this quick response to dietary changes, which differs from horses with PSSM, has not been clearly defined. The response might reflect the role of anxiety as a triggering factor for clinical disease in RER horses, as shown in epidemiologic studies.[153,157] Horses with RER provided a high-energy, high-fat, and low-starch ration showed a lower resting heart rate and packed cell volume concurrently with lower muscle enzyme activities, supporting this hypothesis.[121,158]

Modifying the ration for horses with RER can follow the same steps as for horses with PSSM. However, horses with RER generally seem tolerant of larger amounts of starch than horses with PSSM1, and up to 20% NSC may be acceptable in the total ration. This amount can allow inclusion of up to 2.3 kg (5 pounds) of starch-based concentrate feeds such as grains where moderate caloric supplementation is required. If substantial caloric supplementation is needed, such as for heavy exercise, additional requirements should be met by providing fat-dense sources. Providing additional calories as starch causes substantially higher postexercise serum CK activities in horses with RER, whereas comparable energy intakes provided by rice bran–based feed promotes normal postexercise CK activities in these horses.[121] Ten percent or more of daily DM intake can be provided as vegetable-source fat in high-caloric rations. Horses with RER do not all require fat supplementation in addition to reduction of starch. However, supplementation may be beneficial for particularly nervous horses and is necessary for those with high caloric demands to maintain acceptable amounts of starch in the ration while adequately meeting caloric requirements.

Horses with RER also show a positive response to regular exercise. This response is likely mediated through mechanisms separate to dietary influences. In 1 study, serum CK values, even though significantly lower, declined in a similar fashion throughout a week of regular daily exercise in horses with RER receiving a high-energy–high-fat ration compared with a high-energy–high-carbohydrate ration.[121] In addition, dantrolene sodium has been used in Thoroughbreds with RER to control clinical disease and mitigates increases in serum CK activities in exercised horses.[155,159] Timing of medication should be carefully considered because absorption and subsequent plasma concentrations of dantrolene are enhanced when feeding within 4 hours of dantrolene administration.[160] It is likely most appropriate to provide the drug within 2 hours of exercise when administering to prevent ER. The impact of feeding on dantrolene absorption should also be considered with regard to withdrawal times, because published withdrawal times were established in extensively horses, and therefore are unlikely to be accurate because severely inhibits dantrolene absorption and subsequent plasma concentrations.[161]

Myofibrillar Myopathy

The most recently reported ER disorder, myofibrillar myopathy (MFM), is most prevalent in Arabians and Warmbloods.[162,163] Affected Arabians show ER during training and racing, often at a later age in life, and occasionally have profound biochemical evidence of rhabdomyolysis with mild clinical signs.[164] Affected Warmbloods show similar clinical characteristics to PSSM2, with exercise intolerance, stiffness, nebulous lameness, and reduced performance.[163] Investigation of this disorder in Arabians has confirmed that affected (and healthy) Arabians lack the GYS1 and RYR1 mutations associated with PSSM1, although an underlying heritable disorder is strongly suspected.[164] No scientifically validated genetic test is available, and diagnosis currently must be based on muscle biopsy.[150,165,166] Many affected horses show abnormal accumulations of desmin, a cytoskeletal protein, in mature muscle fibers.[131,132] Metabolic and muscle enzyme responses to submaximal exercise testing are also largely unremarkable, although prerace and postrace evaluations of serum CK activity might help identify affected Arabians that show disproportionately large increases in CK activity than are expected for the distance raced.[164,167]

At present, it is unclear whether nutritional manipulation can influence clinical disease in Arabians or Warmbloods with MFM. Affected Arabians are often already consuming low-starch, fat-supplemented rations when they show clinical disease.[164] The disorder shows characteristics suggestive of disturbed oxidative processes. Therefore, the potential for high-fat diets to exacerbate clinical disease by adding oxidative load must also be considered. Nutritional measures to positively influence oxidative metabolism in muscle cells may be worthy of investigation based on preliminary studies of the pathophysiology of MFM.[168] Similar to other ER disorders, rest periods seem to be a strong triggering factor and should be avoided.

General Considerations

Other general considerations regarding the rations of horses with ER disorders include balancing vitamins and minerals, which might require the addition of a ration balancer pellet that does not contribute substantially to NSC values, when fed in the required amount. Vitamin E supplementation should be considered for any horses that do not have access to fresh green grazing for 6 h/d or more, at a minimum of 2 international units (IU)/kg BW/d.[169] For horses receiving fat supplementation, additional vitamin E can be added at 1 to 1.5 IU/mL or gram of vegetable oil/fat to help offset oxidative load.[114]

Hyperkalemic Periodic Paralysis

HYPP is a well-described hereditary muscular disorder that predominantly affects Quarter horses, Paints, Palominos, Appaloosas, and the Pony of the Americas breed.[170] A prevalence of 4.4% has been reported in the general Quarter horse population but, remarkably, prevalence exceeded 55% in an elite halter horse group.[125] The disease is associated with a point mutation in the SCN4A gene encoding the alpha subunit of the skeletal muscle sodium channel, and is heritable in a codominant autosomal fashion.[151,171] The higher resting membrane potential in muscle fibers containing mutant sodium channels increases their susceptibility to depolarization, particularly in the presence of high serum potassium concentrations.[172] Clinically, this is most often reflected by muscle fasciculations with subsequent weakness. Abnormal muscular activity during clinical episodes promotes efflux of potassium into the extracellular environment in many affected horses, increasing serum potassium concentration. Serum muscle enzymes usually show limited change because muscle necrosis is not typically expected unless concurrent trauma occurs. Diagnosis can be established by scientifically validated genetic testing on whole blood or plucked hair.[151,171]

Dietary manipulation to reduce clinical episodes includes reducing total daily potassium intake and the amount of potassium ingested each meal. A simple, stepwise approach to adjusting the ration for a horse with HYPP is as follows:

- The total ration should not contain greater than 1.5% potassium on a DM basis and should be more stringently restricted for horses with recurrent episodes or severe clinical signs.[132]
- Determine an appropriate forage product to form the ration foundation while permitting achievement of the desired potassium value. Ideally, hay should undergo analysis for potassium content. Green grass (but not clover) is suitable, and grass hays, including Timothy, oat, Bermuda grass, and prairie grass, generally have potassium concentrations between 1% and 2%. Soaking hay (see Megan Shepherd and colleagues' article, "Nutritional Considerations When Dealing with an Obese Adult Equine," in this issue) can reduce potassium concentration as much as 40% within half an hour, and even more substantially over longer periods.[173]
- If forage cannot be identified that permits the desired total potassium value of the ration, or cannot be soaked or fed for other reasons, commercial low-potassium (<1.5%) feed products can substitute some or all forage.
- If additional supplementation is needed to meet caloric demands, low-potassium supplements including cereal grains, nonmolassed beet pulp, vegetable oil/fat sources, or specially formulated commercial feed products can be included. Molasses and nonanalyzed alfalfa sources should be avoided. Supplements should be divided into several meals to reduce the amount of potassium in 1 meal.
- Electrolyte supplementation should be achieved with table salt (sodium chloride) rather than lite salt or products containing potassium, and should be tailored to meet requirements, including exercise.
- Ensure the ration meets vitamin and mineral needs, including vitamin E for horses without green pasture access, and selenium in selenium-deficient areas. Consider specialist nutritional advice.

- Horses that continue to have signs under appropriate dietary management may require daily treatment with acetazolamide, or the drug can be given several days before potentially challenging events such as general anesthesia.

Vitamin E Deficiency Disorders

Vitamin E deficiency can provoke a variety of disorders in horses. Subclinical effects on immune function or reproduction are possible; however, severe or sustained deficiency can cause neuromuscular disorders variably represented by ataxia, fasciculations, weakness, muscle atrophy, and rhabdomyolysis[174] (**Fig. 3**). Specific diseases linked to vitamin E deficiency are summarized in **Table 5**, and are thoroughly described in previous literature.

Vitamin E is a potent antioxidant critical for the maintenance of cell membranes. It is composed of a family of 8 fat-soluble molecules with varying antioxidant properties. There are 4 naturally occurring tocopherols (α-tocopherol, β-tocopherol, γ-tocopherol, and δ-tocopherol) and 4 tocotrienols (α-tocotrienol, β-tocotrienol, γ-tocotrienol, and δ-tocotrienol), all contained at various levels in plant materials. Tocotrienols structure differ from tocopherols because of unsaturated side chains and, because of instability and cost, tocotrienols have limited application in animal feeds. The only molecule that is recognized to have vitamin E activity is α-tocopherol. The other tocopherols (mixed tocopherols) are included in pet foods as natural preservatives. α-Tocopherol is the predominant form of vitamin E found in blood, thus is of greatest significance, and is preferentially bound to α-tocopherol transfer protein (α-TTP) in the liver and transported to extrahepatic tissues. The recognized names for natural α-tocopherol are either RRR-α-tocopherol or D-α-tocopherol, and it is composed of a single molecule. Chemically synthesized α-tocopherol (synthetic) also exists, and is referred to as all-rac-α-tocopherol or D,L-α-tocopherol. Because of α-tocopherol having 3 chiral carbons in the structure, the chemically synthesized form contains a mixture of 8 α-tocopherol isomers, of which only 1 is identical to RRR-α-tocopherol. The other 7 isomers have lower biological activity compared with RRR-α-tocopherol. Because of instability of natural and synthetic α-tocopherols, an ester is attached to α-tocopherol for superior stability in complete feeds. Feed tags typically do not report the source of vitamin E. The only required feed tag for vitamin E in the United States is "vitamin E supplement," which does not identify the source of vitamin E in feeds and supplements. Both naturally derived α-tocopherol and synthetic α-tocopherol

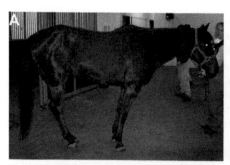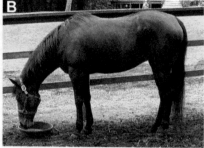

Fig. 3. A 19-year-old Quarter horse mare with advanced signs of equine motor neuron disease and a presenting plasma α-tocopherol concentration of 0.36 μg/mL (reference 1.5–2.0 μg/mL) before (*A*) and after (*B*) 4 months of treatment (5000 IU/d liquid micellized D-α-tocopherol for 2 months, then 2000 IU/d). Ration before onset of signs consisted of grass hay and a senior pellet, estimated to provide less than 100 IU of α-tocopherol per day.

Table 5
Neuromuscular disorders of horses related to vitamin E or selenium deficiency

Disorder	Clinical Signs	Diagnosis	Nutritional Manipulation and Expected Outcome
EDM/neuroaxonal dystrophy	• Spinal ataxia, typically early onset (<1 y)	• Antemortem detection based on clinical signs and ruling out other differentials • Definitive diagnosis requires CNS histopathology	• Prevention: vitamin E at 2–4 IU/kg BW/d may reduce disease severity in susceptible horses from EDM lineage • Treatment: not responsive to vitamin E once signs occur • Prognosis: poor; deficits typically stabilize at 2–3 y but are considered permanent
Equine motor neuron disease	• Weakness, atrophy, and tremors in mature horses • Feet placed close under the body; hindlimb shifting • High CK and AST activities	• Sacrocaudalis dorsalis medialis biopsy (H&E stain for neurogenic atrophy) • Spinal accessory nerve biopsy • Serum or plasma vitamin E concentration typically <1 μg/mL	• Prevention: green pasture access or supplement with vitamin E (≥2 IU/kg BW/d) • Treatment: vitamin E at 10–20 IU/kg BW/d as D-α-tocopherol (natural) for improved CNS absorption • Prognosis: fair; ~20% of horses decline despite treatment, another 40% may have residual deficits
Vitamin E deficiency myopathy	• Weakness, atrophy, and tremors • High CK and AST activities	• Sacrocaudalis dorsalis medialis biopsy: NADH stain for mitochondrial anomalies • Serum or plasma vitamin E concentration can be normal	• Prevention: green pasture access or supplement with vitamin E (≥2 IU/kg BW/d) • Treatment: vitamin E at 10–20 IU/kg BW/d • Prognosis: good; typically treatment responsive
Selenium deficiency disorders	• Weakness, stiffness, atrophy • ± High CK and AST activities, myoglobinuria • Respiratory distress • Ventral edema • Trismus or masseter atrophy • Weak or stillborn foals with high CK activity	• Measurement of blood, plasma, or serum selenium or glutathione peroxidase activity • Muscle biopsy • Echocardiography and cardiac troponin	• Prevention: selenium at minimum 0.1 mg/kg DM/d • Treatment: initial injection of 0.055 mg/kg selenium IM, then supplement orally • Prognosis: good; typically treatment responsive unless chronic, or significant cardiac damage

Abbreviations: CNS, central nervous system; EDM, equine degenerative myeloencephalopathy; H&E, hematoxylin-eosin; IM, intramuscular; NADH, nicotinamide adenine dinucleotide.

are commercially available in liquid and powder acetate esters. Micellization (making water soluble) enhances the bioavailability of RRR-α-tocopherol and feeding nonester sources of vitamin E also enhances bioavailability compared with acetate esters. The recognized biological activity (IU) is highest for natural α-tocopherol (1.49 IU/mg) and lowest for synthetic alpha-tocopheryl acetate (1.0 IU/mg).

Vitamin E is commonly reported in IU for feeding recommendations, and, according to NRC regulations, maintenance, horses should receive at least 1 IU/kg BW/d, although 2 IU/kg BW is likely preferable. Foals, lactating mares, and horses in heavy exercise should receive 3 to 4 IU/kg BW/d. A unit is based on biological activity, and 1 IU = 0.667 mg of D-α-tocopherol or 1.0 mg of D,L-α-tocopherol acetate. Vitamin E is sometimes reported in parts per million (PPM) in feed products, which is equivalent to milligrams per kilogram of feed. It is important to know the volume of feed the PPM value refers to in order to determine how much is being provided to a horse when it is fed a specific amount of a supplemented feed. Micrograms per milliliter (μg/mL) is a common unit of reporting plasma or serum vitamin E in horses, with 2 to 4 μg/mL considered normal, 1 to 2 μg/mL as marginal with possible subclinical effects, and less than 1 μg/mL presenting a strong risk of clinical disease, especially if sustained over time.[174] If results are reported in micromoles per liter (μmol/L), the value can be multiplied by 0.4307 to convert to μg/mL.

Green pasture is the major source of vitamin E to horses, and grazing for at least 6 hours supplies about 500 IU, meeting bare-minimum requirements for mature horses without additional physiologic demands. Aging and processing of hay substantially and rapidly degrades vitamin E (see Nerida Richards and collegaues' article, "Nutritional and Non-Nutritional Aspects of Forage," in this issue). Other sources in equine rations include commercial feed products, vitamin E–fortified oils, and commercial supplements. Foals receive vitamin E in mare's milk.

Horses most at risk of vitamin E deficiency are those without green pasture access, receiving a hay ration, with inadequate supplementation. Exercise and fat supplementation increase oxidative load. Genetics also likely have a strong influence, and individual horses fed and managed similarly can have very different vitamin E status. Furthermore, active supplementation of the ration is not necessarily reliable because of the wide range and variable quality of available products. In a recent study of several hundred horses, more than one-third of the horses had suboptimal plasma vitamin E concentrations, despite greater than 85% of owners providing vitamin E–containing products or supplements.[169] Lack of pasture access was associated with a considerably higher likelihood of deficiency. Periodic blood testing is a convenient way to assess vitamin E status, even if only single sampling is performed. All horses should be managed to ensure appropriate daily intake via adequate green pasture access and/or active supplementation with a suitable product at an appropriate amount to meet individual daily requirements.[169]

Vitamin E can be readily supplemented in the ration of healthy horses by addition of natural or synthetic source products. Synthetic α-tocopherol is stable and often more economical, but has considerably lower potency. Synthetic E transfers less well into nervous tissues, and takes longer to increase blood concentrations, hence naturally derived vitamin E is strongly preferred for treating deficiency-related disorders.[175] Supplementing healthy horses with low vitamin E status can be achieved by providing vitamin E at approximately 10 IU/kg BW for 2 weeks if a naturally derived source is used, and for 4 weeks if a synthetic source is used. Repeat blood testing and reduce supplementation to maintenance rates once plasma values of at least 2 μg/mL have been achieved. When supplementing clinically diseased horses, liquid micellized naturally derived vitamin E is encouraged, provided at 10 to 20 IU/kg BW/d.[175] Long-term high-dose supplementation over many weeks is likely indicated for chronic severe disorders, such as advanced equine motor neuron disease or for neurologic healing, but this can be adjusted depending on clinical progression and reevaluation of plasma/serum concentrations at periodic intervals. Some horses show minimal response in blood concentrations when supplemented with particular products, and, if this is encountered, the product should be changed. Considerations that should be made when selecting a vitamin E supplement include:

- Form: synthetic acetate is acceptable for daily maintenance supplementation, and potentially to increase blood concentrations over time in healthy horses with suboptimal values. Naturally derived forms are more appropriate for treating deficiency-related disorders. Check the ingredient list to determine whether form and potency (IU/mL or IU/g) can be reliably determined for the product in question. If not, choose another supplement.
- Dose: how many IU of vitamin E does the horse in question require each day (discussed earlier). Liquid micellized supplements are often concentrated (eg, 500 IU/mL of naturally derived E in some products compared with 9 IU/g of synthetic E source in some powdered products) and are an efficient and effective means of meeting high requirements in clinical disease.
- Cost: how many horses need how much supplement, and what is the form of the selected supplement?
- Selenium content: excessive selenium intake can occur if using a combination supplement to provide vitamin E at more than maintenance requirements or label recommendations, particularly in areas that have high soil selenium concentrations (see Nerida Richards and collegaues' article, "Nutritional and Non-Nutritional Aspects of Forage," in this issue). However, combined selenium–vitamin E products exist that are appropriate for horses with average requirements for both nutrients.

Selenium Deficiency Disorders

Selenium is a trace element and potent antioxidant compound. Deficiency has traditionally been reported in foals and juvenile horses as the rhabdomyolysis disorder, nutritional myodegeneration (white muscle disease). Affected donkey and horse foals show weakness, recumbency, and poor suckle reflex, in addition to increased serum muscle enzyme activities.[176] Adult horses and donkeys can also develop severe disease from deficiency, with signs variably including trismus and atrophy or swelling of the masseter muscles; cardiac disease reflected by pulmonary edema, ventral edema, and cavitary effusions; and severe rhabdomyolysis reflected by stiffness and myoglobinuria (**Fig. 4**). Clinical signs in severely deficient animals may be as subtle as dropping feed from the mouth, or as profound as fulminant respiratory distress related to myocardial and/or diaphragmatic damage. Increased muscle enzyme activities are often, but not always, observed in clinically affected animals, and range widely. Normal muscle enzyme values do not preclude deficiency-related disease and have been observed in horses with generalized muscle atrophy and whole-blood selenium concentration as low as 25 ng/mL (reference: 160–275 ng/mL).

Selenium deficiency is typically regional, occurring in broad areas of the world where complex interactions between rainfall, soil characteristics, fertilization, and plant factors combine to result in low selenium content in forage.[176] Deficiency arises when horses are fed fresh or preserved forage from deficient areas for a period of time, and are not concurrently adequately supplemented. Foals are susceptible as a result of inadequate status of the mare resulting in poor placental transfer of selenium to the

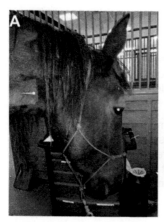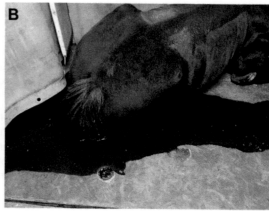

Fig. 4. A 12-year-old Percheron mare with trismus, swollen masseter muscles (*A*), and myoglobinuria (*B*) resulting from selenium deficiency. Presenting serum CK and aspartate aminotransferase values were 63,626 and 12,627 U/L, respectively. Whole blood selenium concentration of 19 ng/mL (reference 160–275 ng/mL). Ration consisted entirely of pasture grass and hay in a selenium-deficient region.

foal, and clinical signs can be evident as early as the first hour of life in foals delivered alive[176] (see Morgane Robles and colleagues' article, "Nutrition of Broodmares," in this issue).

Selenium in feed products is commonly reported as PPM (mg/kg). Selenium can be toxic in small amounts (>20 mg/d for a 500 kg horse), thus the US Food and Drug Administration (FDA) regulations cap selenium at 0.3 PPM in complete feeds and at 120 PPM in salt-mineral mixtures in the United States. Selenium status of horses can be determined from measuring selenium concentration or the selenium-dependent enzyme glutathione peroxidase in whole blood, serum, or plasma. A range of reference intervals exist as a result of the different variables and different sample types, and the most appropriate reference for the sample and test should therefore be applied. Measurement of selenium concentrations in liver tissue represents another method of determining deficiency status.[177]

To prevent deficiency, horses (~500 kg BW) require at least 1 mg of selenium per day[75] or 0.1 mg/kg DM intake. Higher amounts, up to 3 mg/d, may improve specific immune factors, but, ideally, total intake should not exceed a maximum of 1 mg/100 kg BW. Where maintenance supplementation is required, such as for a horse subsisting solely on forage produced from a deficient region, the ration should be supplemented with commercial feed products with appropriate selenium content, or top dressing with selenium-containing supplements. Selenium-containing salt blocks, although theoretically capable of providing adequate selenium, are not reliable because intake is highly variable.[169] In a study of several hundred horses in a deficient area of the United States, nearly 20% of horses had suboptimal blood selenium, and 4% had values that could promote clinical disease. This finding was despite nearly 90% of owners providing some level of selenium supplementation. Horses supplemented only via selenium-containing salt blocks were 20 times more likely to be deficient, underscoring the poor reliability of this method.[169] If supplementation is required for deficiency-related disease, or to increase low blood concentrations, injection with an appropriate parenteral product is recommended, followed by daily oral supplementation.

Selenium can be provided in organic form as selenomethionine or selenium yeast. Alternatively, selenium is also commonly provided as inorganic salt, typically sodium selenite. Although the organic form is reported to have superior bioavailability, both forms are very available to horses, and seem to be similarly effective at preventing deficiency when providing at least 1 mg/d.[169] Supplementation of mares during gestation increases plasma, muscle, and colostrum selenium concentrations, in addition to foal plasma and muscle selenium concentrations.[178] Regardless, in some deficient areas, neonatal foals are supplemented by injection after birth to ensure adequate status is achieved. Periodic testing of blood selenium variables in adult horses is useful to evaluate the efficacy of supplementation practices in individuals or groups.

SUMMARY

Appropriate nutritional management is essential to the development and maintenance of healthy skeletal muscle throughout the lifespan of a horse. Energy is necessary to support muscle growth, maintenance, and activity. Provision of adequate high-quality protein is critical because protein is the major nonwater component of skeletal muscle. Muscle mass can decrease with age as the tissue becomes less sensitive to the anabolic stimuli, and nutritional interventions to prevent this phenomenon are not known for horses. Similarly, feeding protocols that might optimize post-exercise muscle protein synthesis and glycogen repletion in horses have yet to be defined. Horses are prone to several heritable muscular disorders that can be successfully managed by restricting NSC intake for most disorders, or dietary potassium intake for HYPP. Vitamin E and selenium deficiency also remain important causes of muscular disease in horses and deserve appropriate attention in balanced feeding plans.

DISCLOSURE

The authors have nothing to disclose.

REFERENCES

1. Gunn HM. Muscle, bone and fat proportions and muscle distribution of thoroughbreds and other horses. In: Gillespie JR, Robinson NE, editors. Equine exercise physiology 2: proceedings of the Second International Conference on Equine Exercise Physiology. Davis (CA): ICEEP Publications; 1987. p. 253–64.
2. Lorenzo JM, Sarries MV, Tateo A, et al. Carcass characteristics, meat quality and nutritional value of horsemeat: a review. Meat Sci 2014;96:1478–88.
3. Tateo A, De Palo P, Ceci E, et al. Physicochemical properties of meat of Italian Heavy Draft horses slaughtered at the age of eleven months. J Anim Sci 2008; 86:1205–14.
4. Badiani A, Nanni N, Gatta PP, et al. Nutrient profile of horsemeat. J Food Compost Anal 1997;10:254–69.
5. Seong PN, Park KM, Kang GH, et al. The differences in chemical composition, physical quality traits and nutritional values of horse meat as affected by various retail cut types. Asian-Australas J Anim Sci 2016;29:89–99.
6. Frontera WR, Ochala J. Skeletal muscle: a brief review of structure and function. Calcif Tissue Int 2015;96:183–95.
7. Rivero JL, Serrano AL, Barrey E, et al. Analysis of myosin heavy chains at the protein level in horse skeletal muscle. J Muscle Res Cell Motil 1999;20:211–21.

8. Lopez-Rivero JL, Serrano AL, Diz AM, et al. Variability of muscle fibre composition and fibre size in the horse gluteus medius: an enzyme-histochemical and morphometric study. J Anat 1992;181(Pt 1):1–10.

9. Valberg SJ. Muscular causes of exercise intolerance in horses. Vet Clin North Am Equine Pract 1996;12:495–515.

10. Valberg S, Essen Gustavsson B, Skoglund Wallberg H. Oxidative capacity of skeletal muscle fibres in racehorses: histochemical versus biochemical analysis. Equine Vet J 1988;20:291–5.

11. Du M, Tong J, Zhao J, et al. Fetal programming of skeletal muscle development in ruminant animals. J Anim Sci 2010;88:E51–60.

12. Reed SA, Raja JS, Hoffman ML, et al. Poor maternal nutrition inhibits muscle development in ovine offspring. J Anim Sci Biotechnol 2014;5:43.

13. Kawai M, Minami Y, Sayama Y, et al. Muscle fiber population and biochemical properties of whole body muscles in Thoroughbred horses. Anat Rec (Hoboken) 2009;292:1663–9.

14. Rivero JL, Piercy RJ. Muscle physiology: responses to exercise and training. In: Hinchcliff KW, Geor RJ, Kaneps AJ, editors. Equine exercise physiology: the science of exercise in the athletic horse. New York: Saunders Elsevier; 2008. p. 30–80.

15. Latham CM, Fenger CK, White SH. Rapid communication: differential skeletal muscle mitochondrial characteristics of weanling racing-bred horses. J Anim Sci 2019;97:3193–8.

16. Thornton KJ. Triennial growth symposium: the nutrition of muscle growth: impacts of nutrition on the proliferation and differentiation of satellite cells in livestock species1,2. J Anim Sci 2019;97:2258–69.

17. Szczesniak KA, Ciecierska A, Ostaszewski P, et al. Characterisation of equine satellite cell transcriptomic profile response to beta-hydroxy-beta-methylbutyrate (HMB). Br J Nutr 2016;116:1315–25.

18. Gonzalez ML, Jacobs RD, Ely KM, et al. Dietary tributyrin supplementation and submaximal exercise promote activation of equine satellite cells. J Anim Sci 2019;97:4951–6.

19. Yoon MS. mTOR as a key regulator in maintaining skeletal muscle mass. Front Physiol 2017;8:788.

20. van Vliet S, Burd NA, van Loon LJ. The skeletal muscle anabolic response to plant- versus animal-based protein consumption. J Nutr 2015;145:1981–91.

21. Urschel KL, Escobar J, McCutcheon LJ, et al. Effect of feeding a high protein diet following an 18-hour period of feed withholding on mTOR-dependent signaling in skeletal muscle of mature horses. Am J Vet Res 2011;72:248–55.

22. Wagner AL, Urschel KL. Developmental regulation of the activation of translation initiation factors of skeletal muscle in response to feeding in horses. Am J Vet Res 2012;73:1241–51.

23. Loos CMM, McLeod KR, Stratton SC, et al. Short communication: pathways regulating equine skeletal muscle protein synthesis respond in a dose-dependent manner to graded levels of protein intake. J Anim Sci 2020;98:skaa268.

24. Witard OC, Jackman SR, Breen L, et al. Myofibrillar muscle protein synthesis rates subsequent to a meal in response to increasing doses of whey protein at rest and after resistance exercise. Am J Clin Nutr 2014;99:86–95.

25. Gibbs PG, Potter GD, Schelling GT, et al. Digestion of hay protein in different segments of the equine digestive tract. J Anim Sci 1988;66:400–6.

26. Gibbs PG, Potter GD, Schelling GT, et al. The significance of small vs large intestinal digestion of cereal grain and oilseed protein in the equine. J Equine Vet Sci 1996;16:60–5.

27. Suryawan A, Torrazza RM, Gazzaneo MC, et al. Enteral leucine supplementation increases protein synthesis in skeletal and cardiac muscles and visceral tissues of neonatal pigs through mTORC1-dependent pathways. Pediatr Res 2012;71: 324–31.

28. Columbus DA, Steinhoff-Wagner J, Suryawan A, et al. Impact of prolonged leucine supplementation on protein synthesis and lean growth in neonatal pigs. Am J Physiol Endocrinol Metab 2015;309:E601–10.

29. Churchward-Venne TA, Breen L, Di Donato DM, et al. Leucine supplementation of a low-protein mixed macronutrient beverage enhances myofibrillar protein synthesis in young men: a double-blind, randomized trial. Am J Clin Nutr 2014;99:276–86.

30. DeBoer ML, Martinson KM, Pampusch MS, et al. Cultured equine satellite cells as a model system to assess leucine stimulated protein synthesis in horse muscle. J Anim Sci 2018;96:143–53.

31. Phillips SM, Tipton KD, Aarsland A, et al. Mixed muscle protein synthesis and breakdown after resistance exercise in humans. Am J Physiol 1997;273: E99–107.

32. Pennings B, Koopman R, Beelen M, et al. Exercising before protein intake allows for greater use of dietary protein-derived amino acids for de novo muscle protein synthesis in both young and elderly men. Am J Clin Nutr 2011;93:322–31.

33. Moore DR, Robinson MJ, Fry JL, et al. Ingested protein dose response of muscle and albumin protein synthesis after resistance exercise in young men. Am J Clin Nutr 2009;89:161–8.

34. Churchward-Venne TA, Burd NA, Mitchell CJ, et al. Supplementation of a suboptimal protein dose with leucine or essential amino acids: effects on myofibrillar protein synthesis at rest and following resistance exercise in men. J Physiol 2012;590:2751–65.

35. Rennie MJ, Wackerhage H, Spangenburg EE, et al. Control of the size of the human muscle mass. Annu Rev Physiol 2004;66:799–828.

36. Votion DM, Navet R, Lacombe VA, et al. Muscle energetics in exercising horses. Equine Comp Exerc Physiol 2007;4:105–18.

37. Cutmore CM, Snow DH, Newsholme EA. Effects of training on enzyme activities involved in purine nucleotide metabolism in Thoroughbred horses. Equine Vet J 1986;18:72–3.

38. Essen-Gustavsson B, Gottlieb-Vedi M, Lindholm A. Muscle adenine nucleotide degradation during submaximal treadmill exercise to fatigue. Equine Vet J Suppl 1999;(30):298–302.

39. Harris P. Energy sources and requirements of the exercising horse. Annu Rev Nutr 1997;17:185–210.

40. Pethick DW, Rose RJ, Bryden WL, et al. Nutrient utilisation by the hindlimb of thoroughbred horses at rest. Equine Vet J 1993;25:41–4.

41. Snow DH, Harris RC, Gash SP. Metabolic response of equine muscle to intermittent maximal exercise. J Appl Physiol (1985) 1985;58:1689–97.

42. Harris DB, Harris RC, Wilson AM, et al. ATP loss with exercise in muscle fibres of the gluteus medius of the thoroughbred horse. Res Vet Sci 1997;63:231–7.

43. Farris JW, Hinchcliff KW, McKeever KH, et al. Effect of tryptophan and of glucose on exercise capacity of horses. J Appl Physiol 1998;85:807–16.

44. Lacombe VA, Hinchcliff KW, Geor RJ, et al. Muscle glycogen depletion and subsequent replenishment affect anaerobic capacity of horses. J Appl Physiol (1985) 2001;91:1782–90.

45. Snow DH, Kerr MG, Nimmo MA, et al. Alterations in blood, sweat, urine and muscle composition during prolonged exercise in the horse. Vet Rec 1982; 110:377–84.

46. Waller AP, Heigenhauser GJ, Geor RJ, et al. Fluid and electrolyte supplementation after prolonged moderate-intensity exercise enhances muscle glycogen resynthesis in Standardbred horses. J Appl Physiol 2009;106:91–100.

47. Harkins JD, Morris GS, Tulley RT, et al. Effect of added dietary fat on racing performance in thoroughbred horses. J Equine Vet Sci 1992;12:123–9.

48. Geor RJ, Hinchcliff KW, Sams RA. beta-adrenergic blockade augments glucose utilization in horses during graded exercise. J Appl Physiol (1985) 2000;89: 1086–98.

49. McKeever KH. The endocrine system and the challenge of exercise. Vet Clin North Am Equine Pract 2002;18:321–53, vii.

50. Valberg S, Gustavsson BE, Lindholm A, et al. Blood chemistry and skeletal muscle metabolic responses during and after different speeds and durations of trotting. Equine Vet J 1989;21:91–5.

51. Kronfeld DS, Holland JL, Rich GA, et al. Fat digestibility in Equus caballus follows increasing first-order kinetics. J Anim Sci 2004;82:1773–80.

52. Pagan JD, Geor RJ, Harris PA, et al. Effects of fat adaptation on glucose kinetics and substrate oxidation during low-intensity exercise. Equine Vet J Suppl 2002;(34):33–8.

53. Dunnett CE, Marlin DJ, Harris RC. Effect of dietary lipid on response to exercise: relationship to metabolic adaptation. Equine Vet J Suppl 2002;(34):75–80.

54. Treiber KH, Geor RJ, Boston RC, et al. Dietary energy source affects glucose kinetics in trained Arabian geldings at rest and during endurance exercise. J Nutr 2008;138:964–70.

55. Pagan JD, Mesquita VS, Valberg SJ, et al. Effect of non-structural carbohydrate intake on glycogen repletion following intense exercise. J Equine Vet Sci 2015; 38:408–9.

56. Jose-Cunilleras E, Hinchcliff KW, Sams RA, et al. Glycemic index of a meal fed before exercise alters substrate use and glucose flux in exercising horses. J Appl Physiol (1985) 2002;92:117–28.

57. Geor RJ, Hinchcliff KW, Sams RA. Glucose infusion attenuates endogenous glucose production and enhances glucose use of horses during exercise. J Appl Physiol (1985) 2000;88:1765–76.

58. Essen-Gustavsson B, Jensen-Waern M. Effect of an endurance race on muscle amino acids, pro- and macroglycogen and triglycerides. Equine Vet J Suppl 2002;(34):209–13.

59. Trottier NL, Nielsen BD, Lang KJ, et al. Equine endurance exercise alters serum branched-chain amino acid and alanine concentrations. Equine Vet J Suppl 2002;(34):168–72.

60. Bergero D, Assenza A, Schiavone A, et al. Amino acid concentrations in blood serum of horses performing long lasting low-intensity exercise. J Anim Physiol Anim Nutr (Berl) 2005;89:146–50.

61. Glade M. Effects of specific amino acid supplementation lactic acid production by horses exercised on a treadmill. 11th Conference of the Equine Nutrition and Physiology Symposium. Stillwater, OK: May 18-20, 1989. p. 244–8.

62. Stefanon B, Bettini C, Guggia G. Administration of branched-chain amino acids to standardbred horses in training. J Equine Vet Sci 2000;20:115–9.
63. Casini L, Gatta D, Magni L, et al. Effect of prolonged branched-chain amino acid supplementation on metabolic response to anaerobic exercise in standardbreds. J Equine Vet Sci 2000;20:120–3.
64. Hyyppa S, Rasanen LA, Poso AR. Resynthesis of glycogen in skeletal muscle from standardbred trotters after repeated bouts of exercise. Am J Vet Res 1997;58:162–6.
65. Lacombe VA, Hinchcliff KW, Kohn CW, et al. Effects of feeding meals with various soluble-carbohydrate content on muscle glycogen synthesis after exercise in horses. Am J Vet Res 2004;65:916–23.
66. Costill DL, Sherman WM, Fink WJ, et al. The role of dietary carbohydrates in muscle glycogen resynthesis after strenuous running. Am J Clin Nutr 1981;34:1831–6.
67. Jentjens RL, Van Loon LJ, Mann CH, et al. Addition of protein and amino acids to carbohydrates does not enhance postexercise muscle glycogen synthesis. J Appl Physiol 2001;91:839–46.
68. Jose-Cunilleras E, Hinchcliff KW, Lacombe VA, et al. Ingestion of starch-rich meals after exercise increases glucose kinetics but fails to enhance muscle glycogen replenishment in horses. Vet J 2006;171:468–77.
69. Geor RJ, Larsen L, Waterfall HL, et al. Route of carbohydrate administration affects early post exercise muscle glycogen storage in horses. Equine Vet J Suppl 2006;(36):590–5.
70. Brojer JT, Nostell KE, Essen-Gustavsson B, et al. Effect of repeated oral administration of glucose and leucine immediately after exercise on plasma insulin concentration and glycogen synthesis in horses. Am J Vet Res 2012;73:867–74.
71. Pratt SE, Geor RJ, Spriet LL, et al. Time course of insulin sensitivity and skeletal muscle glycogen synthase activity after a single bout of exercise in horses. J Appl Physiol 2007;103:1063–9.
72. Waller AP, Lindinger MI. Nutritional aspects of post exercise skeletal muscle glycogen synthesis in horses: a comparative review. Equine Vet J 2010;42:274–81.
73. Waller AP, Geor RJ, Spriet LL, et al. Oral acetate supplementation after prolonged moderate intensity exercise enhances early muscle glycogen resynthesis in horses. Exp Physiol 2009;94:888–98.
74. Martin-Rosset W. Growth and development in the equine. In: Julliand V, Martin-Rosset W, editors. The growing horse: nutrition and prevention of growth disorders Vol EAAP publication No. 114. Wageningen (the Netherlands): Wageningen Academic Publishers; 2005. p. 15–50.
75. National Research Council. Nutrient requirements of horses. 6th edition. Washington, DC: National Academies Press; 2007.
76. Ott EA, Asquith RL, Feaster JP. Lysine supplementation of diets for yearling horses. J Anim Sci 1981;53:1496–503.
77. Graham PM, Ott EA, Brendemuhl JH, et al. The effect of supplemental lysine and threonine on growth and development of yearling horses. J Anim Sci 1994;72:380–6.
78. Winsco KN, Coverdale JA, Wickersham TA, et al. Influence of dietary methionine concentration on growth and nitrogen balance in weanling Quarter Horses. J Anim Sci 2011;89:2132–8.
79. Bryden WL. Amino acid requirements of horses estimated from tissue composition. Proc Nutr Soc Aust 1991;16:53.

80. Lien KA, Sauer WC, Fenton M. Mucin output in ileal digesta of pigs fed a protein-free diet. Z Ernahrungswiss 1997;36:182–90.

81. Bott RC, Greene EA, Trottier NL, et al. Environmental implications of nitrogen output on horse operations: a review. J Equine Vet Sci 2016;45:98–106.

82. Connysson M, Muhonen S, Lindberg JE, et al. Effects of exercise response, fluid and acid-base balance of protein intake from forage-only diets in Standardbred horses. Equine Vet J Suppl 2006;36:648–53.

83. Meyer H. Nutrition of the Equine Athlete. Paper presented at: Equine Exercise Physiology 2; Aug 7 – 11, 1987, Davis, CA.

84. Graham-Thiers PM, Kronfeld DS. Dietary protein influences acid-base balance in sedentary horses. J Equine Vet Sci 2005;25:434–8.

85. Graham-Thiers PM, Kronfeld DS, Kline KA, et al. Dietary protein restriction and fat supplementation diminish the acidogenic effect of exercise during repeated sprints in horses. J Nutr 2001;131:1959–64.

86. Wysocki AA, Baker JP. Utilization of bacterial protein from the lower gut of the equine. Proceedings of the 4th Equine Nutrition and Physiology Symposium. Pomona, CA: January 16 – 18, 1975. p. 21–43.

87. Woodward AD, Fan MZ, Geor RJ, et al. Characterization of L-lysine transport across equine and porcine jejunal and colonic brush border membrane. J Anim Sci 2012;90:853–62.

88. Woodward AD, Holcombe SJ, Steibel JP, et al. Cationic and neutral amino acid transporter transcript abundances are differentially expressed in the equine intestinal tract. J Anim Sci 2010;88:1028–33.

89. DeBoer ML, Martinson KL, Kuhle KJ, et al. Plasma amino acid concentrations of horses grazing alfalfa, cool-season perennial grasses, and teff. J Equine Vet Sci 2019;72:72–8.

90. Graham-Thiers PM, Bowen LK. Effect of protein source on nitrogen balance and plasma amino acids in exercising horses. J Anim Sci 2011;89:729–35.

91. Ireland JL, Clegg PD, McGowan CM, et al. A cross-sectional study of geriatric horses in the United Kingdom. Part 2: health care and disease. Equine Vet J 2011;43:37–44.

92. McGowan TW, Pinchbeck GP, McGowan CM. Prevalence, risk factors and clinical signs predictive for equine pituitary pars intermedia dysfunction in aged horses. Equine Vet J 2013;45:74–9.

93. Cuthbertson D, Smith K, Babraj J, et al. Anabolic signaling deficits underlie amino acid resistance of wasting, aging muscle. FASEB J 2005;19:422–4.

94. Wagner AL, Urschel KL, Betancourt A, et al. Effects of advanced age on whole-body protein synthesis and skeletal muscle mechanistic target of rapamycin signaling in horses. Am J Vet Res 2013;74:1433–42.

95. Aleman M, Watson JL, Williams DC, et al. Myopathy in horses with pituitary pars intermedia dysfunction (Cushing's disease). Neuromuscul Disord 2006;16:737–44.

96. Mastro LM, Adams AA, Urschel KL. Whole-body phenylalanine kinetics and skeletal muscle protein signaling in horses with pituitary pars intermedia dysfunction. Am J Vet Res 2014;75:658–67.

97. Mastro LM, Adams AA, Urschel KL. Pituitary pars intermedia dysfunction does not necessarily impair insulin sensitivity in old horses. Domest Anim Endocrinol 2015;50:14–25.

98. Matsui A, Ohmura H, Asai Y, et al. Effect of amino acid and glucose administration following exercise on the turnover of muscle protein in the hindlimb femoral region of thoroughbreds. Equine Vet J Suppl 2006;(36):611–6.

99. Jacobs RD, Splan RK, Urschel KL, et al. Post-exercise dietary supplementation leads to improved muscle recovery in fatigued horses. J Equine Vet Sci 2015;35: 395–6.

100. Walker VA, Tranquille CA, Dyson SJ, et al. Association of a subjective muscle score with increased angles of flexion during sitting trot in dressage horses. J Equine Vet Sci 2016;40:6–15.

101. Henneke DR, Potter GD, Kreider JL, et al. Relationship between condition score, physical measurements and body fat percentage in mares. Equine Vet J 1983; 15:371–2.

102. Holecek M. Beta-hydroxy-beta-methylbutyrate supplementation and skeletal muscle in healthy and muscle-wasting conditions. J Cachexia Sarcopenia Muscle 2017;8:529–41.

103. Ostaszewski P, Kowalska A, Szarska E, et al. Effects of β-hydroxy-β-methylbutyrate and γ-oryzanol on blood biochemical markers in exercising Thoroughbred race horses. J Equine Vet Sci 2012;32:542–51.

104. Reiter AS, DeBoer ML, Martinson KL, et al. Effect of β-hydroxy-β-methylbutyrate on protein synthesis of cultured equine myogenic satellite cells. J Equine Vet Sci 2019;76:72.

105. Kreider RB. Effects of creatine supplementation on performance and training adaptations. Mol Cell Biochem 2003;244:89–94.

106. Schuback K, Essen-Gustavsson B, Persson SG. Effect of creatine supplementation on muscle metabolic response to a maximal treadmill exercise test in Standardbred horses. Equine Vet J 2000;32:533–40.

107. D'Angelis FH, Ferraz GC, Boleli IC, et al. Aerobic training, but not creatine supplementation, alters the gluteus medius muscle. J Anim Sci 2005;83:579–85.

108. Teixeira FA, Araujo AL, Ramalho LO, et al. Oral creatine supplementation on performance of Quarter horses used in barrel racing. J Anim Physiol Anim Nutr (Berl) 2016;100:513–9.

109. Fielding R, Riede L, Lugo JP, et al. l-Carnitine supplementation in recovery after exercise. Nutrients 2018;10.

110. van der Kolk JH, Thomas S, Mach N, et al. Serum acylcarnitine profile in endurance horses with and without metabolic dysfunction. Vet J 2020;255:105419.

111. Harris RC, Foster CVL, Snow DH. Plasma carnitine concentration and uptake into muscle with oral and intravenous administration. Equine Vet J Suppl 1995;18:382–7.

112. Rivero JL, Sporleder HP, Quiroz-Rothe E, et al. Oral L-carnitine combined with training promotes changes in skeletal muscle. Equine Vet J Suppl 2002;(34): 269–74.

113. Peters LW, Smiet E, de Sain-van der Velden MG, et al. Acylcarnitine ester utilization by the hindlimb of warmblood horses at rest and following low intensity exercise and carnitine supplementation. Vet Q 2015;35:76–81.

114. Harris PA, Rivero JLL. Nutritional considerations for equine rhabdomyolysis syndrome. Equine Vet Educ 2017;8:459–65.

115. Valberg SJ. Muscle conditions affecting sport horses. Vet Clin North Am Equine Pract 2018;34:253–76.

116. Valberg SJ, McCue ME, Mickelson JR. The interplay of genetics, exercise and nutrition in polysaccharide storage myopathy. J Equine Vet Sci 2011;31:205–10.

117. Carlstrom B. Über die Ätiologie und Pathogenese der Kreuzlähme des Pferdes. (Haemoglobinaemia paralytica). Skand Arch Physiol 1932;63:164–212.

118. Valberg SJ. Muscling in on the cause of tying-up. Frank J Milne State-of-the-Art Lecture. Proceedings, Am Assoc Equine Practitioners 2012;58:85–123.

119. Koterba A, Carlson GP. Acid-base and electrolyte alterations in horses with exertional rhabdomyolysis. J Am Vet Med Assoc 1982;180:303–6.

120. Valberg SJ, Macleay JM, Billstrom JA, et al. Skeletal muscle metabolic response to exercise in horses with 'tying-up' due to polysaccharide storage myopathy. Equine Vet J 1999;31:43–7.

121. McKenzie EC, Valberg SJ, Godden SM, et al. Effect of dietary starch, fat, and bicarbonate content on exercise responses and serum creatine kinase activity in equine recurrent exertional rhabdomyolysis. J Vet Intern Med 2003;17: 693–701.

122. McCue ME, Valberg SJ, Miller MB, et al. Glycogen synthase (GYS1) mutation causes a novel skeletal muscle glycogenosis. Genomics 2008;91:458–66.

123. McCue ME, Valberg SJ, Lucio M, et al. Glycogen synthase 1 (GYS1) mutation in diverse breeds with polysaccharide storage myopathy. J Vet Intern Med 2008; 22:1228–33.

124. McCue ME, Anderson SM, Valberg SJ, et al. Estimated prevalence of the type 1 polysaccharide storage myopathy mutation in selected North American and European breeds. Anim Genet 2010;41(Suppl 2):145–9.

125. Tryon RC, Penedo MC, McCue ME, et al. Evaluation of allele frequencies of inherited disease genes in subgroups of American Quarter Horses. J Am Vet Med Assoc 2009;234:120–5.

126. Naylor RJ, Livesey L, Schumacher J, et al. Allele copy number and underlying pathology are associated with subclinical severity in equine type 1 polysaccharide storage myopathy (PSSM1). PLoS One 2012;7:e42317.

127. Valberg SJ, MacLeay JM, Mickelson JR. Exertional rhabdomyolysis and polysaccharide storage myopathy in horses. Compend Contin Educ Vet 1997;19: 1077–86.

128. Valentine BA, Credille KM, Lavoie JP, et al. Severe polysaccharide storage myopathy in Belgian and Percheron draught horses. Equine Vet J 1997;29: 220–5.

129. Firshman AM, Baird JD, Valberg SJ. Prevalences and clinical signs of polysaccharide storage myopathy and shivers in Belgian draft horses. J Am Vet Med Assoc 2005;227:1958–64.

130. Quiroz-Rothe E, Novales M, Aguilera-Tejero E, et al. Polysaccharide storage myopathy in the M. longissimus lumborum of showjumpers and dressage horses with back pain. Equine Vet J 2002;34:171–6.

131. Lewis SS, Nicholson AM, Williams ZJ, et al. Clinical characteristics and muscle glycogen concentrations in warmblood horses with polysaccharide storage myopathy. Am J Vet Res 2017;78:1305–12.

132. Finno CJ, Spier SJ, Valberg SJ. Equine diseases caused by known genetic mutations. Vet J 2009;179:336–47.

133. McCue ME, Valberg SJ, Jackson M, et al. Polysaccharide storage myopathy phenotype in quarter horse-related breeds is modified by the presence of an RYR1 mutation. Neuromuscul Disord 2009;19:37–43.

134. Aleman M, Nieto JE, Magdesian KG. Malignant hyperthermia associated with ryanodine receptor 1 (C7360G) mutation in Quarter Horses. J Vet Intern Med 2009;23:329–34.

135. Firshman AM, Valberg SJ, Bender JB, et al. Epidemiologic characteristics and management of polysaccharide storage myopathy in Quarter Horses. Am J Vet Res 2003;64:1319–27.

136. De La Corte FD, Valberg SJ, MacLeay JM, et al. Glucose uptake in horses with polysaccharide storage myopathy. Am J Vet Res 1999;60:458–62.

137. De La Corte FD, Valberg SJ, Mickelson JR, et al. Blood glucose clearance after feeding and exercise in polysaccharide storage myopathy. Equine Vet J Suppl 1999;(30):324–8.

138. Valentine BA, Van Saun RJ, Thompson KN, et al. Role of dietary carbohydrate and fat in horses with equine polysaccharide storage myopathy. J Am Vet Med Assoc 2001;219:1537–44.

139. Ribeiro WP, Valberg SJ, Pagan JD, et al. The effect of varying dietary starch and fat content on serum creatine kinase activity and substrate availability in equine polysaccharide storage myopathy. J Vet Intern Med 2004;18:887–94.

140. Harris PA, Geor RJ. Nutrition for the equine athlete: nutrient requirements and key principles in ration design. In: Hinchcliff KW, Kaneps AJ, Geor RJ, editors. Equine sports medicine and surgery. New York: Saunders Elsevier; 2014. p. 797–818.

141. Johlig L, Valberg SJ, Mickelson JR, et al. Epidemiological and genetic study of exertional rhabdomyolysis in a Warmblood horse family in Switzerland. Equine Vet J 2011;43:240–5.

142. Schroder U, Licka TF, Zsoldos R, et al. Effect of diet on Haflinger horses with GYS1-mutation (polysaccharide storage myopathy type 1). J Equine Vet Sci 2015;35:1281–90.

143. Borgia L, Valberg S, McCue M, et al. Glycaemic and insulinaemic responses to feeding hay with different non-structural carbohydrate content in control and polysaccharide storage myopathy-affected horses. J Anim Physiol Anim Nutr (Berl) 2011;95:798–807.

144. Argo CM, Dugdale AH, McGowan CM. Considerations for the use of restricted, soaked grass hay diets to promote weight loss in the management of equine metabolic syndrome and obesity. Vet J 2015;206:170–7.

145. Borgia LA, Valberg SJ, McCue ME, et al. Effect of dietary fats with odd or even numbers of carbon atoms on metabolic response and muscle damage with exercise in Quarter Horse-type horses with type 1 polysaccharide storage myopathy. Am J Vet Res 2010;71:326–36.

146. Hunt LM, Valberg SJ, Steffenhagen K, et al. An epidemiological study of myopathies in Warmblood horses. Equine Vet J 2008;40:171–7.

147. Williams ZJ, Bertels M, Valberg SJ. Muscle glycogen concentrations and response to diet and exercise regimes in Warmblood horses with type 2 Polysaccharide Storage Myopathy. PLoS One 2018;13:e0203467.

148. Stanley RL, McCue ME, Valberg SJ, et al. A glycogen synthase 1 mutation associated with equine polysaccharide storage myopathy and exertional rhabdomyolysis occurs in a variety of UK breeds. Equine Vet J 2009;41:597–601.

149. McCue ME, Armien AG, Lucio M, et al. Comparative skeletal muscle histopathologic and ultrastructural features in two forms of polysaccharide storage myopathy in horses. Vet Pathol 2009;46:1281–91.

150. Valberg SJ, Finno CJ, Henry ML, et al. Commercial genetic testing for type 2 polysaccharide storage myopathy and myofibrillar myopathy does not correspond to a histopathological diagnosis. Equine Vet J 2020. Available at: https://beva.onlinelibrary.wiley.com/doi/full/10.1111/evj.13345.

151. Mickelson JR, Valberg SJ. The genetics of skeletal muscle disorders in horses. Annu Rev Anim Biosci 2015;3:197–217.

152. Isgren CM, Upjohn MM, Fernandez-Fuente M, et al. Epidemiology of exertional rhabdomyolysis susceptibility in standardbred horses reveals associated risk factors and underlying enhanced performance. PLoS One 2010;5:e11594.

153. MacLeay JM, Sorum SA, Valberg SJ, et al. Epidemiologic analysis of factors influencing exertional rhabdomyolysis in Thoroughbreds. Am J Vet Res 1999; 60:1562–6.

154. Lentz LR, Valberg SJ, Balog EM, et al. Abnormal regulation of muscle contraction in horses with recurrent exertional rhabdomyolysis. Am J Vet Res 1999;60: 992–9.

155. McKenzie EC, Valberg SJ, Godden SM, et al. Effect of oral administration of dantrolene sodium on serum creatine kinase activity after exercise in horses with recurrent exertional rhabdomyolysis. Am J Vet Res 2004;65:74–9.

156. Norton EM, Mickelson JR, Binns MM, et al. Heritability of recurrent exertional rhabdomyolysis in standardbred and thoroughbred racehorses derived from SNP genotyping data. J Hered 2016;107:537–43.

157. Bulmer L, McBride S, Williams K, et al. The effects of a high-starch or high-fibre diet on equine reactivity and handling behavior. Appl Anim Behav Sci 2015;165: 95–102.

158. MacLeay JM, Valberg SJ, Pagan JD, et al. Effect of ration and exercise on plasma creatine kinase activity and lactate concentration in Thoroughbred horses with recurrent exertional rhabdomyolysis. Am J Vet Res 2000;61:1390–5.

159. Edwards JG, Newtont JR, Ramzan PH, et al. The efficacy of dantrolene sodium in controlling exertional rhabdomyolysis in the Thoroughbred racehorse. Equine Vet J 2003;35:707–11.

160. McKenzie EC, Garrett RL, Payton ME, et al. Effect of feed restriction on plasma dantrolene concentrations in horses. Equine Vet J Suppl 2010;(38):613–7.

161. DiMaio Knych HK, Arthur RM, Taylor A, et al. Pharmacokinetics and metabolism of dantrolene in horses. J Vet Pharmacol Ther 2011;34:238–46.

162. Valberg SJ, McKenzie EC, Eyrich LV, et al. Suspected myofibrillar myopathy in Arabian horses with a history of exertional rhabdomyolysis. Equine Vet J 2016;48:548–56.

163. Valberg SJ, Nicholson AM, Lewis SS, et al. Clinical and histopathological features of myofibrillar myopathy in Warmblood horses. Equine Vet J 2017;49: 739–45.

164. Wilberger MS, McKenzie EC, Payton ME, et al. Prevalence of exertional rhabdomyolysis in endurance horses in the Pacific Northwestern United States. Equine Vet J 2015;47:165–70.

165. Williams ZJ, Velez-Irizarry D, Petersen JL, et al. Candidate gene expression and coding sequence variants in Warmblood horses with myofibrillar myopathy. Equine Vet J 2020. Available at: https://beva.onlinelibrary.wiley.com/doi/abs/ 10.1111/evj.13286.

166. Myofibrillar Myopathy. The College of Veterinary Medicine at Michigan State University. Available at: https://cvm.msu.edu/research/faculty-research/comparative-medical-genetics/valberg-laboratory/myofibrillar-myopathy. Accessed October 19, 2020.

167. McKenzie EC, Eyrich LV, Payton ME, et al. Clinical, histopathological and metabolic responses following exercise in Arabian horses with a history of exertional rhabdomyolysis. Vet J 2016;216:196–201.

168. Valberg SJ, Perumbakkam S, McKenzie EC, et al. Proteome and transcriptome profiling of equine myofibrillar myopathy identifies diminished peroxiredoxin 6 and altered cysteine metabolic pathways. Physiol Genomics 2018;50:1036–50.

169. Pitel MO, McKenzie EC, Johns JL, et al. Influence of specific management practices on blood selenium, vitamin E, and beta-carotene concentrations in horses and risk of nutritional deficiency. J Vet Intern Med 2020;34(5):2132–41.

170. Naylor JM. Hyperkalemic periodic paralysis. Vet Clin North Am Equine Pract 1997;13:129–44.
171. Naylor JM, Nickel DD, Trimino G, et al. Hyperkalaemic periodic paralysis in homozygous and heterozygous horses: a co-dominant genetic condition. Equine Vet J 1999;31:153–9.
172. Pickar JG, Spier SJ, Snyder JR, et al. Altered ionic permeability in skeletal muscle from horses with hyperkalemic periodic paralysis. Am J Physiol 1991;260: C926–33.
173. Owens TG, Barnes M, Gargano VM, et al. Nutrient content changes from steaming or soaking timothy-alfalfa hay: effects on feed preferences and acute glycemic response in Standardbred racehorses. J Anim Sci 2019;97:4199–207.
174. Finno CJ, Valberg SJ. A comparative review of vitamin E and associated equine disorders. J Vet Intern Med 2012;26:1251–66.
175. Brown JC, Valberg SJ, Hogg M, et al. Effects of feeding two RRR-alpha-tocopherol formulations on serum, cerebrospinal fluid and muscle alpha-tocopherol concentrations in horses with subclinical vitamin E deficiency. Equine Vet J 2017;49:753–8.
176. Delesalle C, de Bruijn M, Wilmink S, et al. White muscle disease in foals: focus on selenium soil content. A case series. BMC Vet Res 2017;13:121.
177. Hosnedlova B, Kepinska M, Skalickova S, et al. A summary of new findings on the biological effects of selenium in selected animal species-a critical review. Int J Mol Sci 2017;18:2209.
178. Karren BJ, Thorson JF, Cavinder CA, et al. Effect of selenium supplementation and plane of nutrition on mares and their foals: selenium concentrations and glutathione peroxidase. J Anim Sci 2010;88:991–7.

Nutrition of Broodmares

Morgane Robles, PhD[a,b,c],*, Carolyn Hammer, DVM, PhD[d],
Burt Staniar, PhD[e], Pascale Chavatte-Palmer, DVM, PhD, HDR[b,c]

KEYWORDS

- Nutrition - Developmental origins of health and diseases (DOHaD) - Critical periods
- Gestation - Broodmare

KEY POINTS

- Under normal conditions, forage availability can match mares' energy and protein needs but low forage quality or breeding out of season requires nutritional supplementation.
- Micronutrient availability, however, should be verified and often requires supplementation.
- Attention needs to be placed not only on the quantity of energy and nutrients, but also on their quality and characteristics.
- Mare nutrition and adiposity can influence the foal's long-term health and metabolism (developmental origins of health and disease); excess nutrition can be as deleterious as feed restriction.
- There is a need for more research on broodmare nutrition, taking into consideration genetics, breed, breeding conditions, and environment.

INTRODUCTION

Nutrition and reproduction are central facets of life, highlighting the critical importance of optimal nutrition for the broodmare. Our goal with this review is to provide the reader with a solid foundation of knowledge regarding:

1. Core broodmare and fetal physiology, as well as maternal nutritional requirements, and
2. The influence broodmare nutrition can have on the future health and performance of the foal.

[a] Institut National de la Recherche Scientifique (INRS), Centre Armand Frappier, 532 Boul. des Prairies, Laval, Quebec, Canada H7V 1B7; [b] Université Paris-Saclay, UVSQ, INRAE, BREED, Jouy-en-Josas 78350, France; [c] Ecole Nationale Vétérinaire d'Alfort, BREED, Maisons-Alfort 94700, France; [d] Department of Animal Sciences, North Dakota State University, 1300 Albrecht Boulevard, Fargo, ND 58102, USA; [e] Penn State University, 316 Agricultural Sciences & Industries Building, University Park, PA 16802, USA
* Corresponding author.
E-mail address: morgane.robles@gmail.com

Vet Clin Equine 37 (2021) 177–205
https://doi.org/10.1016/j.cveq.2021.01.001
0749-0739/21/© 2021 Elsevier Inc. All rights reserved.
vetequine.theclinics.com

This review should enable readers to move beyond the basic dietary energy and nutrient requirements and consider a more precise formulation of diets for broodmares being kept in a wide range of different environments.

The first step in any nutritional evaluation should be to evaluate the mare and the performance sought. Once this point has been well-characterized, the diet and management best suited to that scenario can be formulated. Gestation and lactation result in substantial increases in nutritional requirements. Estimates of energy and nutrient requirements developed by equine nutritionists represent an excellent starting point for formulating a broodmare's diet.[1–3]

Nutrition, along with day length and ambient temperature, are important environment variables. Over tens of millions of years of evolution, horses have developed a seasonally polyestrous reproductive physiology that resulted in most foals being born in late spring and early summer, thereby synchronizing the nutrient requirements of late gestation and early lactation with environmental energy and nutrient availability.

Although those caring for broodmares can easily evaluate the mare and her environment (day length, ambient temperature, and forage and diet characteristics), it is more challenging to know the condition of the fetus or modify its environment. A primary histotrophic nutrition (based on uterine secretions) transitions to hemo (based on exchange between maternal and fetal bloods) and histotrophic nutrition after implantation.[4] The fetus progresses through various developmental stages, all of which may be influenced by the dam's nutrition. A growing body of research highlights the importance of the link between maternal nutrition and developmental programming of the fetus.

Nutrition is customarily evaluated as a balance between the requirements of the horse and the dietary supply. The objective is to find a balance that optimizes the long-term health and performance of the broodmare and her foal. Finding this balance requires an understanding of overnutrition and undernutrition, as well as the changes in requirements according to physiologic status. Furthermore, we now appreciate that optimal nutrition goes beyond simple quantities and requires consideration of the quality and form of the dietary energy and nutrients.

With the increasing incidence of obesity and the metabolic syndrome in horses, in addition to effects on mare fertility,[5] unforeseen effects may result, especially in terms of offspring health and metabolism. Conversely, under moderate maternal undernutrition, foal birth weight is not affected but long-term metabolic consequences may still be observed in offspring. There is a relatively clear connection between glucose and insulin homeostasis and metabolic consequences. However, other dietary components should also be considered, despite the fact that current knowledge is limited.

Key points

- Recommendations for dietary energy, protein, vitamins, minerals, and water are available, but these should be considered a starting point, from which the unique characteristics of each breeding operation should be further considered.

- Practitioners should consider the environment that a broodmares' physiology has been well adapted to as they make choices regarding diet and management during different stages of gestation.

- Knowledge of the negative implications of overnutrition and undernutrition, the metabolic and developmental impact of fiber, nonstructural carbohydrates, and fats as dietary energy sources, and the potential benefits of precision feeding using supplements or ration balancers is invaluable when formulating diets for broodmares.

CURRENT NUTRITION RECOMMENDATIONS
General Estimation of Broodmare Needs

Intake during gestation needs to meet mare plus fetal growth requirements. Studies on fetal growth, however, are limited. Fetal growth curve data are based on aborted or stillborn animals,[6–8] thus potentially underestimating fetal growth at the end of gestation.[1]

Historically, mare gestational nutritional requirements have been calculated based on the following assumptions:

- Accretion of uterine and placental tissues takes place in midgestation.[7,8] It is assumed that fetal adnexal tissue (placenta, amnion) and mammary development are linear to that of the fetus, as observed in the cow,[9] but this point has not been demonstrated in the horse.[10]
- Fetal growth is best represented by an exponential growth curve with rapid fetal development occurring from day 240 of gestation to parturition.[10]
- The foal's weight at birth is assumed to be approximately 10% of the dam's nonpregnant mature body weight.
- Uterine and placental tissues are metabolically more active (66.6 kcal/kg) than the rest of the body (33.3 kcal/kg body weight) and therefore have higher energy needs.[10]
- The efficiency of using digestible energy (DE) for depositing fetal and placental tissue during gestation is assumed to be 60%.[11]

Most of these factors are considered in the estimate of energy and nutrient requirements for pregnant broodmares that have been developed around the world. Differences between the various estimates are often owing to variation in interpretations of fetal, placental, and uterine growth data and estimates of changes in mare metabolism during gestation[12] (personal communication, Manfred Coenen, 2020).

Energy and Protein Requirements and Recommendations

Lactation and rapid fetal development in late gestation represent periods of high nutritional requirements for broodmares.[1,10] Nonlactating mares in early and even midgestation have energy and protein requirements either at or close to maintenance levels (**Fig. 1**). Estimated energy requirements in late gestation increase to between 1.3 and 1.5 times maintenance levels, and lactation can result in a doubling of energy requirements.

Horses obtain energy effectively from their environment, primarily from forages. Total dry matter intake (DMI) will likely range from 1.5% to 3.0% body weight, and in most cases at the higher end of this range in pregnant or lactating broodmares. Forages have most of their potential energy stored in the chemical bonds of structural and nonstructural carbohydrates and horses have evolved for the optimal use of this particular environmental dietary energy source. Therefore, caregivers should focus first on providing dietary energy from forages. Based on a host of published information, a rough approximation of the DE content of most forages is between 1.5 and 2.5 Mcal/kg, with more mature forages usually providing less DE.[1–3] For most mares, forages should make up at least 50% of their daily DMI, and in many cases may be close to 100%, if no energy rich concentrate/complementary feed or vitamin and mineral supplement is needed. Once dietary forage has been optimized, attention can shift to concentrates and/or vitamin and mineral supplements.

Mares in late gestation provided concentrates, in addition to grass forage, maintain body condition and weight better than those on forage alone.[13] Grains and

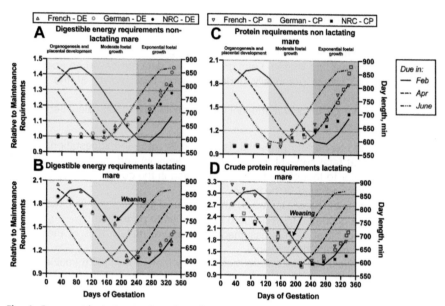

Fig. 1. Pregnant lactating and nonlactating mares' energy and protein requirements relative to maintenance, according to time of gestation and compared with day length. The symbols represent the DE (A, B) or CP (C, D) requirements relative to maintenance of broodmares with (B, D) or without (A, C) a foal at their side during gestation as determined using the French, German, and North American feeding standards for horses.[1–3] The lines represent the calculated day length at any point during gestation for foals due in February, April, or June for a north- ern latitude of 35, as an indicator of ambient temperature and forage availability. The colored regions represent important stages of gestation, represented by preimplantation, endometrial cups, and organogenesis (0–120 d), moderate fetal and organ growth (120– 240 d), and rapid fetal development (240–340 d). Those interpreting this figure should consider the synchrony between day length, a proxy for the broodmare's environment, and energy and nutrient requirements during gestation. (*Data from* Refs.[1–3])

concentrates should really be viewed as a complement or supplement to the energy and nutrients provided in the base forage diet (see Patricia Harris and Megan Shepherd's article, "What Would Be Good for All Veterinarians to Know About Equine Nutrition"; and Myriam Hesta and Megan Shepherd's article, "How to Perform a Nutritional Assessment in a First Line/General Practice"; and Nerida Richards and colleagues' article, "Nutritional and Non-Nutritional Aspects of Forage," in this issue). Grains contain high concentrations of starch, a nonstructural carbohydrate that can be a valuable dietary energy source for broodmares. An approximation of the DE content of grains is 2.5 to 3.8 Mcal/kg of DM,[1–3] with some high-fat grains providing even more. The DE in most commercial concentrates containing mixtures of nonstructural carbohydrates, fiber, and vegetable oil or fat will range from 3.0 to 3.8 Mcal/kg DM. In the vast majority of scenarios, grains and concentrates should not constitute more than 50% of the daily DMI. A range of 5% to 30% is probably appropriate in most cases, depending on the body condition score (BCS) of the mare, her health, and the quality and availability of the forage. More details on starch intake are developed in the section discussing the developmental origins of health and diseases.

Horses are somewhat unique as a grazing species owing to their gastrointestinal anatomy and their ability to digest and use dietary fats.[14] The location of the small intestine before the cecum and colon, allows the horse digestive and absorptive capabilities for fats before those fats reach the primary microbial populations in the cecum and colon. Adding dietary fat, therefore, can be an effective strategy to increase dietary calories for broodmares[15] while limiting the potential negative effects of excess starch on offspring health (see Part 3). Research indicates that horses are likely capable of digesting and absorbing dietary fat at concentrations of up to 200 g/kg DM density.[14] The increased energy density of added vegetable fat/oil provides several possible benefits, including flexibility to maximize fiber without sacrificing energy intake, especially when energy requirements are high and DMI may be limited, and potential improvements in fat soluble vitamin absorption[14,16] While horses may be capable of digesting and absorbing upwards of 15% to 20% dietary fat, forage contains only 2% to 4% fat/lipid. In the authors' opinion, the potential benefits of adding fat are more likely to be seen in the range of 5% to 10% dietary fat on a DM basis, calculated by evaluating both forage and concentrate fat intake. The quantity and ratio of dietary omega-6 and omega-3 fatty acids may influence inflammation, alter cell membrane fluidity, and gene expression but much more work is needed in this area.[17] Most forages are rich in omega-3 fatty acids (eg, alpha linolenic acid), so diets that contain at least 50% forage are more likely to have a relatively low omega-6-to-omega-3 ratio.[17] If additional omega-3 fatty acids are desired, flaxseed or flax oil would likely be the most practical to incorporate into the ration, but other sources such as fish and algae oils can also be used depending on the budget and the palatability of the oil for the individual animal.

The pattern of change in crude protein (CP) requirements during gestation is similar to that of DE (see **Fig. 1**). The CP requirements for nonlactating early gestation mares are near or at maintenance levels and increase exponentially in the last third of gestation, and then increase again during lactation. The estimated CP requirements vary around the world, likely owing to different assumptions of protein use for fetal, placental, and uterine development, as well as protein as an energy source in late gestation.

Of greater importance is protein quality, specifically its digestibility and amino acid composition. Under most circumstances, feeding the broodmare a higher quality protein will improve the mare's and developing fetus's ability to use amino acids for tissue development. The amount of available protein can be estimated by subtracting the acid detergent insoluble nitrogen and the nonprotein nitrogen from the CP to provide a better estimate of the protein available for absorption in the horse's small intestine.[1] This information can be provided on demand by most laboratories. The quality of the dietary protein is also improved by providing a composition of essential amino acids that most closely meets the requirements of tissue development.[18] More research is needed to uncover knowledge of broodmare's amino acid requirements, but it is assumed that lysine is the first limiting amino acid and its concentration is approximately 4.3% of the CP requirement.[1] Quality protein sources include soybean meal, alfalfa, and certain milk byproducts, owing to their amino acid composition.

Vitamins, Minerals, and Water Requirements and Recommendations

Essential vitamin and mineral requirements needed to support optimal embryo and fetal development are not clear. Vitamins A and E are normally high in fresh forages (**Table 1**).[19,20] Vitamin D requirements should be met by the horse having sunlight exposure; thus, mares maintained predominantly indoors may require additional vitamin D from the diet (see also Nerida Richards and colleagues' article, "Nutritional and Non-Nutritional Aspects of Forage," in this issue). Horses maintained in an environment where they have sufficient access to immature fresh forages during

Table 1
Ability of forage to meet broodmare fat soluble vitamin requirements

	National Research Council Requirement (500 kg of Body Weight)				Fresh Forage Content (U/d)[a]	Hay Content (U/d)[a]	Is Forage Adequate?[b]
Vitamin	0–120 d Gestation	120–250 d Gestation	250–340 d Gestation	0–30 d Lactation			
Vitamin A (kIU)	30	30	30	30	55–2418[c]	3.6–593.0[c]	Likely inadequate in preserved forage/hay
Vitamin D (IU)	3300	3300	3300	3300	341–19,800	990–61,160	Yes, if sun-exposure is not greatly limited. Higher values found in sun-dried forage/hay compared with fresh pasture.
Vitamin E (IU)	800	800	800	1000	147.5–6556[d]	164–3458[d]	Likely inadequate in preserved forage/hay

[a] Forage and hay calculations based on 500 kg body weight horse and 2% body weight (DM basis) consumption of forage only.
[b] For more information, see Nerida Richards and colleagues' article, "Nutritional and Non-Nutritional Aspects of Forage," in this issue (Forage).
[c] Calculated using the conversion 1 mg β-carotene = 333 IU vitamin A during pregnancy.[20]
[d] Calculated using the conversion 1 mg α-tocopherol = 1.49 IU vitamin E.[1]

late gestation and early lactation will likely be meeting their requirements. In contrast, dried hay (and especially hay that has been stored for a long time) will not be sufficient to maintain adequate vitamin A and E levels in pregnant mares when fed for several months.[21] Serum vitamins A and E concentrations are higher in summer when pregnant mares are in pasture, compared with in winter, when they are typically stabled and fed preserved forage.[19,22] Various B vitamins are found in forage and are also produced by microbes within the equine digestive tract. However, little is known regarding B vitamin requirements during gestation or their relative concentrations in forages.

Mineral supply from the pasture and hay is influenced by soil factors, plant species, state of vegetative growth, and fertilization and irrigation.[23,24] Therefore, specific recommendations regarding the need for mineral supplementation are difficult to state because they depend on the grass type, geographic location, and season of the year. Many fresh forages will meet the macromineral needs (see also Patricia Harris and Megan Shepherd's article, "What Would Be Good for All Veterinarians to Know About Equine Nutrition"; and Nerida Richards and colleagues' article, "Nutritional and Non-Nutritional Aspects of Forage," in this issue) of the mare during gestation for calcium (Ca), phosphorus (P), and potassium (K), but may be low in sodium (Na) and some trace minerals, including copper (Cu), zinc (Zn), and selenium (Se)[23,25–27] **(Table 2)**.

Table 2
Ability of forage to meet broodmare mineral requirements

Mineral	National Research Council Requirement (500 kg)				Cool Season Grass Content (U/d)[a]	Warm Season Grass Content (U/d)[a]	Is Forage Adequate?[b]
	0–120 d Gestation	120–250 d Gestation	250–340 d Gestation	0–30 d Lactation			
Calcium (g)	20.0	28.0	36.0	59.1	20–86	24–89	Yes, although supplementation may be needed during early lactation.
Phosphorus (g)	14.0	20.0	26.3	38.3	12–31	15–98	Yes, although supplementation may be needed during late gestation or early lactation if consuming mature (seed heads present) cool season grass.
Potassium (g)	25.0	25.0	25.9	47.8	37–269	63–298	Yes
Sodium (g)	10.0	10.0	10.0	12.8	0–36.8[c]	Not reported	Supplementation is often needed.
Chloride (g)	40.0	40.0	40.0	45.5	19.6–144.0[c]	Not reported	May require supplementation.
Copper (mg)	100.0	100.0	125.0	125.0	39–87	43–143	Most cool season grasses are too low in Cu to meet the requirements throughout gestation. Some warm season grasses may provide adequate levels.
Zinc (mg)	400.0	400.0	400.0	500.0	149–273	196–634	Supplementation needed.
Selenium (mg)	1.0	1.0	1.0	1.25	0.5–0.7	0.3–4.0	Depends on geographic region.

[a] Grass value calculations based on 500 kg body weight horse and 2% body weight (DM basis) consumption of forage only.
[b] For more information, see Nerida Richards and colleagues' article, "Nutritional and Non-Nutritional Aspects of Forage," in this issue (Forage).
[c] Values for general grass pasture obtained from https://equi-analytical.com/common-feed-profiles/.

Water requirements during gestation seem to be similar to that of maintenance. Observed intakes range from 5.1 L/100 kg body weight[28] to 6.9 L/100 kg body weight[29] in pregnant mares and from 11.9 L/100 kg body weight to 13.9 L/100 kg body weight in lactating mares[1] and are influenced by several factors, including DMI and the environmental temperature. The availability of water is especially important for horses consuming dried preserved forage, such as during cold seasons and when stalled.[30,31] Water restriction during pregnancy results in decreased feed intake and loss of body weight.[29] Thus, water restriction should be avoided.

Key points

- Published energy and nutrient recommendations are best viewed as starting values, which can be tailored to meet individual scenarios.
- Mares' requirements are continuously changing based on stage of gestation and lactation.

NUTRITION OF THE BROODMARE: ADDITIONAL FACTORS TO CONSIDER
Gestation: A Unique Physiologic Status Affecting Metabolism

In early gestation, mares have more efficient glucose absorption, which results in a higher postprandial blood glucose.[32] They also have an enhanced endocrine pancreatic response, resulting in increased postprandial insulin secretion and basal hyperinsulinemia compared with nonpregnant mares.[32] Therefore, mares dedicate the first part of gestation to glucose storage as fat or glycogen in peripheral tissues (adipose tissue, muscles, and liver), to stock up for when fetal needs will increase. This is called "facilitated anabolism."[33] At the end of gestation, mares become more insulin resistant, have a decreased peripheral tissue glucose tolerance, and decreased pancreatic β-cell sensitivity, limiting the glucose storage in maternal tissues.[32,34–36] These changes are associated with a pronounced increase in glucose absorption after meals[32,36,37] (**Fig. 2**). These physiologic adaptations coincide with a strong increase in fetoplacental glucose requirements at the end of gestation; almost 75% of the circulating maternal glucose is used by the uterus and fetal tissues.[38]

Age and parity may alter these metabolic changes in mares. For instance, primiparous mares have been shown to have higher insulin responses to feeding compared with multiparous mares in late gestation, which could mean impaired metabolic adaptation to gestation in primiparous dams.[35]

In late gestation, mares have an increase in lipid mobilization, as observed through the following:

- Increased serum β-hydroxy-butyric acid[39] concentrations, a ketone that serves as an alternate adenosine triphosphate or energy substrate when glucose availability is low.[40]
- Some authors observed an increase in the plasma triglyceride concentration reaching a plateau from the seventh month of gestation onward[41,42]; however, not all investigators have observed such a change.[39,43]
- Plasma cholesterol concentrations are stable during gestation[44] and lower than in nonpregnant mares,[39] which may result from use of cholesterol for steroid synthesis.[45,46]

Nitrogen metabolism also adapts to the pregnant state. During gestation, the plasma total protein concentration varies,[39,41–43,47] although it remains lower than in nonpregnant mares.[39,42,43] Plasma urea concentrations are higher in late gestion

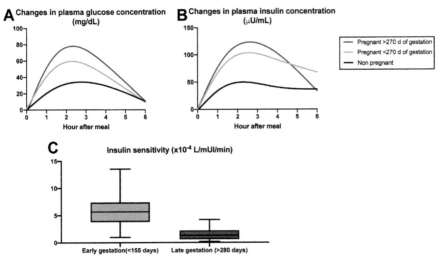

Fig. 2. Evolution of glucose metabolism during pregnancy in mares. (*A*) Changes in plasma glucose concentration after a meal in nonpregnant (*black*, n = 4) and pregnant mares at less than 270 days (*green*, n = 6) or greater than 270 days (*red*, n = 5) pregnancy. Pregnant and especially late pregnant mares are more efficient in absorbing sugar ingested. (*B*) Changes in plasma insulin concentration after a meal in nonpregnant (*black*) and pregnant mares at less than 270 days (*green*) or greater than 270 days (*red*) gestation. Pregnant mares produce more insulin in response to plasma glucose increase, but this response does not change between early and late gestation. (*C*) Insulin sensitivity in early (<155 days, n = 12) and late (>280 days, n = 37) gestation in French-Anglo Arabian mares. Insulin sensitivity decreases as gestation progresses. (Courtesy of Abigail L. Fowden, Development and Neuroscience University of Cambridge; with permission.)

mares than in nonpregnant mares, reflecting the increased need for amino acids to support anabolic processes during gestation.[39,43] Metabolic changes are summarized in **Fig. 3**.

Key points

- During the end of gestation, maternal metabolism allows for maximum glucose redirection to the fetus to meet its needs for full growth.

- The high use of glucose by the fetus leads the mare to use mainly her lipid reserves to meet both her own and fetal needs. This factor highlights the importance of the first months of gestation for the buildup of lipid reserves. A BCS of 5 (1–9 scale), however, should be targeted to avoid the detrimental effects of overweight and obesity on both maternal and fetal health.

- If there has been insufficient lipid storage earlier in pregnancy, the mare will need to also draw on her protein reserves to meet her own energy needs, as well as those of the fetus.

Considering the Season in Mare's Nutrition

Providing optimal nutrition for broodmares requires consideration of multiple factors, each likely to be changing daily over the approximately 340 days of gestation. Feral and semiferal horses manage excellent reproductive performance without human intervention,[48–50] even though body condition loss is often observed in late gestation.[48,49,51] Their success may be attributed to reproductive and feeding strategies

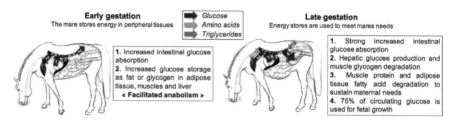

Fig. 3. Evolution of the mare's metabolism during gestation. Changes in carbohydrate, protein, and lipid metabolism allow the mare to provide for the needs of the fetus while having limited food availability in winter.

that evolved over 30 to 40 million years in temperate grassland environments, enabling adaptation to an environment that changed in a predictable manner with each season. Feral and semiferal horse herds today still foal and breed during some of the longest days of the year.[48,50] The connection of reproductive patterns with day length and nutrition are well-recognized,[52] with an evolutionary benefit to synchronizing reproduction, growth, and lactation needs with the environmentally available energy sources.

The diet is the primary source of energy, with adipose (and muscle) tissue serving as a supplementary source when the diet is limited. For domesticated broodmares, the responsibility for nutritional and reproductive management is that of the caregivers. In addition to gestational needs, changes in energy requirements owing to thermoregulation, feed acquisition, and disease in broodmares have been poorly studied. Optimal broodmare nutrition can be achieved by understanding and accounting for each of these factors.

In **Fig. 1**, the DE and CP requirements of broodmares during gestation are overlaid on day length, one of the primary environmental variables that leads to changes in ambient temperature and forage growth and availability. The day length curves represent day length experienced by mares that were due in mid to late winter (February), early to midspring (April), or early summer (June) in the northern hemisphere. Those feeding broodmares can examine this figure and not only consider what the broodmare's requirements are, but also the environmental energy and nutrient sources and sinks by which she is being influenced. Here are a few examples.

- A broodmare at 320 days of gestation and due in February has both high DE and CP requirements, yet day length is short, and ambient temperatures and fresh forage availability are low. Her caregiver should provide high-quality preserved forage and consider a complementary concentrate feed to provide the required DE and CP (including essential amino acids). Another broodmare at the same stage in gestation, but instead due in June has identical requirements, but is in an environment where day length is long, and the ambient temperatures and fresh forage availability are high. In this case, the caregiver can provide significantly less complementary feeds, based on what the mare's environment provides.
- A lactating broodmare at 40 days of gestation and due in February has high DE and CP requirements, primarily related to lactation. Day length is increasing, but the ambient temperature and fresh forage availability are just beginning to increase. To meet the nutritional demands of early lactation, she will require high-quality preserved forage and possibly a complementary concentrate. Another broodmare at the same stage in gestation, but instead due in June, has identical requirements, but is in an environment where day length has already

peaked, leading to higher ambient temperatures and likely plentiful fresh forage availability.

- Finally, **Fig. 1** highlights a nutritional opportunity during early and midgestation to increase a broodmare's BCS when energy and nutrient requirements are low (in a natural environment, that is, if the mare is not overweight or obese). Obviously, this period is shorter for the lactating mare, extending from late lactation to the last third of gestation. An example would be a mare who foaled in midspring, was bred 1 month later, and her foal had been weaned at the end of the summer. She should be able to take advantage of good fall forage and relatively low energy and nutrient requirements of midgestation to increase her BCS. Another example would be a mare with no foal at her side, bred in March, taking advantage of spring forage to improve BCS. It will be much more challenging to increase BCS during early lactation, even with good spring forage, or in late gestation, because energy will be partitioned away from the mare and to the rapidly developing fetus.

The BCS is an indicator of energy balance. The BCS is a standardized subjective evaluation of subcutaneous fat stores. The evidence seems to indicate a moderate BCS of 5 (1–9 scale[53]) and 3 (1–5 scale[54,55]) in the broodmare as a target through gestation. Fat stores provide energy when the less predictable short-term environmental patterns of dietary energy result in a deficit. Maintaining sufficient energy savings can help to weather some of the unpredictability in other energy sources and sinks. The majority of evidence indicates that domesticated broodmares are best managed by maintaining a moderate BCS, but there remains some lack of clarity regarding how changing planes of nutrition, and even a changing BCS, may have positive or negative impacts on reproductive performance and progeny success.[5] Future work should focus on investigating how dietary energy and stored energy are communicated to the gonadotropic and somatotropic axes to influence reproduction and growth.[56] The knowledge uncovered here might allow for more precise and nuanced modifications of the diet through gestation to optimize health and performance of the offspring, but also the continued reproductive performance of the broodmare.

Key points

- Feral mares are bred and foal in the longest days, which coincides with increased nutrient availability from grazing. In midgestation (120–250 days of gestation), the fiber content of the forage increases and nutrient availability, as well as day length decrease. Late gestation (250–340 days of gestation) begins with low nutrient availability and short day lengths, but rapidly increasing nutrient availability coincides with exponential fetal growth.

- The body condition of the mare represents her energy savings, and hence her ability to provide for a rapidly developing fetus in late gestation and reproduce in the subsequent breeding season. In most situations it is prudent to maintain a moderate BCS (5/9) throughout gestation, with the understanding that, during lactation and late gestation, energy partitioning will first direct resources to milk and fetal development.

Fetal Nutrition During Pregnancy

Development and role of the placenta

During the first 40 days of the embryo's life, histotrophic secretions (endometrial glands secretions) are the main source of nutrients for the embryo.[4] Briefly, the embryo enters the uterus around 6 to 7 days after ovulation.[57] At this time and for the next 20 to 25 days, the embryo is surrounded by a capsule composed of glycoproteins, which regulates the assimilation of uterine secretions.[4,58] Between 20 and 30 days, the embryo capsule disintegrates so that the trophectoderm (precursor of placenta) is directly in contact with the endometrium.[59] Trophoblastic cells (placental epithelial cells involved in feto-maternal exchanges) develop and protrude into the endometrial glands, which facilitates histotrophic nutrition before implantation.[60,61] Thus, the embryo solely depends on the uterine environment for its development during this period.

The following nutrition and metabolic factors affect the uterine environment in the mare:

- Maternal obesity and excessively increased insulin resistance (knowing that insulin resistance is increased physiologically in response to gestation) in mares has been shown to increase the expression of genes and/or proteins involved in inflammation, lipid homeostasis, growth factors, and cell stress in uterine secretions, the endometrium, and embryos.[62,63] Moreover, alterations in the concentration of lipids involved in cell membrane integrity and signal transduction was observed in embryos of obese mares.[62]
- Conversely, supplementing the diet of overweight mares with omega-3 fatty acids–rich fat sources has been shown to increase the expression of genes involved in embryo and trophoblast development[64] and to decrease expression of proteins involved in inflammation.[63] Nevertheless, this has not been shown to overcome adverse effects of maternal obesity.

Although there is so far little knowledge on specific nutritional needs in early gestation in the mare, the quality of maternal nutrition should not be neglected at this stage.

The placenta is a complex organ involved in gestation maintenance, fetomaternal exchange, metabolism, hormones synthesis and immunity. In the mare, 2 different placentas develop during gestation (**Fig. 4**):

- A transient trophoblast (chorionic girdle) from 30 to 120 to 140 days of gestation.[4]
- A definitive noninvasive placenta that forms close interdigitations (microcotyledons) with the endometrium from 40 days. Two trophoblasts are involved in fetomaternal exchanges. The hemotrophic trophoblast lines the microcotyledons in close contact with the endometrium[65] and ensures exchanges between maternal and fetal bloods. The histotrophic trophoblast is located at the basis of microcotyledons and collects uterine gland secretions. Therefore, both hemotrophic and histotrophic nutrition play essential roles for fetal development.

Of interest is that the placental microvilli lengthen and branch out throughout gestation[66] and can adapt to a certain extent to adverse maternal nutritional conditions. For instance, in moderately undernourished mares, normal fetal growth was observed[67] thanks to placental adaptations:

- Increased volume of microcotyledonary vessels and
- Increased expression of genes involved in amino and fatty acids catabolism as well as vitamin transport.[68]

However, placental structural adaptations cannot overcome severe undernutrition.[69]

Developmental origins of health and diseases and critical periods of embryo and fetal development

The concept of developmental origins of health and diseases stipulates that fetal adaptations to an adverse in utero environment induce permanent changes in the fetus that are revealed as the individual ages or in the presence of an adverse postnatal

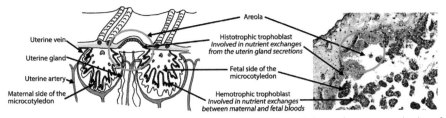

A **The transient invasive placenta**

Allantois

Amnios

Yolk sac

Chorionic girdle   **38 d embryo**

1. Apical cells become binucleated
2 to 4. Binucleated cells penetrate the endometrial stroma

The chorionic girdle produces equine Chorionic Gonadotropin (eCG), involved in maintenance of pregnancy.
Chorionic girdle is observed from 30 to 140 dpo.

B **The definitive non-invasive placenta**

Areola

Uterine vein

Uterine gland

Uterine artery

Maternal side of the microcotyledon

Histotrophic trophoblast
Involved in nutrient exchanges from the uterin gland secretions

Fetal side of the microcotyledon

Hemotrophic trophoblast
Involved in nutrient exchanges between maternal and fetal bloods

Fig. 4. Transient invasive and definitive noninvasive placentas. (*A*) Development and roles of the chorionic girdles. (*B*) Structure of the definitive chorioallantois. ([*A*] *Adapted from* Allen WR, Wilsher S. A Review of Implantation and Early Placentation in the Mare. *Placenta.* 2009;30(12):1005-1015; and Allen WR, Stewart F. Equine placentation. *Reproduction, Fertility and Development.* 2001;13(8):623-634; and Wooding FBP, Burton G. *Comparative Placentation: Structures, Functions and Evolution.*, Springer, 2008; and [*B*] *From* Steven DH, Samuel CA. Anatomy of the placetal barrier in the mare. *J Reprod Fert.* 1975;Suppl. 23:579-582; with permission.)

environment. First demonstrated in humans,[70,71] this phenomenon has also been shown in animal models and domestic animals,[72,73] including horses.[74–77]

The adverse effects on fetal and postnatal development have been shown to differ, depending on the gestational stage at which they were applied.[71] This finding implies the existence of critical periods of development that are directly correlated with the timeline of fetal organ development and maturation. Mechanisms underlying these effects involve modification of gene expression without changing of DNA structure (epigenetic mechanisms[78]), which are sensitive to the environment and can persist until adulthood.

Critical periods of development can be defined depending on the organ concerned (**Fig. 5**). In the horse, by day 35, the embryo has completed most of its organogenesis[4,79] and is referred to as a fetus.[4] This time of gestation also coincides with the onset of placentation. These differences between organs have an important impact on fetal development in response to maternal feeding as the embryo and fetal organ development and maturation depend on the maternal environment (metabolism and nutrition). For more detailed information and references, see **Fig. 6**.

Although the developmental origins of health and diseases and the importance of critical periods have been well-described in animal models and some domestic species, so far, few data are available in horses. Nevertheless, maternal nutrition has been demonstrated to affect foal metabolism, onset of osteochondrosis, and the maturation of reproductive organs (**Fig. 7**).[77]

Key points

- The horse embryo depends solely on nutrients from uterine glands until 30 to 40 days after ovulation. Uterine environment may vary depending on maternal nutrition and metabolism.

- Obese mares may have a more inflammatory endometrial environment, which could impact embryo health and development in the first month of gestation.

- Organogenesis is largely completed at 40 days after ovulation, but organs continue to mature afterward, and critical periods of development vary between organs.

- Maternal environment (and nutrition) from early gestation has long term effects on offspring development.

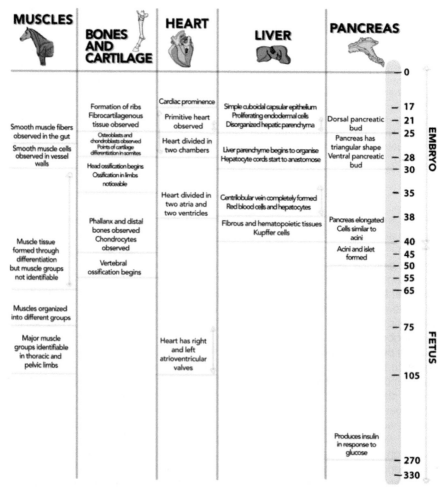

Fig. 5. The timing of organ development in the equine embryo and fetus. *Horizontal lines* indicate the specific day of gestation and *vertical arrows* indicate periods of gestation where observations were made.

EQUINE FETAL DEVELOPMENT

TEETH

0   120   140   160   220

- Ossification of alveolar cavities
- Dental germs in the alveolar groove
- Alveolar septa development

- Early appearance of P3 dental germ (140)
- Cusps of P3 visible
- P2, P3, P4 germs visible (146)

- Appearance of incisor teeth germ (160-224)

Soana et al (1998). The teeth of the horse: evolution and anatomo-morphological and radiographic study of their development in the foetus

PANCREAS

0   25   30   40   50

- Appearance of the dorsal pancreatic bud
- Strong Oct4 staining

- Pancreas as a triangular shape
- Located between intestinal loops
- Ventral pancreatic buds form parts of pancreatic heads

- Pancreas elongated
- Cells similar to acini

- Acini and pancreatic islets formed

Rodrigues et al (2014). Prenatal development of the digestive system in the horse

	175-230 DAYS	290-327 DAYS
Basal insulin (µU/mL)	6 ± 1.1	9.05 ± 1.4
Basal glucose (nmol/L)	2.79 ± 0.36	3.09 ± 0.22
Insulin after glucose infusion	No effect	Increased insulin release (even more in more mature fetuses)

Less mature => cortisol < 15ng/mL
More mature => cortisol > 15ng/mL

Fowden et al (2005). Maturation of pancreatic b-cell function in the foetal horse during late gestation

INSULIN RELEASE AFTER GLUCOSE INJECTION

	150-210 D	240-270 D	270-300 D	>300 D
Basal insulin (µU/mL)	8.0 ± 1.0	7.0 ± 1.5	6.5 ± 1.0	9.0 ± 2.0
Basal glucose (nmol/L)	2.41 ± 0.19	3.09 ± 0.24	2.59 ± 0.21	2.77 ± 0.33
Insulin after glucose infusion	No effect	No effect	Small rise	High rise

Fowden and Silver (1995). Pancreatic b-cell function in the foetal foal and mare

+ From 260 d equine pancreatic α cells are functional but are unresponsive to variations in glycaemia until after birth

Fowden et al (1998). Pancreatic α-cell function in the foetal foal during late gestation

LIVER

0   21-25   30   35-38   40

- Simple cuboidal capsular epithelium (21)
- Proliferating endodermal cells (21)
- Disorganized hepatic parenchyma (25)
- Hepatoblasts (25)
- Strong Oct4 staining

- Liver parenchyma begins to organise
- Hepatocyte cords start to anastomose

- Canalicular vein completely formed
- Red blood cells and hepatocytes

- Fibrous and hematopoietic tissues
- Kupffer cells
- Oct4 restricted to the hepatocytes

Rodrigues et al (2014). Prenatal development of the digestive system in the horse
Franciolli et al (2011). Characteristics of the equine embryo from days 15 to 107 of pregnancy

The liver is an active site of hematopoiesis at 100 days (but maybe before)

Barbosa et al (2014). Haematopoiesis in the equine foetal liver suggests immune preparedness

HEART

0   17-19   24-25   21-28   38   75-115

Cardiac prominence

Primitive heart observed

Heart divided in two chambers

Heart divided in two atria and two ventricles

Heart has right and left atrioventricular valves

Beating and discernible from 20 d in the ventral quadrant

Rodrigues et al (2014). Prenatal development of the digestive system in the horse
Franciolli et al (2011). Characteristics of the equine embryo from days 15 to 107 of pregnancy
Aben and Webster (2005). A review of legislation and early placentation in the mare
Rodrigues et al (2014). Embryonic and fetal development of the aortic respiratory apparatus in horses from 20 to 115 days of gestation

BONES AND CARTILAGE

0   25   30   35   45   55

- Formation of ribs
- Fibrocartilagenous tissue observed

- Osteoblasts, chondroblasts and fibroblasts observed
- Points of cartilage differentiation in somites

- Head ossification begins
- Ossification in limbs noticeable

- Phalanx and distal bones observed
- Chondrocytes observed

- Vertebral ossification begins

Barreto et al (2018). Organogenesis of the musculoskeletal system in horse embryo and early fetuses
Franciolli et al (2011). Characteristics of the equine embryo and fetus from days 15 to 107 of pregnancy
Acker et al (2001). Morphologic stages of the equine embryo proper on day 17 to 40 after ovulation

MUSCLES

0   28   30   65   75   105

Smooth muscle fibers observed in the gut

Smooth muscle cells observed in vessel walls

Muscle tissue is formed through differentiation but muscle groups are not identifiable

Muscles organised into different groups

Major muscle groups identifiable in thoracic and pelvic limbs

Barreto et al (2018). Organogenesis of the musculoskeletal system in horse embryo and early fetuses

GONADS

0   25   270

Ovary containing primordial follicles and unorganized primordial cells is observed

Inguinal migration begins

+ Fetal gonads grow rapidly and peak between the 6th and 8th months of gestation when they reach the weight of adult gonads before regressing

Cole and Hart (1930). The development and hormonal content of fetal horse gonads.
Gaian (1955). Studies on the development of the embryonic ovary in swine, cattle and horse.
Franciolli et al (2011). Characteristics of the equine embryo and fetus from days 15 to 107 of pregnancy.
Bergin et al (1970). A developmental concept of equine cryptorchism.

MISCELLANEOUS

- Onset of neurulation at 13 d
- Lung buds are observable at 24 d
- Formation of the pituitary gland between 31 and 48 d   (depending on the study)
- Formation of the mammary gland at 80 d

0   22   26   28   30

- Urogenital ridges observed
- Pronephric gut observed
- Nephric vesicles contain tubules

Glomeruli observed

- Ureter identified
- Mesonephric vesicles opened in mesonephric ducts

Mesonephros fully formed

Acker et al (2001). Morphologic stages of the equine embryo proper on day 17 to 40 of ovulation
Franciolli et al (2014). Characteristics of the equine embryo and fetus from days 15 to 107 of pregnancy
Galeas et al (2014). Contribution and the establishment of the three germ layers in the early horse conceptus.

DEVELOPMENTAL ORIGINS OF HEALTH AND DISEASE

The nutrition of the broodmare during gestation and lactation is not only important for her own health and fertility, but also for the development and health of her foal. The limited information available in horses is detailed here.

Maternal Energy Restriction

Moderate (70%–80% of energy requirements) undernutrition does not seem to affect in utero or preweaning postnatal growth of the foal.[67,80,81] Placental[68] (increased vascularization and nutrient transport) and maternal[67] (decreased insulin secretion following a glucose challenge, lipid mobilization) adaptive mechanisms seem to be sufficient to sustain fetal growth. However, moderate maternal undernutrition is associated with delayed testicular maturation at 12 months of age (beginning of puberty), decreased insulin sensitivity at 19 months of age, and decreased cannon width from 19 months of age.[82] Furthermore, severe undernutrition leads to in utero growth retardation.[69]

Energy Overfeeding and Obesity

Because horses are herbivorous, their body condition varies according to season and the nutritional availability of pasture.[51] A healthy horse in outdoor conditions will generally have a higher BCS in summer than in winter.[83] A horse is considered overweight when its BCS exceeds 6[53] (or 3.5 if using the 1–5 scale[54,55]) and obese when its BCS exceeds 7[84] (or 4 using the 1–5 scale). Obesity can also be chronic, as some horses maintain a high BCS throughout the year, with no seasonal variation[83]; see Megan Shepherd and colleagues' article, "Nutritional Considerations When Dealing with an Obese Adult Equine," in this issue.

A mare can be overweight owing to short-term overnutrition during pregnancy (or excess gestational fat deposition). Alternatively, obesity can result from long-term overnutrition and/or metabolic disease. These 2 scenarios may have different effects on foal health and development:

- *Obesity in late gestation*: Overnutrition during pregnancy, leading to obesity in late gestation, does not affect a foal's birthweight.[80,85] Nevertheless, decreased weight and thoracic perimeter at 2 months of age have been described when excess maternal nutrition is continuous from 2 months gestation.[86] This finding may be due to decreased milk production in overnourished mares during the first 2 months of lactation.[86] When overnutrition begins later (eighth month of gestation), a foal's growth between birth and 3 months of age was not affected[81] (later effects have not been studied).
- *Long-term obesity*: Maternal obesity from the time of insemination, together with decreased insulin sensitivity and increased plasma concentrations of

Fig. 6. The timing of organ development in the equine embryo and fetus, detailed version. Each organ is separated by *horizontal lines* and represented by an icon. Part 1 features the teeth, pancreas, liver, and heart. Part 2 features the bones and cartilage, muscles, gonads, and a summary of neurons, lungs, pituitary gland, mammary glands, and kidneys. For each organ, a timeline expressed in days after ovulation presents the major developmental events, described in brown boxes. Detailed results in fetal insulin production are also provided for pancreas (tables and figures). For muscles, the *blue line* over the timeline highlights a period more than a set point. References are written directly in the figure for clarity.

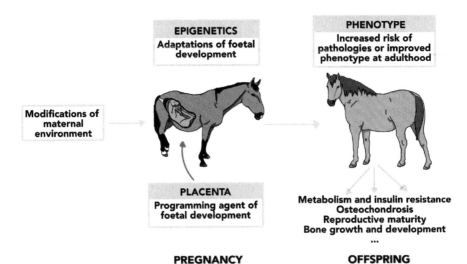

Fig. 7. The principles of the developmental origins of health and disease in the horse.

inflammatory biomarkers in late gestation, did not affect the birth weight or the growth of foals when monitored until at least 18 months of age.[87,88]

- Nevertheless, maternal obesity was associated with increased systemic inflammation, decreased insulin sensitivity, and an increased incidence of osteochondrosis in foals.[87] Maternal adiposity at the base of the tail, as measured by ultrasound assessment, has also been positively correlated to the same measurement in 4-month-old foals.[89]

The Source of Energy Matters

The use and effects of starch

Epidemiologic observations demonstrated that the risks for a foal to develop osteochondrosis were 11-fold higher when the broodmare's diet included "concentrated feeds" during gestation, compared with forage only.[90] This study, however, did not consider the quantity or the source of the concentrates given to the mares, albeit experimental studies performed using starch-rich barley as a concentrate validated this observation.[67] Nevertheless, in field conditions, forage is sometimes not available in sufficient quantity and quality to cover the mare's needs and the provision of an energy-rich concentrated feed remains a practical necessity. To decrease the potential detrimental effects of starch on foal development, starch quantity per meal and per day has to be closely monitored.

The results from several experimental studies, where the source of energy used was known can help to build these recommendations:

- *Study 1[67]:* Mares received 1.7 g of starch/kg body weight per meal as barley in addition to hay and haylage, or hay and haylage only during the last 4.5 months of gestation. Mares fed with barley produced more foals affected with osteochondrosis lesions at 6 months of age (45%) compared with mares fed with hay and haylage only (17%). This difference was not observed at 12 and 18 months of age, with some lesions spontaneously resolved and some new lesions in different individuals.[82]
- *Study 2 (MR, PCP personal communication):* Mares were fed with either a maximum of 0.75 g of starch/kg body weight per meal (range, 0.40–0.75,

n = 5) or a minimum of 1.1 g of starch/kg body weight per meal (range, 1.1–1.6, n = 5) during the last 2 months of gestation. Both groups received the same amount and type of forage during gestation. As a result, 12-month-old foals born to mares fed the high-starch meals experienced a higher incidence (80%) of osteochondrosis lesions, as compared with foals of mares fed low-starch meals (20%) (**Fig. 8**). Unfortunately, the foals were not monitored further.

These results indicate that excess starch provided to mares per meal has an impact on the osteoarticular development of foals. However, the role of starch source has not been fully investigated. Regardless, for now, the authors recommend that the starch plus sugar intake in pregnant mares should not exceed 1 g/kg of body weight per meal. Limits per day are currently unknown.

Feeding the broodmare with starch-rich concentrates may also affect colostrum quality; it has been shown to decrease the IgG colostrum concentration at birth, in comparison with mares fed with forage only.[12,91] A French epidemiologic study showed that mares producing foals with osteochondrosis lesions had colostrum that was poorer in IgG compared with mares that produced foals that remained healthy.[92]

The use and effects of fats

Because the diets richer in starch were also more energy dense in the previously mentioned studies, discrimination between the effect of starch and that of energy content per se on the foals' osteoarticular development is impossible. Feeding pregnant mares with a diet rich in starch (corn, >1 g starch/kg body weight per meal) was shown to alter the glucose metabolism of foals during preweaning growth compared with a diet rich in lipids (corn oil, <0.15 g starch/kg body weight per meal, 14% DM fat). These results indicate that vegetable oil or fat may be a good way to increase the energetic density of the diet of pregnant mares, without increasing the starch content, thus limiting detrimental effects on foal's development.[93]

The fatty acid composition may be important, because some fatty acids have immunomodulatory properties and could, therefore, affect the pathways involved not only in fertility, but also in inflammation. Essential fatty acids are also involved in fetal neuronal development. Thus, dietary fatty acids could affect maternal and uterine environment quality and, subsequently, embryo and fetal development. This point is particularly important for mares fed dry forage and concentrates, because the omega-3 to

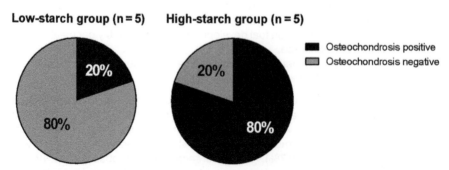

Fig. 8. The incidence of osteochondrosis at 12 months of age was higher in foals born to mares fed with high-starch meals (>110 g/100 kg body weight) compared with foals born to mares fed with low-starch meals (<75 g/100 kg body weight) (*MR, PCP personal communication*).

omega-6 ratios are low in dry forage and especially in cereals, in contrast with grass and fresh forage.[17,94,95] Because horses evolved grazing on fresh grass, the dietary omega-3 contents and omega-3 to omega-6 ratio are most probably important, especially around conception. However, there is little confirmed information regarding the exact quantities and ratios that might be optimal.

For now, supplementing mares with fat sources rich in omega-3 fatty acids has only been shown to increase the total omega-3 and docosahexaenoic acid transfer from the dam to the fetus at birth[96,97] and to increase lymphocyte proliferation in 7-day-old foals.[98] No other effects on colostrum quality or foal growth have been demonstrated.[96–98] The effects of maternal supplementation with omega-3 fatty acid during gestation on maternal and foal metabolism remain unknown. Both fish/algae and flax-seed oils have been studied independently, but more studies are needed to compare the efficiency of both sources. For now, we recommend flaxseed oil because it is more practical.

The use and effects of proteins

Protein needs are increased during gestation in mares. The quality of proteins, and especially the content of essential amino acids, such as lysine and threonine, is crucial for foal development.[1] It must be noted that, although the role of protein excess in foals in the development of osteochondrosis lesions has been ruled out,[99] to the best of our knowledge, no studies have been performed on the effect of overall protein quality fed to broodmares on the long-term health of the foals.

As an example, L-arginine is an essential amino acid during pregnancy and growth in the horse. The particular abundance of arginine in mare's milk seems to indicate that L-arginine may be needed in much greater proportions in foals than in the offspring of other species.[100] Supplementation with L-arginine (100 g/d) during the last 4 months of gestation to primiparous mares improved their glucose metabolism and increased the placental expression of genes involved in glucose and fatty acid transport, but did not affect placental and birth weights or the growth of foals monitored until 2 months of age.[47] In a study where mares' parity was not described, supplementation with 100 g of L-arginine/day from 21 days before foaling increased uterine arterial blood flow and shortened the gestational length by 12 days, without affecting the placental and foal weight at birth.[101] The effects on gestational duration were, however, not observed in another study supplementing 50 g of L-arginine per day in pregnant mares from 90 days before foaling.[102]

Further studies are needed to determine the effect of protein deficiency or excess, as well as the effect of protein quality during gestation, on foals' long-term health. Interestingly, alteration of protein intake in other species has been shown to affect the behavior, health and lifespan of the offspring.[103] Because some amino acids can affect absorption and cell use of other amino acids, dietary amino acid contents should be checked in accordance to the known optimal ratios, which may change between the different physiologic states.[1]

Key points

- Overnutrition and undernutrition of the mare are detrimental to foal's health. The energy content of the mare's feed should be considered according to mare's BCS and DMI.

- Forage should be the basis of a broodmare's diet.

- Broodmares should not receive more than 1 g of starch plus sugar/kg body weight per meal to limit the detrimental effects of nonstructural carbohydrates on a foal's metabolic and osteoarticular health.

- Vegetable oil or fat may be a good way to increase the energy content of the diet.
- The quantity (and ratio to omega-6 fatty acids) of omega-3 fatty acids may be important.

Feed Supplements: Useful for Improving the Health of the Future Foal?

As presented in section 1.3, the geographic location, season, soil factors, plant species, state of vegetative growth, and fertilization and irrigation can affect the amino acid and fatty acid profiles, as well as the vitamin and mineral content of the forage. Moreover, using cereal grains to provide additional energy can alter the balance between minerals. Depending on these factors, supplementation is not always needed and should be carefully thought out.

Some vitamins and minerals easily cross the placenta to be delivered to the fetus during gestation. In contrast, some are weakly transported through the placenta and their storage in colostrum is therefore essential for the newborn foal. For instance, vitamins A and E are poorly transferred through the placenta but are concentrated in colostrum,[104] whereas iodine is actively transferred through placenta and is also rich in colostrum and milk.[105] Some other nutrients, like copper, are stored in the fetal liver during gestation and used during fetal growth to compensate for low milk concentrations.[106]

Vitamins

Studies on the effects of vitamin excess and deficiency on the health of foals are lacking. In other species, it has been shown that maternal imbalance in D and B group vitamins could affect not only in utero growth, but also long-term growth, metabolism diseases and behavior of the offspring.[107] As presented in Section 1.3, vitamins E and D, as well as β-carotene, concentrations are high in fresh grass in spring and summer, implying that supplementation may not be needed if mares are kept in pasture and bred between spring and summer.[21] Conversely, mares bred out of season or fed dried forage would benefit from vitamin supplementation as observed in the following studies.

Natural vitamin E (RRR-α-tocopherol) oral supplementation, fed above the National Research Council (NRC) requirements (200%–300%)[1] has been shown to increase the concentration of vitamin E in the colostrum, milk, and plasma of neonatal foals as well as the immunoglobulin concentration in colostrum and plasma of 3-day-old foals, compared with mares fed a diet deficient in vitamin E (15%–30% of the NRC requirements).[108] Moreover, oral supplementation with β-carotene (1000 mg/d) to mares fed with hay and concentrates from 2 weeks before foaling, increased the concentration of β-carotene in colostrum and plasma of foals at 1 day of age.[109] To our knowledge, long-term effects of these supplements on foal health and development have not been studied yet. The observed increased insemination success with β-carotene supplementation, however, may imply an effect on the uterine environment, and then, on embryo and fetal development.[109]

Minerals and microminerals

Calcium and phosphorus. The effects of an inverse calcium:phosphorus ratio during pregnancy have not been studied, but may negatively impact the foal's bone and articular development. Mares consuming diets providing 80% of the NRC requirement for calcium (Ca:P = 1.1, lower limit) during late gestation gave birth to foals with thinner and weaker cannon bones, which persisted through the period of observation (10 months of age).[110]

Copper. Copper is a micromineral essential for the development of cartilage and bone. Although pregnant mare copper supplementation above NRC requirements (200%–300%) have been shown to decrease the prevalence of articular cartilage lesions in growing foals,[111,112] there is, so far, no substantial evidence that pregnant mares should be supplemented over the recommendations if the diet is correctly balanced (especially the Cu:Zn ratio).[1,113] Maternal copper supplementation does not affect milk copper concentration or foal plasma copper concentrations, but increases the foal's liver copper storage.[106] These results imply that fetal liver copper storage is essential for a foal's osteoarticular health, especially because supplementing the foal after birth will not counter the detrimental effects of in utero deficiencies.[112]

Selenium. Selenium deficiencies during gestation have been associated with white muscle disease in foals, a myodegenerative pathology, affecting skeletal and cardiac muscles and leading to the death of the foal in most cases.[114] The form of selenium distributed to pregnant mares is potentially important, as inorganic and organic selenium are not absorbed and incorporated into body tissues equally.[115,116] In fact, supplementing the mares with selenium yeast in the 2 last months of gestation increased the expression of genes involved in the proliferation and cellular immune response in lymphocytes of growing foals, compared with mares supplemented with sodium selenite,[117] which may imply improved foal immunity. Moreover, supplementation with selenium yeast (0.65 ppm vs. 0.35 ppm Se in total diet [650% vs. 350% of NRC requirements]) during the last 4 months of gestation has been shown to increase the selenium concentration in the plasma and muscle of foals, but without affecting the glutathione peroxidase activity in the foal's plasma.[118] Special caution must be paid to selenium excess because the optimal range is narrow, that is, the level of toxicity close to the recommended amounts (0.2 mg/100 kg body weight is recommended in pregnancy, and the safe upper limit is considered to be 1 mg/100 kg body weight[1]). Organic forms of selenium may have a stronger beneficial effect on foal development compared with inorganic selenium, but more studies are needed to confirm these effects.

Iodine. Thyroid function is involved in metabolism, bone development and growth. Foals have a very high iodine serum concentration at birth that slowly decreases during growth,[105] which correlates to tri-iodothyronine and thyroxine plasma concentrations.[87] Transplacental iodine transport may therefore be efficient. A strong excess or deficiency in iodine in the maternal diet have been linked to congenital hypothyroidism in foals, which can be characterized by thyroid gland hyperplasia and musculoskeletal abnormalities in foals, as well as an increased gestational duration.[119] More work is needed to study the effects of iodine intake on long-term foal development. Seaweed supplementation can cause iodine excess; therefore, iodine levels in seaweed supplements have to be carefully considered before feeding seaweed to pregnant mares.

Other minerals and microminerals. Other minerals and microminerals are also involved in metabolism regulation (chromium), inflammation and oxidation (iron), as well as bone and teeth development (fluorine), and their imbalances may also impact the long-term health of the offspring. Mineral supplementation should be developed in accordance with the balance between minerals and microminerals, because it can affect their absorption and cell use.[1] More work is needed to develop specific recommendations for pregnant mares.

The use of probiotics. The intestinal microbiota in early life can impact metabolic health, growth, and behavior of the individual.[120] The equine microbiota influences the risk of resistance to endoparasites,[118] colic[121] and metabolic syndrome.[122] However, few studies have focused on the effect of the mare's gut microbiota on foal health. Few prebiotics have been tested in pregnant mares so far, despite a large number of yeast and bacteria strains available on the market. Effects observed from one strain of probiotics cannot be extrapolated to other strains. Safety of strains and effective dosing are unknown, which calls for a cautious use of these nutraceuticals in mares (see also Ruth Bishop and David A. Dzanis' article, "Staying on the Right Side of the Regulatory Authorities"; and Ingrid Vervuert and Meri Stratton-Phelps' article, "The Safety and Efficacy in Horses of Certain Nutraceuticals that Claim to Have Health Benefits," in this issue).

Pregnant mare probiotic supplementation, however, has shown some beneficial effects on foal health and development. Pregnant mares were supplemented with live yeast (*Saccharomyces cerevisiae* CNCM-I1079, 7.10^{10} colony-forming units per day) from 8 days before to 4 days after foaling. Their foals had a decreased quantity of *Escherichia coli* and enterobacteria in the feces at 10 days of age, an increased proportion of normal-looking feces, and a tendency to an increase in the average daily gain from birth until 20 days of age.[123] In another study, the supplementation of pregnant mares with fermented feed products from 45 days before foaling until 60 days after did not affect the fecal pH of mares or the fecal concentration of culturable bacteria, but increased the maternal fecal proportion of acetate. Moreover, foals born to supplemented mares had an earlier establishment of gut microbiota and gut function, possibly leading to an increased weight between 19 and 60 days of age.[124]

In conclusion, studies on the long-term effect of probiotics during pregnancy and/or growth are needed to help develop recommendations on the use of these supplements in breeding horses. It is also worth noting that safety in pregnant animals has not been tested for most supplements. The effects of other nutritional supplements on other aspects, such as muscular and cardiovascular development as well as bone strength and resistance, remain to be studied in the horse.

Key points

- Supplementation must be carefully thought out because some supplements have not been tested for safety.
- Vitamins and minerals in excess can be as detrimental as deficiencies for the health of both the mare and the foal.
- Nutritional balance is important when supplementing amino acids, vitamins and minerals.
- More studies are needed to confirm beneficial effects of supplements in pregnant mares on long-term health of the foals.

SUMMARY

Although the basic recommendations for broodmare nutrition are known, as described in the first part of this article, there are many variations in the needs of mares according to season and possibly breed, age, or even parity. Combined with the discordant studies, more research is therefore needed. The mare's diet can positively or negatively affect her foal's health. Limiting the intake of starch and sugar rich concentrates especially and maximizing the intake of forage may help prevent nontransmittable diseases such as osteochondrosis and possibly, the in longer term, equine metabolic syndrome. Long-term studies are urgently needed to answer these questions.

ACKNOWLEDGMENTS

The authors thank Manfred Coenen and Sue McDonnell for their help in writing this article through discussions and scientific exchanges with the authors.

DISCLOSURE

The authors have nothing to disclose.

REFERENCES

1. National Research Council. Nutrient requirements of horses. Sixth Revised Edition. Washington, DC: National Academies Press; 2007.
2. Gesellschaft für Ernährungsphysiologie. Empfehlungen zur Energie- und Nährstoffversorgung von Pferden (Energie- und Nährstoffbedarf landwirtschaftlicher Nutztiere). Frankfurt, Germany: DLG-Verlag GmbH; 2014.
3. Martin-Rosset W. Nutrition et alimentation des chevaux. Versailles, France: Editions Quae; 2012.
4. Allen WR, Wilsher S. A review of implantation and early placentation in the mare. Placenta 2009;30(12):1005–15.
5. Morley SA, Murray J-A. Effects of body condition score on the reproductive physiology of the broodmare: a review. J Equine Vet Sci 2014;34(7):842–53.
6. Dusek J. Notes on the problem of the prenatal development of horse. Vedecke Prace Výzkumné Stanice pro Chov Koni Slatińany. 1966;2:1–25.
7. Meyer H, Ahlswede L. Über das intrauterine Wachstum und die Körperzusammensetzung von Fohlen. Übersichten Tierernährung. 1976;4:263–92.
8. Platt H. Growth and maturity in the equine fetus. J R Soc Med 1978;71:658–61.
9. Bell AW, Slepetis R, Ehrhardt UA. Growth and accretion of energy and protein in the gravid uterus during late pregnancy in Holstein cows. J Dairy Sci 1995; 78(9):1954–61.
10. Coenen M, Kienzle E, Vervuert I, et al. Recent German developments in the formulation of energy and nutrient requirements in horses and the resulting feeding recommendations. J Equine Vet Sci 2011;31(5–6):219–29.
11. National Research Council. Nutrient requirements of horses. Fifth Revised Edition. Washington, DC: National Academies Press; 1989.
12. Robles M. Influence du métabolisme maternel sur la fonction placentaire et la santé du poulain. Published online October 19. 2017. Available at: http://www.theses.fr/2017SACLA029. Accessed August 16, 2020.
13. Winsco KN, Coverdale JA, Wickersham TA, et al. Influence of maternal plane of nutrition on mares and their foals: determination of mare performance and voluntary dry matter intake during late pregnancy using a dual-marker system. J Anim Sci 2013;91(9):4208–15.
14. Kronfeld DS, Holland JL, Rich GA, et al. Fat digestibility in Equus caballus follows increasing first-order kinetics. J Anim Sci 2004;82(6):1773–80.
15. Davison KE, Potter GD, Greene LW, et al. Lactation and reproductive performance of mares fed added dietary fat during late gestation and early lactation. J Equine Vet Sci 1991;11(2):111–5.
16. White WS, Zhou Y, Crane A, et al. Modeling the dose effects of soybean oil in salad dressing on carotenoid and fat-soluble vitamin bioavailability in salad vegetables. Am J Clin Nutr 2017;106(4):1041–51.
17. Warren L, Vineyard K. Fat and fatty acids. In: Equine applied and clinical nutrition. Saunders, Elsevier; 2013. p. 136–55.
18. Urschel KL, Lawrence LM. Amino acids and protein. In: Equine applied and clinical nutrition. Saunders, Elsevier; 2013. p. 113–35.
19. Ballet N, Robert JC, Williams PEV. Vitamins in forages. In: Givens DI, Owen E, Axford RFE, et al, editors. Forage evaluation in ruminant nutrition. CABI; 2000. p. 399–431.

20. McDowell L. Vitamins in animal and human nutrition. 2nd edition. Ames, Iowa: Iowa State University Press; 2000.

21. Mäenpää PH, Koskinen T, Koskinen E. Serum profiles of Vitamins A, E and D in mares and foals during different seasons. J Anim Sci 1988;66(6):1418.

22. Greiwe-Crandell KM, Kronfeld DS, Gay LA, et al. Seasonal Vitamin A depletion in grazing horses is assessed better by the relative dose response test than by serum retinol concentration. J Nutr 1995;125(10):2711–6.

23. Grings EE, Haferkamp MR, Heitschmidt RK, et al. Mineral dynamics in forages of the northern great plains. J Range Management 1996;49(3):234.

24. Sprinkle JE, Baker SD, Church JA, et al. Case study: regional assessment of mineral element concentrations in Idaho forage and range grasses. Prof Anim sci 2018;34(5):494–504.

25. Jones GB, Tracy BF. Evaluating seasonal variation in mineral concentration of cool-season pasture herbage. Grass Forage Sci 2015;70(1):94–101.

26. Greene LW, Hardt PF, Herd DB. Mineral composition of bermudagrass and native forages in Texas. Tex J Agric Nat Resour 1998;11:96–109.

27. Kappel LC, Morgan EB, Kilgore L, et al. Seasonal changes of mineral content of southern forages. J Dairy Sci 1985;68(7):1822–7.

28. Freeman DA, Cymbaluk NF, Schott HC, et al. Clinical, biochemical, and hygiene assessment of stabled horses provided continuous or intermittent access to drinking water. Am J Vet Res 1999;60(11):1445–50.

29. Houpt KA, Eggleston A, Kunkle K, et al. Effect of water restriction on equine behaviour and physiology. Equine Vet J 2000;32(4):341–4.

30. Brinkmann L, Gerken M, Riek A. Seasonal changes of total body water and water intake in Shetland ponies measured by an isotope dilution technique1. J Anim Sci 2013;91(8):3750–8.

31. Williams S, Horner J, Orton E, et al. Water intake, faecal output and intestinal motility in horses moved from pasture to a stabled management regime with controlled exercise: gastrointestinal changes in horses moved from pasture to stabled management. Equine Vet J 2015;47(1):96–100.

32. Fowden AL, Comline RS, Silver M. Insulin secretion and carbohydrate metabolism during pregnancy in the mare. Equine Vet J 1984;16(4):239–46.

33. Freinkel N, Metzger BE, Nitzan M, et al. Facilitated anabolism in late pregnancy: some novel maternal compensations for accelerated starvation. Proceedings of the VIIIth congress of the international diabetes federation. 1974:474–88.

34. George LA, Staniar WB, Cubitt TA, et al. Evaluation of the effects of pregnancy on insulin sensitivity, insulin secretion, and glucose dynamics in Thoroughbred mares. Am J Vet Res 2011;72(5):666–74.

35. Robles M, Couturier-Tarrade A, Derisoud E, et al. Effects of dietary arginine supplementation in pregnant mares on maternal metabolism, placental structure and function and foal growth. Sci Rep 2019;9(1):1–19.

36. Fowden AL, Barnes RJ, Comline RS, et al. Pancreatic β-cell function in the fetal foal and mare. J Endocrinol 1980;87(2):293–301.

37. Hoffman RM, Kronfeld DS, Cooper WL, et al. Glucose clearance in grazing mares is affected by diet, pregnancy, and lactation. J Anim Sci 2003;81(7):1764–71.

38. Fowden AL, Taylor PM, White KL, et al. Ontogenic and nutritionally induced changes in fetal metabolism in the horse. J Physiol 2000;528(1):209–19.

39. Bazzano M, Giannetto C, Fazio F, et al. Metabolic profile of broodmares during late pregnancy and early post-partum. Reprod Domest Anim 2014;49(6):947–53.

40. Fukao T, Lopaschuk GD, Mitchell GA. Pathways and control of ketone body metabolism: on the fringe of lipid biochemistry. Prostaglandins Leukot Essent fatty Acids 2004;70(3):243–51.
41. Harvey JW, Pate MG, Kivipelto J, et al. Clinical biochemistry of pregnant and nursing mares. Vet Clin Pathol 2005;34(3):248–54.
42. Vincze B, Kutasi O, Baska F, et al. Pregnancy-associated changes of sérum biochemical values in Lipizzaner Broodmares. Acta Vet Hung 2015;63(3): 303–16.
43. Mariella J, Pirrone A, Gentilini F, et al. Hematologic and biochemical profiles in Standardbred mares during peripartum. Theriogenology 2014;81(4):526–34.
44. Bonelli F, Rota A, Corazza M, et al. Hematological and biochemical findings in pregnant, postfoaling, and lactating jennies. Theriogenology 2016;85(7): 1233–8.
45. Legacki EL, Scholtz EL, Ball BA, et al. The dynamic steroid landscape of equine pregnancy mapped by mass spectrometry. Reproduction 2016;151(4):421–30.
46. Chavatte P, Holtan D, Ousey J, et al. Biosynthesis and possible biological roles of progestagens during equine pregnancy and in the newborn foal. Equine Vet J 1997;29(S24):89–95.
47. Satué K, Muñoz A, Blanco O. Pregnancy influences the hematological profile of Carthusian broodmares. Pol J Vet Sci 2010;13(2):393.
48. Keiper R, Houpt K. Reproduction in feral horses: an eight-year study. Am J Vet Res 1984;45(5):991–5.
49. Whitesell KMJ, Sertich PL, McDonnell SM. Endometrial histology of mares from a semi-feral pony herd of known lifelong high fertility and fecundity. J Equine Vet Sci 2019;74:65–7.
50. Ransom JI, Hobbs NT, Bruemmer J. In: Sorci G, editor. Contraception can lead to trophic asynchrony between birth pulse and resources. PLoS ONE 2013;8(1): e54972.
51. Dawson MJ, Hone J. Demography and dynamics of three wild horse populations in the Australian Alps. Austral Ecol 2012;37(1):97–109.
52. Dini P, Ducheyne K, Lemahieu I, et al. Effect of environmental factors and changes in the body condition score on the onset of the breeding season in mares. Reprod Domest Anim 2019;54(7):987–95.
53. Henneke DR, Potter GD, Kreider JL, et al. Relationship between condition score, physical measurements and body fat percentage in mares. Equine Vet J 1983; 15(4):371–2.
54. Carroll CL, Huntington PJ. Body condition scoring and weight estimation of horses. Equine Vet J 1988;20(1):41–5.
55. Martin-Rosset W, Vernet J, Dubroeucq H, et al. Variation of fatness and energy content of the body with body condition score in sport horses and its prediction. In: Saastamoinen MT, Martin-Rosset W, editors. Nutrition of the exercising horse. Wageningen: Wageningen Academic Publishers; 2008. pp. 167–176.
56. Chagas LM, Bass JJ, Blache D, et al. Invited review: new perspectives on the roles of nutrition and metabolic priorities in the subfertility of high-producing dairy cows. J Dairy Sci 2007;90(9):4022–32.
57. Battut I, Colchen S, Fieni F, et al. Success rates when attempting to nonsurgically collect equine embryos at 144, 156 or 168 hours after ovulation. Equine Vet J 1997;29(S25):60–2.
58. Oriol JG, Betteridge KJ, Hardy J, et al. Structural and developmental relationship between capsular glycoproteins of the horse (Equus caballus) and the donkey (Equus asinus). Equine Vet J 1993;25(S15):14–8.

59. Stout TA. Embryo–maternal communication during the first 4 weeks of equine pregnancy. Theriogenology 2016;86(1):349–54.

60. Amoroso E. Placentation. In: Parkes A, editor. Marshall's Physiology of Reproduction. Boston, USA: Little Brown & Co.; 1952. p. 127–311.

61. Allen WR, Stewart F. Equine placentation. Reprod Fertil Dev 2001;13(8):623–34.

62. Sessions-Bresnahan DR, Heuberger AL, Carnevale EM. Obesity in mares promotes uterine inflammation and alters embryo lipid fingerprints and homeostasis. Biol Reprod 2018;99(4):761–72.

63. Pennington PM, Splan RK, Jacobs RD, et al. Influence of metabolic status and diet on early pregnant equine histotroph proteome: preliminary findings. J Equine Vet Sci 2020;88:102938.

64. Jacobs RD, Ealy AD, Pennington PM, et al. Dietary supplementation of algae-derived omega-3 fatty acids influences endometrial and conceptus transcript profiles in mares. J Equine Vet Sci 2018;62:66–75.

65. Samuel CA, Allen WR, Steven DH. Studies on the equine placenta. I. Development of the microcotyledons. J Reprod Fertil 1974;41(2):441–5.

66. Macdonald AA, Chavatte P, Fowden AL. Scanning electron microscopy of the microcotyledonary placenta of the horse (equus caballus) in the latter half of gestation. Placenta 2000;21(5):565–74.

67. Peugnet P, Robles M, Mendoza L, et al. In: Crocker DE, editor. Effects of moderate amounts of barley in late pregnancy on growth, glucose metabolism and osteoarticular status of pre-weaning horses. PLoS One 2015;10(4):e0122596.

68. Robles M, Peugnet P, Dubois C, et al. Placental function and structure at term is altered in broodmares fed with cereals from mid-gestation. Placenta 2018;64: 44–52.

69. Wilsher S, Allen WR. Effects of a Streptococcus equi infection-mediated nutritional insult during mid-gestation in primiparous Thoroughbred fillies. Part 1: placental and fetal development. Equine Vet J 2006;38(6):549–57.

70. Barker DJP, Fall C, Osmond C, et al. Fetal and infant growth and impaired glucose tolerance: authors' reply. BMJ : Br Med J 1991;303(6815):1474–5.

71. Hanson MA, Gluckman PD. Early developmental conditioning of later health and disease: physiology or pathophysiology? Physiol Rev 2014;94(4):1027–76.

72. Wu G, Bazer FW, Wallace JM, et al. Intrauterine growth retardation: implications for the animal sciences. J Anim Sci 2006;84(9):2316–37.

73. Chavatte-Palmer P, Tarrade A, Kiefer H, et al. Breeding animals for quality products: not only genetics. Reprod Fertil Dev 2016;28(2):94.

74. Rossdale PD, Ousey JC. Fetal programming for athletic performance in the horse: potential effects of IUGR. Equine Vet Educ 2010;14(2):98–112.

75. Fowden AL, Jellyman JK, Valenzuela OA, et al. Nutritional programming of intrauterine development: a concept applicable to the horse? J Equine Vet Sci 2013; 33(5):295–304.

76. Chavatte-Palmer P, Peugnet P, Robles M. Developmental programming in equine species: relevance for the horse industry. Anim Front 2017;7(3):48–54.

77. Peugnet P, Robles M, Wimel L, et al. Management of the pregnant mare and long-term consequences on the offspring. Theriogenology 2016;86(1):99–109.

78. Jammes H, Junien C, Chavatte-Palmer P. Epigenetic control of development and expression of quantitative traits. Reprod Fertil Dev 2011;23(1):64–74.

79. Franciolli ALR, Cordeiro BM, da Fonseca ET, et al. Characteristics of the equine embryo and fetus from days 15 to 107 of pregnancy. Theriogenology 2011; 76(5):819–32.

80. Banach MA, Evans JW. Effects of inadequate energy during gestation and lactation on the oestrus cycle and conception rates of mares and of their foals weights. Seventh Equine Nutrition and Physiology Symposium, Warrenton, Virginia: Equine Nutrition and Physiology Society; 1981;97–100.
81. Henneke DR, Potter Gd, Kreider JL. Body condition during pregnancy and lactation and reproductive efficiency of mares. Theriogenology 1984;21(6): 897–909.
82. Robles M, Gautier C, Mendoza L, et al. Maternal nutrition during pregnancy affects testicular and bone development, glucose metabolism and response to overnutrition in weaned horses up to two years. PloS One 2017;12(1):e0169295.
83. Giles SL, Rands SA, Nicol CJ, et al. Obesity prevalence and associated risk factors in outdoor living domestic horses and ponies. PeerJ 2014;2:e299.
84. Dugdale AHA, Grove-White D, Curtis GC, et al. Body condition scoring as a predictor of body fat in horses and ponies. Vet J 2012;194(2):173–8.
85. Kubiak JR, Evans JW, Potter GD, et al. Parturition in the multiparous mare fed to obesity. J Equine Vet Sci 1988;8(2):135–40.
86. Kubiak JR, Evans JW, Potter GD, et al. Milk yield and composition in the multiparous mare fed to obesity. J Equine Vet Sci 1991;11(3):158–62.
87. Robles M, Nouveau E, Gautier C, et al. Maternal obesity increases insulin resistance, low-grade inflammation and osteochondrosis lesions in foals and yearlings until 18 months of age. PloS One 2018;13(1):e0190309.
88. Mousquer MA, Pereira AB, Finger IS, et al. Glucose and insulin curve in pregnant mares and its relationship with clinical and biometric features of newborn foals. Pesquisa Veterinária Brasileira 2019;39(9):764–70. https://doi.org/10. 1590/1678-5150-pvb-6227.
89. Kasinger S, Brasil CL, Santos AC, et al. Influence of adiposity during pregnancy of Crioulo mares on the fat accumulation in their foals. Arquivo Brasileiro de Medicina Veterinária e Zootecnia 2020;72(2):411–8.
90. Vander Heyden L, Lejeune J-P, Caudron I, et al. Association of breeding conditions with prevalence of osteochondrosis in foals. Vet Rec 2013;172(3):68.
91. Thorson JF, Karren BJ, Bauer ML, et al. Effect of selenium supplementation and plane of nutrition on mares and their foals: foaling data. J Anim Sci 2010;88(3): 982–90.
92. Caure S, Lebreton P. Ostéochondrose chez le trotteur au sevrage et corrélation avec divers paramètres. Pratique vétérinaire équine 2004;36:47–57.
93. George LA, Staniar WB, Treiber KH, et al. Insulin sensitivity and glucose dynamics during pre-weaning foal development and in response to maternal diet composition. Domest Anim Endocrinol 2009;37(1):23–9.
94. Ryan E, Galvin K, O'Connor TP, et al. Phytosterol, squalene, tocopherol content and fatty acid profile of selected seeds, grains, and legumes. Plant Foods Hum Nutr 2007;62(3):85–91.
95. Dewhurst RJ, Scollan ND, Youell SJ, et al. Influence of species, cutting date and cutting interval on the fatty acid composition of grasses. Grass Forage Sci 2001; 56(1):68–74.
96. Adkin AM, Warren LK, Mortensen CJ, et al. Maternal supplementation of docosahexaenoic acid and its effect on fatty acid transfer to the foal. J Equine Vet Sci 2013;5(33):336.
97. Kouba JM, Burns TA, Webel SK. Effect of dietary supplementation with long-chain n-3 fatty acids during late gestation and early lactation on mare and foal plasma fatty acid composition, milk fatty acid composition, and mare reproductive variables. Anim Reprod Sci 2019;203:33–44.

98. Hodge LB, Rude BJ, Dinh TN, et al. Effect of omega-3 fatty acid supplementation to gestating and lactating mares: on milk IgG, mare and foal blood concentrations of IgG, insulin and glucose, placental efficiency, and fatty acid composition of milk and serum from mares and foals. J equine Vet Sci 2017; 51:70–8.

99. Savage CJ, McCarthy RN, Jeffcott LB. Effects of dietary energy and protein on induction of dyschondroplasia in foals. Equine Vet J 1993;25(S16):74–9.

100. Davis TA, Nguyen HV, Garcia-Bravo R, et al. Amino acid composition of human milk is not unique. J Nutr 1994;124(7):1126–32.

101. Mortensen CJ, Kelley DE, Warren LK. Supplemental L-arginine shortens gestation length and increases mare uterine blood flow before and after parturition. J Equine Vet Sci 2011;31(9):514–20.

102. Mesa AM, Warren LK, Sheehan JM, et al. L-Arginine supplementation 0.5% of diet during the last 90 days of gestation and 14 days postpartum reduced uterine fluid accumulation in the broodmare. Anim Reprod Sci 2015;159:46–51.

103. Jahan-Mihan A, Rodriguez J, Christie C, et al. The role of maternal dietary proteins in development of metabolic syndrome in offspring. Nutrients 2015;7(11): 9185–217.

104. Gay LS, Kronfeld DS, Grimsley-Cook A, et al. Retinol, β-carotene and β-tocopherol concentrations in mare and foal plasma and in colostrum. J Equine Vet Sci 2004;24(3):115–20.

105. Lopez-Rodriguez MF, Cymbaluk NF, Epp T, et al. A field study of serum, colostrum, milk iodine, and thyroid hormone concentrations in postpartum draft mares and foals. J Equine Vet Sci 2020;90:103018.

106. Pearce SG, Grace ND, Wichtel JJ, et al. Effect of copper supplementation on copper status of pregnant mares and foals. Equine Vet J 1998;30(3):200–3.

107. Pannia E, Cho CE, Kubant R, et al. Role of maternal vitamins in programming health and chronic disease. Nutr Rev 2016;74(3):166–80.

108. Bondo T, Jensen SK. Administration of RRR-α-tocopherol to pregnant mares stimulates maternal IgG and IgM production in colostrum and enhances vitamin E and IgM status in foals. J Anim Physiol Anim Nutr 2011;95(2):214–22.

109. Kuhl J, Aurich JE, Wulf M, et al. Effects of oral supplementation with β-carotene on concentrations of β-carotene, vitamin A and α-tocopherol in plasma, colostrum and milk of mares and plasma of their foals and on fertility in mares: effects of oral β-carotene supplementation to mares. J Anim Physiol Anim Nutr 2012; 96(3):376–84.

110. Glade MJ. Effects of gestation, lactation, and maternal calcium intake on mechanical strength of equine bone. J Am Coll Nutr 1993;12(4):372–7.

111. Knight D, Weisbrode SE, Schmall LM, et al. The effects of copper supplementation on the prevalence of cartilage lesions in foals. Equine Vet J 1990;22(6): 426–32.

112. Pearce SG, Firth EC, Grace ND, et al. Effect of copper supplementation on the evidence of developmental orthopaedic disease in pasture-fed New Zealand Thoroughbreds. Equine Vet J 1998;30(3):211–8.

113. Kavazis AN, Kivipelto J, Ott EA. Supplementation of broodmares with copper, zinc, iron, manganese, cobalt, iodine, and selenium. J Equine Vet Sci 2002; 22(10):460–4.

114. Löfstedt J. White muscle disease of foals. Vet Clin North Am Equine Pract 1997; 13(1):169–85.

115. Calamari L, Ferrari A, Bertin G. Effect of selenium source and dose on selenium status of mature horses. J Anim Sci 2009;87(1):167–78.

116. Richardson SM, Siciliano PD, Engle TE, et al. Effect of selenium supplementation and source on the selenium status of horses. J Anim Sci 2006;84(7):1742–8.
117. Montgomery JB, Wichtel JJ, Wichtel MG, et al. The effects of selenium source on measures of selenium status of mares and selenium status and immune function of their foals. J Equine Vet Sci 2012;32(6):352–9.
118. Clark A, Sallé G, Ballan V, et al. Strongyle infection and gut microbiota: profiling of resistant and susceptible horses over a grazing season. Front Physiol 2018; 9:272.
119. Koikkalainen K, Knuuttila A, Karikoski N, et al. Congenital hypothyroidism and dysmaturity syndrome in foals: first reported cases in Europe. Equine Vet Educ 2014;26(4):181–9.
120. Stiemsma LT, Michels KB. The role of the microbiome in the developmental origins of health and disease. Pediatrics 2018;141(4)::e20172437.
121. Weese JS, Holcombe SJ, Embertson RM, et al. Changes in the faecal microbiota of mares precede the development of post partum colic. Equine Vet J 2015; 47(6):641–9.
122. Elzinga SE, Weese JS, Adams AA. Comparison of the fecal microbiota in horses with equine metabolic syndrome and metabolically normal controls fed a similar all-forage diet. J Equine Vet Sci 2016;44:9–16.
123. Betsch J, Chaucheyras Durand F, Sacy A, et al. Etude de la cinétique de l'installation de la flore du poulain et effets d'une levure vivante administrée à la jument ou au poulain nouveau-né. 40ème Journée de La Recherche Equine, Paris: Institut Français du Cheval et de l'Equitation; 2014;16–25.
124. Faubladier C, Julliand V, Danel J, et al. Bacterial carbohydrate-degrading capacity in foal faeces: changes from birth to pre-weaning and the impact of maternal supplementation with fermented feed products. Br J Nutr 2013; 110(6):1040–52.

The Safety and Efficacy in Horses of Certain Nutraceuticals that Claim to Have Health Benefits

Ingrid Vervuert, DVM[a],*, Meri Stratton-Phelps, DVM[b]

KEYWORDS

- Supplements • Research • Evidence • Health • Horse

KEY POINTS

- Before a supplement is selected for use, it is important to first ensure that the horse is being fed a balanced ration appropriate to its individual needs.
- Different models (in vitro and in vivo) have been used to test the efficacy of dietary supplements.
- In vivo models that demonstrate how the ingredients are absorbed and metabolized to achieve a particular health benefit in the horse are preferred versus results obtained in a laboratory setting.
- Only a few nutraceuticals have shown potential to improve health above and beyond the provision of a well-balanced diet.

INTRODUCTION

The term nutraceutical was developed from the words "nutrition" and "pharmaceutical" in the early 1990s and although it is often used in the marketing of equine complementary feeds or supplements, it has no regulatory definition (see Ruth Bishop and David A. Dzanis' article, "Staying on the Right Side of the Regulatory Authorities," in this issue). Nutraceuticals are commonly described as feed ingredients that may have a beneficial effect on the health of horses. Dietary supplements discussed in this article follow the definition provided by the US National Research Council (NRC) as:

[a] Institute of Animal Nutrition, Nutrition Diseases and Dietetics, Faculty of Veterinary Medicine, Leipzig University, An den Tierkliniken 9, Leipzig 04103, Germany; [b] All Creatures Veterinary Nutrition Consulting, 3407 Millbrook Court, Fairfield, CA 94534, USA
* Corresponding author.
E-mail address: ingrid.vervuert@vetmed.uni-leipzig.de

Vet Clin Equine 37 (2021) 207–222
https://doi.org/10.1016/j.cveq.2020.11.002
0749-0739/21/© 2020 Elsevier Inc. All rights reserved.
vetequine.theclinics.com

*a substance for oral consumption by horses whether in/on feed or offered sepa-
rately, intended for the specific benefit to the animal by means other than provision of nutrients recognized as essential or for provision of essential nutrients
for intended effect on the animal beyond normal nutritional needs, but not
including legally defined drugs.[1]*

The use of equine dietary supplements has undergone a rapid expansion in the past
10 to 15 years. Owners can easily purchase a variety of different products for their
horses, designed to support the health of all possible body systems. Any determination of safety and/or efficacy is difficult owing to the limited peer-reviewed studies on
individual supplement ingredients or on multi-ingredient products.

The primary challenge of the equine veterinarian is to be able to critically evaluate a
product to determine that it is not only safe to use, but also potentially effective and
likely to result in a desired health response.

Before a supplement is selected for use in a horse at any age or life stage, it is important to first ensure that a well-balanced diet is being fed. The ration should be based on
forages ($\geq$1.5 – % of body weight, as dry matter) and then may also include manufactured equine feeds and/or single ration ingredients such as oil, rice bran, or beet pulp
to help meet individual nutrient requirements. Rations that only include forage, with or
without such single ration ingredients, often require a vitamin and mineral supplement
or a ration balancer as discussed elsewhere in this issue. In some cases, extra protein
is required as forages may be low in protein and essential amino acids.

It can be confusing to determine if a dietary supplement is necessary or when a particular product may be helpful in maintaining, supporting or improving health. When dietary
supplements are used concurrently with any pharmacotherapy; assessment should be
made regarding potential nutrient–drug interactions that may alter the bioavailability
and metabolism of either the drug or the supplement ingredients. This point is especially
important with botanic ingredients. Some equine supplements contain potentially toxic
ingredients (garlic, pyrrolizidine alkaloids) and use should be approached with caution
or avoided completely.[2,3] Many common ingredients in equine supplements may result
in a positive drug test in an equine athlete (see Ruth Bishop and David A. Dzanis' article,
"Staying on the Right Side of the Regulatory Authorities," in this issue).

SUPPLEMENT EVALUATION

Before a supplement is selected for use, the following product related points should
be evaluated:

1. Is species-specific research available to support marketing claims, either on the
   product formulation, or on well-defined active ingredients? Or is research available
   in other species to support the supplement claim or function and can this be
   reasonably extrapolated to horses?
2. Can the source of the active ingredient and the delivery per dose be justified by
   quoted supportive research?
3. Are active ingredients quantified by analysis, for example, 20 mg biotin per provided scoop?
4. Is there scientific evidence that the feeding of the active ingredients, is safe?
5. Is there the potential for any cross-reactivity, for example, herbs with other supplements or medicines?
6. Are the active ingredients considered allowable by any relevant regulations (eg, the
   Fédération Équestaire Internationale and the United States Equestrian Federation)?
7. What are the contamination risks for prohibited substances?

Nutraceutical Supplements to Support Metabolic Health

In recent years, the equine metabolic syndrome has become a widely recognized clinical condition.[4] A primary strategy to manage the equine metabolic syndrome is to ensure any required weight loss by calorie restriction (see Megan Shepherd and colleagues' article, "Nutritional Considerations When Dealing with an Obese Adult Equine," in this issue). Furthermore, the intake of hydrolysable carbohydrates (also known as nonstructural carbohydrates) should be limited to prevent high postprandial insulin responses. In an attempt to improve systemic insulin regulation, many commercial products have been developed with the aim of improving glucose regulation at the cellular level. The most popular ingredients being used are magnesium (typically either as an organic or an inorganic chelate) and chromium (as chromium yeast or chromium propionate). Evidence to support their use has largely been extrapolated from studies in humans with type 2 diabetes.[5] Dietary chromium showed minimal benefit on glucose regulation[6–8] in earlier work, but a recent study showed that oral chromium propionate (2 or 4 mg chromium/d) could potentially increase insulin sensitivity in healthy horses.[9] Data in horses with insulin dysregulation are, however, lacking. Additionally, in Europe, chromium is not approved as a feed additive; therefore, chromium-containing supplements for equines are prohibited. In horses, magnesium as a single nutrient has only limited evidence of improving insulin regulation.[10]

In humans with metabolic disorders, especially type 2 diabetes, L-carnitine supplementation can improve glucose tolerance and insulin sensitivity.[11] In obese ponies, on an energy restriction diet, L-carnitine did not improve insulin sensitivity.[12] The authors suggested that endogenous L-carnitine synthesis was sufficient to facilitate lipid and glucose metabolism in adult ponies. A variety of other ingredients have been suggested to provide metabolic support including vitamin E, selenium, iodine, biotin, grape seed extract, cinnamon, chasteberry (*Vitex agnus-castus*), and fish oil. However, robust published research to support the use of these ingredients to manage insulin dysregulation in horses is currently lacking.

Ingredients with some limited support for a beneficial effect on either insulin sensitivity or circulating glucose and insulin concentrations include short-chain fructo-oligosaccharides, psyllium, and resveratrol (a natural polyphenol with antioxidant properties), in combination with leucine.[13] However, more work is needed to confirm these findings and the doses required.

Key points

- Limited evidence available currently to support the potential to improve insulin regulation through dietary supplementation and further work is needed to confirm the potential of ingredients such as resveratrol.
- It is unlikely that any dietary supplement can replace dietary restriction, and increased exercise where possible, in managing obesity in horses, especially in so-called easy keepers.

Nutraceutical Supplements to Improve Gastric Health

Erosive and ulcerative diseases of the stomach are described by the term equine gastric ulcer syndrome.[14] However, it is recommended to specify between the squamous and glandular region as equine squamous gastric disease (ESGD) and equine glandular gastric disease as terms that more specifically describe the affected region anatomically.[14]

Several studies have confirmed an improvement of gastric ulcers by administering the drugs, cimetidine, ranitidine,[15] and particularly omeprazole.[16] In addition, to medical treatment, optimizing feeding and housing management are highly recommended. For example, forage should be provided ad libitum or at least to a daily minimum of 1.5% of body weight as dry matter[17] (see Myriam Hesta and Marcio Costa's article, "How Can Nutrition Help with Gastrointestinal Tract-Based Issues," in this issue). In exercising horses, grain intake should be limited to a maximum of 1 g starch/kg body weight per meal.[18] Several dietary supplements claiming to support gastric mucosa health are commercially available.

Antacid-buffering supplements

It is postulated that gastric mucosal injury will be less likely in a more alkaline environment. The oral application of 30 g of aluminum hydroxide combined with 15 g of magnesium hydroxide resulted in a significantly higher gastric pH (>4) for at least 2 hours in healthy horses.[19] However, a single administration of an antacid drug combination containing 5.4 g or 8.1 g of aluminum hydroxide and 4.8 g or 7.2 g of magnesium hydroxide only very transiently increased gastric pH to 6 in just 2 of 6 horses.[20] In both studies, horses were not evaluated for gastric ulcers. Furthermore, in foals, 16-day supplementation with magnesium oxide, fortified with herbs of unknown origin, did not improve gastric mucosa health, using the weaning process as a model to induce gastric mucosal lesions[20].

Pectin–lecithin complex

Pectin is a soluble complex polysaccharide derived from the cell wall of fruits or the sugar beet. Lecithin is a phospholipid derived from soybeans. It has been postulated that lecithin is an emulsifying, lubricating agent with surfactant properties.[21] It is speculated that pectin acts with lecithin as a hydrophobic barrier on the gastric mucosal membranes, thereby having some protective function against gastric acids.

Supplementing a commercial pectin–lecithin supplement to horses fed hay (1.5% of body weight) and a starch-containing complementary feed (1% of body weight) did not affect stomach pH[22] in 1 study. However, supplementation for 10 days apparently resulted in improved healing of gastric mucosal lesions under field conditions, with uncontrolled feeding and management conditions.[23] Ferrucci and colleagues[24] also found significant improvements in gastric mucosa lesions after feeding the same pectin–lecithin supplement for 30 days (horses fed daily 5 kg hay and 5–7 kg concentrate), although there was no control group. In contrast, Murray and Grady[25] and Sanz and colleagues[26] could not find any protective effect of feeding the same commercial pectin–lecithin supplement in a gastric ulceration model using an intermittent fasting protocol.

From the published studies, beneficial effects of supplementing a pectin–lecithin containing supplement are unlikely.

Dietary oils

In humans and rats, the supplementation of arachidonic acid precursors such as linoleic acid increase endogenous prostaglandin production and decrease gastric acid output.[27] Ponies on a forage-based diet supplemented with corn oil (rich in linoleic acid; 0.3–0.4 mL/kg body weight) showed a significant decrease in maximal gastric acid output induced by a pentagastrin challenge.[28] However, gastroscopic examinations were not performed. Furthermore, supplementation of corn oil, refined rice bran oil, or crude rice bran oil (0.5–0.6 mL/kg of body weight) did not have any beneficial effects on the development of nonglandular gastric ulcers using an intermittent fasting protocol.[28]

Currently, the potential of adding dietary oils to improve gastric mucosa health needs more evidence.

Sea buckthorn berries

Sea buckthorn berries are rich in phenols, vitamins, flavonoids, fatty acids, plant sterols, lignans, and minerals.[29] These compounds have antioxidant and immunoactive properties, which might be beneficial in mucosal healing. Sea buckthorn berries do not seem to be effective in the treatment or prevention of ESGD.[30,31] Furthermore, Sea buckthorn berries–treated horses were approximately 5 times more likely to develop hyperkeratosis in the squamous mucosa than control horses, although the significance of hyperkeratosis to stomach health is not fully understood.[30,31] However, horses with equine glandular gastric disease were improved, when compared with untreated controls in stall-confined horses fed a different extract of sea buckthorn berries and pulp.[30,31] Sea buckthorn berries may have some potential to promote healing, but further work is needed especially in spontaneously occurring clinical cases.

Herbs

Herbs may also have beneficial effects owing to their anti-inflammatory properties. Six weeks of supplementation with an herbal blend in adult horses or donkeys with spontaneously occurring gastric mucosal lesions resulted in complete ESGD healing or significant improvement compared with the blinded placebo group.[32] However, information about the feeding and management was not provided.

Supplementing a Chinese herbal formulation (2 traditional herbal formulas: Xiao Yao San and Er Chen Tang) did not decrease the severity, compared with a placebo of experimentally induced ESGD, undergoing intermittent feeding.[33] The data about herb supplementation to improve gastric mucosa health is limited; thus, more equine studies are needed for further elucidation.

Mixed supplements

A blend of sea buckthorn, pectin, lecithin, L-glutamine and other ingredients,[34] when mixed with grain, decreased the number of ESGD present 14 days after omeprazole treatment was discontinued and during a week of intermittent feed-deprivation compared with unsupplemented control horses.

A 90-day blinded randomized clinical trial compared the efficacy of oral omeprazole with a dietary supplement containing oat oil rich in polar lipids, oat flour rich in β-glucan, L-glutamine, and L-threonine and extracts of the cell wall of *Saccharomyces cerevisiae* for the management of ESGD in racehorses.[35] In the first 30 days, omeprazole treatment was more effective at decreasing the squamous ulcer score by 2 or more grades than the dietary supplement. However, at day 90 both treatments were similar with respect to the changes in the squamous ulcer score. However, complete resolution of the squamous ulcers was less than 20% at day 60 and 90 of the study in both treatment groups.

Hellings and Larsen[36] fed either a placebo or a supplement consisting of organic acid-salts and B-vitamins in trotting racehorses with endoscopically verified ESGD (severity grade 2 out of 4 or higher). No significant differences were detected between supplement or placebo on ulcer score within 3 weeks of treatment. Interestingly, there was a significant improvement in ulcer severity in the placebo group (58.1%) from 3 weeks to the end of additionally 2 to 4 weeks of treatment. These findings support the requirement for a placebo group in studies evaluating dietary supplement efficacy. Sykes and colleagues[37] reported in a placebo-controlled study that a combination of pectin-lecithin complex, *S cerevisiae* and magnesium hydroxide, when supplemented 1 to 4 hours before exercise was prophylactic in preventing the development or exacerbation of existing squamous and glandular gastric ulcers in Thoroughbred horses in race training.

Woodward and colleagues[38] found that the supplementation of antacids did not prevent gastric ulceration of the squamous mucosa. However, such supplementation may have some beneficial effects on the healing process in Thoroughbred horses using the feed deprivation model to induce gastric ulcers.

Feeding a mineral or vitamin supplement containing a zinc–methionine complex resulted in lower gastric ulcer scores in horses after omeprazole treatment had been finished than feeding zinc sulfate.[39]

Key points

- Different models have been used to test efficacy of dietary supplements, which makes it difficult to compare studies.
- Supplements that work under experimental conditions may not work under field conditions where multifactorial risk factors may be present with nonstandardized feeding and housing conditions.
- A few products may have some potential to support mucosal healing processes. However, no current supplements have achieved complete mucosal damage resolution nor have been consistently able to prevent ulcer formation.

Hoof Supplements

In a recent UK study on hoof management, 89% of horse owners (n = 345) reported hoof problems in the past 5 years, such as abscesses, cracks, and bruising.[40] Thirty-five percent used nutritional products targeted at the hoof and the majority were willing to try new hoof products and treatments.

Horn quality, hoof growth, and strength are influenced by several factors such as age, breed, genetics, metabolic rate, exercise, external temperature, environmental moisture, illness, trimming, shoeing, and nutrition.[41–45] Hoof horn is produced by a complex process of differentiation (keratinization) of epidermal cells that depends on the appropriate provision of nutrients such as amino acids, minerals, and vitamins.[41]

Protein and amino acids

Hoof contains high levels of amino acids, especially cystine, arginine, leucine, lysine, proline, serine, glycine, and valine, and lower levels of methionine, phenylalanine, and histidine.[42,43] The sulfur-containing amino acids cystine and methionine are crucial for the structural integrity of the keratinocyte.[44] Cystine is the oxidized dimer form of the amino acid cysteine. During keratinization and cornification, the formation of disulfide bonds between cystine units are essential in the final stages, providing cell wall rigidity and high resistance against a variety of proteolytic enzymes.[45]

Most commercially available hoof supplements add methionine as the sole sulfur-containing amino acid (personal communication Vervuert, 2020). However, it is unclear whether the synthesis of cysteine in the liver from its precursor methionine is a rate-limiting step in the keratinization process or not. The provision of cysteine might be beneficial, because this amino acid is preferentially incorporated into the epidermal lamina.[46] Surprisingly, poor hoof horn quality was related to higher methionine levels in the sole horn, compared with good horn quality.[43] From this study, the role of methionine as a sulfur source in keratinization process remains open. Hoof horn contains other amino acids, but the value of other amino acids on hoof health have not been investigated.

Calcium

Despite the relative low calcium content in hooves, calcium plays an essential role in the keratinization and cornification processes through the activation of enzymes that initiate and regulate the terminal differentiation of the epidermal cells. Kempson[47] found improvements in hoof horn defects after the addition of calcium in combination with protein by feeding alfalfa or by adding 7.5 g limestone in 2 horses that failed to respond to a biotin supplementation. From this case report, it remains unclear whether it was the calcium and/or the provision of essential amino acids via the alfalfa that improved hoof health. Most equine diets provide sufficient calcium to cover or to exceed calcium requirements. However, the concentration and bioavailability across feeds varies.

Trace elements

Interactions and synergistic effects exist between several trace minerals; therefore, supplying a combination of trace minerals would seem potentially to be more beneficial. However, little work has been undertaken to date and many of the studies have significant limitations.

Zinc has been identified as a key mineral in the keratinization process via (i) the activation of catalytic zinc metalloenzymes, (ii) the formation of zinc finger structural proteins and, (iii) the regulation of proteins that are involved in the differentiation processes of keratinocytes.[41] Coenen and Spitzlei[43] reported lower hoof horn zinc levels in hooves of poorer quality.

No relationship between hoof horn zinc levels and biomechanical variables, such as strength or elasticity, were found in ponies fed 2 different diets.[48] However, even the restricted diet met zinc requirements. No beneficial effects on hoof horn quality were found in a field study where horses were fed 1 mg zinc/kg body weight as zinc sulfate for 12 months, although basal zinc intake was not reported.[49]

Copper activates the enzyme responsible for the formation of the disulfide bonds between the cystine links of the keratin filaments, which contribute to the structural strength by giving rigidity to the keratinized cell matrix.[41] Higami[50] found a higher incidence of white line disease in horses fed long-term diets low in zinc and copper. Over a 9-month period, the hoof wall growth rate was lower in the horses fed the zinc- and copper-deficient basal diet, compared with those where additional amino acid chelated (ie, organic) zinc and copper was added to meet requirements.[50] Copper and zinc absorption may have been enhanced by intestinal amino acid transporters. However, Siciliano and colleagues[51] compared the supplementation of inorganic and organic sources (50% intake supplied by amino acid complexes) of zinc, copper, and manganese in horses. Both diets met the respective requirements; however, hoof horn quality and growth rates were not influenced by mineral source.

Manganese is needed for the activation of enzymes involved in the synthesis of chondroitin-sulfate side chains of proteoglycans, which are essential for the formation of normal cartilage and bone. Manganese also has several indirect functions in the keratinization process.[52] Manganese also activates several enzymes that play a role in the provision of cellular energy, which is important for horn metabolism. Furthermore, manganese-containing superoxide dismutase provides a crucial defense mechanism against free radicals. However, equine diets, especially when forage-based rations are provided, are rarely deficient in manganese. There is little scientific evidence to support the provision of additional manganese.

Selenium is an essential cofactor in several enzymes including glutathione peroxidase and thioredoxin reductase.[52] The importance of selenium for membrane integrity, growth, reproduction, and immune response is well-established in horses.[52] Excessive intake of selenium results in high selenium hoof horn levels, coronary band disease, and substantial horn cracks in horses.[53] High selenium levels disrupt the disulfide bonds between cystine units, the key step for cell wall rigidity and resistance. Selenium intake therefore should be strictly controlled according to requirements and caution is needed with respect to selenium addition through hoof products. Regional differences in soil selenium influence risk.

Role of vitamins

Biotin. During keratin formation, biotin is essential for the formation of complex lipid molecules in the intercellular cementing substance.[54] Furthermore, biotin directly stimulates the differentiation of epidermal cells.[55] Most research, therefore, has focused on biotin supplementation to improve hoof growth and hoof horn quality in several species, and is often associated with a positive effect.[56–60] However, the effects on poor hoof horn quality strongly depend on sufficient duration (>9 months) and dosage (3–4 mg/100 kg body weight/d) of biotin supplementation. Healthy horses fed forage-based diets may meet biotin requirements by hindgut microbial production. Therefore, factors that negatively impact on the intestinal microbiota, such as starch overload, may reduce microbial biotin synthesis. Beneficial effects of biotin on poor hoof horn quality have been found only when high dosages were provided, versus relying on microbial production alone. It is important to note that not all hoof problems are biotin responsive.

Other vitamins such as vitamin A, vitamin D, and vitamin E are essential in developing the integrity, structure, and quality of keratinized horn tissue. However, scientific data about the effects of supplementation on hoof growth and hoof quality are lacking in the horse.

Key points

- Research suggests that horn strength and quality are mostly improved by balancing energy and nutrient intake according to requirements rather than focusing on one single nutrient such as biotin, calcium, or zinc.
- Because copper and zinc intake can be quite variable in equine diets, the provision of these trace elements may have some beneficial potential in a hoof supplement if the current diet is deficient.
- Except for biotin, scientific data regarding the role of vitamins in hoof health are lacking.

Joint Supplements

Oral joint supplements are one of the most popular category of equine supplements in the United States[61] and Europe.[62]

Currently available equine oral joint supplements commonly use a blend of different 'active' components, often referred to as chondroprotective agents.[63] The main desired potential of chondroprotective substances can be summarized as:

- Increase collagen and proteoglycan synthesis of chondrocytes
- Increase hyaluronic acid synthesis in synovial cells
- Inhibit enzymes that destroy cartilage
- Inhibit fibrin synthesis in synovial and subchondral vessels

The main ingredients provided in supplements and their role in cartilage metabolism are summarized in **Table 1**.

Table 1	
Ingredients which are frequently used in oral joint supplements	
Ingredients	**Rational Role**
Chondroitin sulfate	Component of glycosaminoglycan chains
Hyaluronate	Cartilage component
Glucosamine	Precursor of glycosaminoglycan chains
Methylsulphonylmethane	Source of sulfur, a component of cartilage
Unsaponified avocado soy	Inflammation modulation
Omega 3 fatty acids	Inflammation modulation
Cetyl myristoleate	Inflammation modulation
Selenium, vitamin E	Antioxidants
Manganese, vitamin A	Co-factors in glycosaminoglycan synthesis
Copper, vitamin C, gelatin	Collagen synthesis
Herbs such as devil's claw or Indian celery	Inflammation modulation

Glucosamine and chondroitin sulfate

Glucosamine and chondroitin sulfate are probably the most commonly used chondroprotective ingredients. Pearson and Lindinger[64] conducted an extensive review of published in vivo research on glucosamine and/or chondroitin sulfate based nutraceuticals for horses. They concluded that many supplement studies were confounded by several major limitations related to the study design (eg, missing control or placebo groups, low horse numbers, undiagnosed lameness, suboptimal diagnostic parameters, or statistical interpretation), which did not allow a clear conclusion to be made about the efficacy of glucosamine and/or chondroitin sulfate–based nutraceuticals for joint health. A similar conclusion was reached in 2013, by McIlwraith[65] owing to a lack of well-designed studies.

Another major limitation of such supplements relates to their very low oral bioavailability (0%–5.9%, and 0%–32%, for glucosamine and chondroitin sulfate, respectively[66–68]). Welch and colleagues[68] did not find any blood response despite frequent blood collection after the oral intake of glucosamine (5.5–8.5 g/horse) or chondroitin sulfate (2–3.5 g/horse) in adult horses. They suggested that orally fed glucosamine and chondroitin sulfate were not absorbed owing to rapid fermentation or degradation by mucosa-associated enzymes. There is also limited published clinical evidence of efficacy; for example, in a study by Higler and colleagues,[69] supplementation for 3 months with glucosamine, chondroitin sulfate, and methylsulphonylmethane in aged horses did not improve gait kinematic data assessed on a treadmill.

In addition, it should be emphasized that high dosages of glucosamine and chondroitin sulfate were used in vitro to investigate potential mechanism and pathways on cartilage metabolism. Those high levels of glucosamine and/or chondroitin sulfate achieved with in vitro studies are not found in vivo.[70]

Perhaps owing to the lack of conclusive data on the effective dosage of oral glucosamine and/or chondroitin sulfate supplementation, there is a considerable variation in the concentration of glucosamine and/or chondroitin sulfate in commercial products. For example, Oke and colleagues[71] reported a range of glucosamine concentrations from 1.7 to 29.6 mg/50 mg product. According to information provided on the product labels, the average recommended daily dose ranged from 1800 to 12,000 mg glucosamine for an average sized mature horse.[71]

Dietary oils

Omega 3 fatty acids such as eicosapentaenoic acid (EPA) and docosahexaenoic acid (DHA) have gained interest as potential modifiers of inflammation.[72] The supplementation of either a marine derived omega 3 fatty acid source (alpha linolenic acids 2 g, EPA 7.6 g, docosapentaenoic acid 1.7 g, and DHA 26.6 g) or a vegetable source (flaxseed with 38 g alpha linolenic acids) did not impact synovial prostaglandin E2 levels in healthy horses.[73] However, there is some evidence that the metabolism of the flaxseed alpha linolenic acids to EPA and DHA might be restricted, suggesting a possible advantage of direct EPA and DHA supplementation, for example, by feeding a marine-derived omega 3 fatty acid source. However, in an experimentally induced synovitis model in horses, the supplementation of a marine-derived omega 3 fatty acids source (per 100 kilograms of body weight: alpha linolenic acids 0.36 g, docosapentaenoic acid 0.36 g, EPA 1.93 g, and DHA 5.43 g) did not modify synovial inflammation processes, despite higher synovial levels of EPA and DHA acid compared with the control group.[73]

Conjugated linoleic acid has been shown to have anti-inflammatory effects in several animal species.[74] Plasma and synovial omega-6 arachidonic levels were decreased in horses after feeding 1% of a conjugated linoleic acid–containing supplement. However, the degree of inflammation after an intraarticular lipopolysaccharide challenge, as indicated by joint temperature and synovial prostaglandin E2, remained unchanged.[75]

Cetyl myristoleate is another fatty acid that may have beneficial effects on the modification of inflammatory responses by cytokines and the arachidonic acid cascade.[76] Cetyl myristoleate is included in several commercial joint supplements; however, well-designed studies are lacking to be able to give recommendations according to the efficacy.

Vegetable extracts
Resveratrol. Resveratrol (3,4,5-trihydroxystilbene) is a natural polyphenolic compound found in many plants such as red grapes, peanuts, blueberries, some pines, and the roots and stalks of Japanese knotweed. Resveratrol has been proposed to have anti-oxidative properties owing to its free radical scavenging.[77] In a placebo-controlled study, feeding 3 weeks of a commercially available oral resveratrol (450 mg twice per day for 3 weeks, per the manufacturer's recommendation) did not affect phagocytic activity, oxidative burst function, or cytokine production in horses.[78]

Ememe and colleagues[79] reported some beneficial effects of the supplementation of a product (30 g) containing resveratrol, hyaluronic acid and *S cerevisiae* (2000 mg of resveratrol, 200 mg of sodium hyaluronic acid, and the carrier *S cerevisiae*) on blood antioxidative capacity in lame horses; lameness was not evaluated.

A combined therapy with resveratrol supplementation (containing 1000 mg of resveratrol and the carrier *S cerevisiae*) for 4 months after intra-articular injection of triamcinolone in the centrodistal and tarsometatarsal joints improved lameness assessed by an objective sensory system and subjective rider's assessment.[80] However, only 8 of 21 supplemented horses and 7 or 20 placebo horses had returned to full work at the end of the 4-month observation period. In addition, the lameness examination by an experienced veterinarian still identified 15 of 21 and 15 of 20 horses in the supplementation or placebo groups, respectively, with a lameness grade of 3 out of 3 at the end of the study.

From the present data, beneficial effects of resveratrol on equine osteoarthritis are questionable.

Avocado and soybean unsaponifiables
Vegetable extracts from avocado and soybean oils have been considered for the treatment of OA. Avocado and soybean unsaponifiables are complex mixture of compounds, such as fat-soluble vitamins, sterols, and triterpene alcohols.[81] An extensive meta-analysis suggested some beneficial effects of avocado and soybean unsaponifiables treatment in humans, but not in horses.[82]

Other substances

A blend of lipids from the New Zealand green lipped mussel (*Perna canaliculus*), shark cartilage (*Galorhinus galeus*), abalone (*Haliotis sp*), and *Biota orientalis* lipid extract have been shown to decreased inflammation in a cartilage explant model in vitro.[83] A supplement containing glucosamine sulfate, shark chondroitin sulfate, methylsulphonylmethane, boswellic acid dry extract 65%, *Ananasus comosus* extract, L-glutamine, feverfew dry extract, and hyaluronic acid fed to horses before induced joint inflammation (intra-articular lipopolysaccharide) resulted in lower synovial prostaglandin E2 levels and total nucleated cell counts compared with the placebo group.[84] However, it remains still unclear whether such results obtained in a joint inflammation–induced model are comparable with naturally occurring joint inflammation in horses.

Feeding a commercial product containing chondroitin sulfate 162 g/kg, glucosamine 190 g/kg, vitamin C 80 g/kg, methylsulphonylmethane 256 g/kg, DHA 66 g/kg, and EPA 34 g/kg improved lameness grade, ridden and groundwork scores, and "ease of movement," when compared with feeding a placebo.[85] However, a main limitation of this study was that 30% of the horses were not lame and the rest of the horses had a low lameness score with an unknown lameness diagnosis. Furthermore, dosage of the product was not mentioned in the study.

Herbs

As an alternative to drug treatments, popular herbs include devil's claw (*Harpagophytum procumbens*), Indian celery (*Apium graveolens*),[86] and blue green algae.[87]

Devil's claw (*H procumbens*) for example, is widely used owing to its potential anti-inflammatory properties.[88] Devil's claw is an extract obtained from the root of the *H procumbens*. A clear mechanism for any anti-inflammatory action still needs to be established, although it is purported to inhibit the arachidonic, and subsequently the inflammatory cyclo-oxygenase, and the lipo-oxygenase pathways.[89] Despite the high number of supplements containing devil's claw, other than the pharmacokinetics of its active chemical constituent harpagoside,[90] the results of clinical studies have not been published in horses. Furthermore, devil's claw is a banned substance in competing horses. Currently, the results are very inconclusive, and more research is necessary to give recommendations about their efficacy.

Key points

- Despite the global use of joints supplements, scientific evidence is limited regarding their efficacy on naturally occurring osteoarthritis in horses.
- Currently, it is not possible to come to a conclusion regarding the efficacy of oral joint supplements in horse.

DISCLOSURE

The authors declare that they have no financial conflicts of interest.

REFERENCES

1. National Research Council. Safety of dietary supplements for horses, dogs, and cats. Washington, DC: National Academies Press; 2009.
2. Saastamoinen M, Särkijärvi S, Hyyppä S. Garlic (Allium Sativum) supplementation improves respiratory health but has increased risk of lower hematologic values in horses. Animals (Basel) 2019;9(1):13.
3. Rückert C, Emmerich I, Hertzsch R, et al. Pyrrolizidine alkaloids in commercial feedstuffs for horses. Equine Vet J 2019;51(4):495–9.

4. Durham AE, Frank N, McGowan CM, et al. ECEIM consensus statement on equine metabolic syndrome. J Vet Intern Med 2019;33(2):335–49.

5. Dubey P, Thakur V, Chattopadhyay M. Role of minerals and trace elements in diabetes and insulin resistance. Nutrients 2020;12(6):1–17.

6. Chameroy KA, Frank N, Elliott SB, et al. Effects of a supplement containing chromium and magnesium on morphometric measurements, resting glucose, insulin concentrations and insulin sensitivity in laminitic obese horses. Equine Vet J 2011;43(4):494–9.

7. Vervuert I, Klein S, Coenen M. Short-term effects of a moderate fish oil or soybean oil supplementation on postprandial glucose and insulin responses in healthy horses. Vet J 2010;184(2):162–6.

8. Cartmill JA, Thompson DL, Storer WA, et al. Effect of dexamethasone, feeding time, and insulin infusion on leptin concentrations in stallions. J Anim Sci 2005; 83(8):1875–81.

9. Spears JW, Lloyd KE, Siciliano P, et al. Chromium propionate increases insulin sensitivity in horses following oral and intravenous carbohydrate administration. J Anim Sci 2020;98(4).

10. Winter JC, Liertz S, Merle R, et al. Oral supplementation of magnesium aspartate hydrochloride in horses with Equine Metabolic Syndrome. Pferdeheilkunde 2016; 32(4):372–7.

11. Ringseis R, Keller J, Eder K. Role of carnitine in the regulation of glucose homeostasis and insulin sensitivity: evidence from in vivo and in vitro studies with carnitine supplementation and carnitine deficiency. Eur J Nutr 2012;51(1):1–18.

12. Schmengler U, Ungru J, Boston R, et al. Effects of L-carnitine supplementation on body weight losses and metabolic profile in obese and insulin-resistant ponies during a 14-week body weight reduction programme. Livest Sci 2013;155(2–3): 301–7.

13. Manfredi JM, Stapley ED, Nadeau JA, et al. Investigation of the effects of a dietary supplement on Insulin and Adipokine concentrations in Equine Metabolic Syndrome/Insulin Dysregulation. J Equine Vet Sci 2020;88:102930.

14. Sykes BW, Hewetson M, Hepburn RJ, et al. European College of Equine Internal Medicine consensus statement-equine gastric ulcer syndrome in adult horses. J Vet Intern Med 2015;29(5):1288–99.

15. Lester GD, Smith RL, Robertson ID. Effects of treatment with omeprazole or ranitidine on gastric squamous ulceration in racing Thoroughbreds. J Am Vet Med Assoc 2005;227(10):1636–9.

16. Birkmann K, Junge HK, Maischberger E, et al. Efficacy of omeprazole powder paste or enteric-coated formulation in healing of gastric ulcers in horses. J Vet Intern Med 2014;28(3):925–33.

17. Coenen M, Kienzle E, Vervuert I, et al. Recent German developments in the formulation of energy and nutrient requirements in horses and the resulting feeding recommendations. J Equine Vet Sci 2011;31(5):219–29.

18. Vervuert I, Voigt K, Hollands T, et al. Effect of feeding increasing quantities of starch on glycaemic and insulinaemic responses in healthy horses. Vet J 2009; 182(1):67–72.

19. Clark AK, Rakes AH. Effect of Methionine Hydroxy analog supplementation on dairy cattle hoof growth and composition1, 2. J Dairy Sci 1982;65(8):1493–502.

20. Murray MJ, Grodinsky C. The effects of famotidine, ranitidine and magnesium hydroxide/aluminium hydroxide on gastric fluid pH in adult horses. Equine Vet J 1992;24(11):52–5.

21. Aramaki K, Adachi K, Maeda M, et al. Formulation of bicelles based on Lecithin-Nonionic Surfactant Mixtures. Materials (Basel) 2020;13(14):3066.

22. Damke C, Snyder A, Uhlig A, et al. Impact of diet on 24-hour intragastric pH profile in healthy horses. Berl Munch Tierarztl Wochenschr 2015;128(9–10):345–9.

23. Venner M, Lauffs S, Deegen E. Treatment of gastric lesions in horses with pectin-lecithin complex. Equine Vet J 1999;(29):91–6.

24. Ferrucci F, Zucca E, Croci C, et al. Treatment of gastric ulceration in 10 standardbred racehorses with a pectin-lecithin complex. Vet Rec 2003;152(22):679–81.

25. Murray MJ, Grady TC. The effect of a pectin-lecithin complex on prevention of gastric mucosal lesions in ponies. Equine Vet J 2002;34(2):195–8.

26. Sanz MG, Viljoen A, Saulez MN, et al. Efficacy of a pectin-lecithin complex for treatment and prevention of gastric ulcers in horses. Vet Rec 2014;175(6):147.

27. Grant HW, Palmer KR, Kelly RW, et al. Dietary linoleic acid, gastric acid, and prostaglandin secretion. Gastroenterology 1988;94(4):955–9.

28. Frank N, Andrews FM, Elliott SB, et al. Effects of rice bran oil on plasma lipid concentrations, lipoprotein composition, and glucose dynamics in mares. J Anim Sci 2005;83(11):2509–18.

29. Yang BR, Kallio H. Composition and physiological effects of sea buckthorn (Hippophae) lipids. Trends Food Sci Technol 2002;13(5):160–7.

30. Reese R, Andrews F, Elliott S, et al. The effect of seabuckthorn extract in the treatment and prevention of gastric ulcers in horses. J Vet Intern Med 2008;22(3):815.

31. Huff NK, Auer AD, Garza F, et al. Effect of Sea Buckthorn Berries and Pulp in a liquid emulsion on gastric ulcer scores and gastric juice pH in horses. J Vet Intern Med 2012;26:1186–91.

32. Bonelli F, Busechian S, Meucci V, et al. pHyloGASTRO in the treatment of equine gastric ulcer lesions. J Equine Vet Sci 2016;46:69–72.

33. Munsterman AS, Dias Moreira AS, Marqués FJ. Evaluation of a Chinese herbal supplement on equine squamous gastric disease and gastric fluid pH in mares. J Vet Intern Med 2019;33(5):2280–5.

34. Andrews FM, Camacho-Luna P, Loftin PG, et al. Effect of a pelleted supplement fed during and after omeprazole treatment on nonglandular gastric ulcer scores and gastric juice pH in horses. Equine Vet Educ 2016;28(4):196–202.

35. Kerbyson NC, Knottenbelt DK, Carslake HB, et al. A comparison between Omeprazole and a dietary supplement for the management of squamous gastric ulceration in horses. J Equine Vet Sci 2016;40:94–101.

36. Hellings IR, Larsen S. ImproWin® in the treatment of gastric ulceration of the squamous mucosa in trotting racehorses. Acta Vet Scand 2014;56(1):13.

37. Sykes BW, Sykes KM, Hallowell GD. Efficacy of a combination of a unique Pectin-Lecithin Complex (Apolectol®), Live Yeast and Magnesium Hydroxide in the prevention of EGUS and faecal acidosis in Thoroughbred Racehorses: a randomised, blinded, placebo controlled clinical trial. Equine Vet J 2013;45:13.

38. Woodward MC, Huff NK, Garza F, et al. Effect of pectin, lecithin, and antacid feed supplements (Egusin®) on gastric ulcer scores, gastric fluid pH and blood gas values in horses. BMC Vet Res 2014;10(Suppl 1):S4.

39. Loftin P, Woodward M, Bidot W, et al. Evaluating replacement of supplemental inorganic minerals with zinpro performance minerals on prevention of gastric ulcers in horses. J Vet Intern Med 2012;26(3):737–8.

40. Thirkell J, Hyland R. A preliminary review of equine hoof management and the client–farrier relationship in the United Kingdom. J Equine Vet Sci 2017;59:88–94.

41. Tomlinson DJ, Mülling CH, Fakler TM. Invited review: formation of keratins in the bovine claw: roles of hormones, minerals, and vitamins in functional claw integrity. J Dairy Sci 2004;87(4):797–809.

42. Samata T, Matsuda M. Studies on the amino acid compositions of the equine body hair and the hoof. Nihon Juigaku Zasshi 1988;50(2):333–40.

43. Coenen M, Spitzlei S. Zur Zusammensetzung des Hufhorns in Abhängigkeit von Alter, Rasse und Hufhornqualität. Pferdeheilkunde 1996;12(3):279–83.

44. Ekfalck A. Amino acids in different layers of the matrix of the normal equine hoof. J Vet Med 1990;37(1-10):1–8.

45. Fraser RD, Macrae TP. Molecular structure and mechanical properties of keratins. Symp Soc Exp Biol 1980;34:211–46. Available at: https://pubmed.ncbi.nlm.nih.gov/6166998/.

46. Grosenbaugh DA, Hood DM. Keratin and associated proteins of the equine hoof wall. Am J Vet Res 1992;53(10):1859–63.

47. Kempson SA. Scanning electron microscope observations of hoof horn from horses with brittle feet. Vet Rec 1987;120(24):568–70.

48. Butler KD, Hintz HF. Effect of level of feed intake and gelatin supplementation on growth and quality of hoofs of ponies. J Anim Sci 1977;44(2):257–61.

49. Philipp M, Kienzle E. A double blind placebo controlled field study on the effect of biotin or zinc on the state of poor hoof horn quality. In: Proceedings of the 12th Congress of the European Society of Veterinary and Comparative Nutrition, Vienna, Austria: September 25–27, 2008:45.

50. Higami A. Occurrence of white line disease in performance horses fed on low-zinc and low-copper diets. J Equine Sci 1999;10(1):1–5.

51. Siciliano PD, Culley KD, Engle TE, et al. Effect of trace mineral source (inorganic vs organic) on hoof wall growth rate, hardness and tensile strength. In: Proceedings of the 17th Equine Nutrition and Physiology Symposium. Lexington Kentucky: 2001. p. 143–44.

52. Combs GF, Combs SB. The role of Selenium in nutrition. Orlando (FL): Academic Press; 1986.

53. Coenen M, Landes E, Assmann G. Selenium toxicosis in the horse — case report. J Anim Physiol Anim Nutr (Berl) 1998;80(1-5):153–7.

54. Geyer H. The influence of biotin on horn quality of hooves and claws. In: 10th International Symposium on Lameness in Ruminants. Lucerne, Switzerland. p. 1998:192–99.

55. Fritsche A, Mathis GA, Althaus FR. Pharmakologische Wirkungen von Biotin auf Epidermiszellen. Schweiz Arch Tierheilkd 1991;133(6):277–83.

56. Comben N, Clark RJ, Sutherland DJ. Clinical observations on the response of equine hoof defects to dietary supplementation with biotin. Vet Rec 1984;115(25–26):642–5.

57. Buffa EA, van den Berg SS, Verstraete FJ, et al. Effect of dietary biotin supplement on equine hoof horn growth rate and hardness. Equine Vet J 1992;24(6):472–4.

58. Josseck H, Zenker W, Geyer H. Hoof horn abnormalities in Lipizzaner horses and the effect of dietary biotin on macroscopic aspects of hoof horn quality. Equine Vet J 1995;27(3):175–82.

59. Zenker W, Josseck H, Geyer H. Histological and physical assessment of poor hoof horn quality in Lipizzaner horses and a therapeutic trial with biotin and a placebotherapeutic trial with biotin and a placebo. Equine Vet J 1995;27(3):183–91.

60. Reilly JD, Cottrell DF, Martin RJ, et al. Effect of supplementary dietary biotin on hoof growth and hoof growth rate in ponies: a controlled trial. Equine Vet J 1998;(26):51–7.

61. McIlwraith CW, Frisbie DD, Kawcak CE. The horse as a model of naturally occurring osteoarthritis. Bone Joint Res 2012;1(11):297–309.

62. Murray C, Marshall M, Rathod T, et al. Population prevalence and distribution of ankle pain and symptomatic radiographic ankle osteoarthritis in community dwelling older adults: a systematic review and cross-sectional study. PLoS ONE 2018;13(4):e0193662.

63. Gosh P, Smith M, Wells C. Second-line agents in osteoarthritis. In: Dixon J, Furst D, editors. Second line agents in the treatment of rheumatic diseases. New York: Marcel Dekker; 1992. p. 363–427.

64. Pearson WN, Lindinger MI. Critical review of research evaluating glucosamine-based nutraceuticals for treatment of joint pain and degenerative joint disease in horses. In: Proceedings of the 4th European Equine Nutrition & Health Congress. Netherlands: 2008. p. 81–91.

65. McIlwraith CW. Oral joint supplements in the management of osteoarthritis. In: Geor RJ, Harris PA, Coenen M, editors. Equine applied and clinical nutrition: health, welfare and performance. 2013. p. 549–57.

66. Du J, White N, Eddington ND. The bioavailability and pharmacokinetics of glucosamine hydrochloride and chondroitin sulfate after oral and intravenous single dose administration in the horse. Biopharm Drug Dispos 2004;25:109–16.

67. Laverty S, Sandy JD, Celeste C, et al. Synovial fluid levels and serum pharmacokinetics in a large animal model following treatment with oral glucosamine at clinically relevant doses. Arthritis Rheum 2005;52(1):181–91.

68. Welch CA, Potter GD, Gibbs PG, et al. Plasma concentration of Glucosamine and Chondroitin Sulfate in horses after an oral dose. J Equine Vet Sci 2012; 32(1):60–4.

69. Higler MH, Brommer H, L'Ami JJ, et al. The effects of three-month oral supplementation with a nutraceutical and exercise on the locomotor pattern of aged horses. Equine Vet J 2014;46(5):611–7.

70. Meulyzer M, Vachon P, Beaudry F, et al. Joint inflammation increases glucosamine levels attained in synovial fluid following oral administration of glucosamine hydrochloride. Osteoarthr Cartil 2009;17(2):228–34.

71. Oke S, Aghazadeh-Habashi A, Weese JS, et al. Evaluation of glucosamine levels in commercial equine oral supplements for joints. Equine Vet J 2006;38(1):93–5.

72. Moosavian SP, Arab A, Mehrabani S, et al. The effect of omega-3 and vitamin E on oxidative stress and inflammation: systematic review and meta-analysis of randomized controlled trials. Int J Vitam Nutr Res 2020;90(5–6):553–63.

73. Ross-Jones T, Hess T, Rexford J, et al. Effects of omega-3 long chain polyunsaturated fatty acid supplementation on equine synovial fluid fatty acid composition and Prostaglandin E2. J Equine Vet Sci 2014;34(6):779–83.

74. Haghighatdoost F, Nobakht MGh BF. Effect of conjugated linoleic acid on blood inflammatory markers: a systematic review and meta-analysis on randomized controlled trials. Eur J Clin Nutr 2018;72(8):1071–82.

75. Bradbery AN, Coverdale JA, Vernon KL, et al. Evaluation of conjugated linoleic acid supplementation on markers of joint inflammation and cartilage metabolism in young horses challenged with lipopolysaccharide. J Anim Sci 2018;96(2): 579–90.

76. Hunter KW, Gault RA, Stehouwer JS, et al. Synthesis of cetyl myristoleate and evaluation of its therapeutic efficacy in a murine model of collagen-induced arthritis. Pharmacol Res 2003;47(1):43–7.
77. Singh AP, Singh R, Verma SS, et al. Health benefits of resveratrol: evidence from clinical studies. Med Res Rev 2019;39(5):1851–91.
78. Martin LM, Johnson PJ, Amorim JR, et al. Effects of orally administered Resveratrol on TNF, IL-1β, leukocyte phagocytic activity and oxidative burst function in horses: a prospective, randomized, double-blinded, placebo-controlled study. Int J Mol Sci 2020;21(4):1453.
79. Ememe MU, Mshelia WP, Ayo JO. Ameliorative effects of Resveratrol on oxidative stress biomarkers in horses. J Equine Vet Sci 2015;35(6):518–23.
80. Watts AE, Dabareiner R, Marsh C, et al. A randomized, controlled trial of the effects of resveratrol administration in performance horses with lameness localized to the distal tarsal joints. J Am Vet Med Assoc 2016;249(6):650–9.
81. Lippiello L, Nardo JV, Harlan R, et al. Metabolic effects of avocado/soy unsaponifiables on articular chondrocytes. Evid Based Complement Alternat Med 2008; 5(2):191–7.
82. Simental-Mendía M, Sánchez-García A, Acosta-Olivo CA, et al. Efficacy and safety of avocado-soybean unsaponifiables for the treatment of hip and knee osteoarthritis: a systematic review and meta-analysis of randomized placebo-controlled trials. Int J Rheum Dis 2019;22(9):1607–15.
83. Pearson W, Orth MW, Karrow NA, et al. Anti-inflammatory and chondroprotective effects of nutraceuticals from Sasha's Blend in a cartilage explant model of inflammation. Mol Nutr Food Res 2007;51(8):1020–30.
84. van de Water E, Oosterlinck M, Dumoulin M, et al. The preventive effects of two nutraceuticals on experimentally induced acute synovitis. Equine Vet J 2017;49: 532–8.
85. Murray RC, Walker VA, Tranquille CA, et al. A randomized blinded crossover clinical trial to determine the effect of an oral joint supplement on equine limb kinematics, orthopedic, physiotherapy, and handler evaluation scores. J Equine Vet Sci 2017;50:121–8.
86. Battaglia B, Angelone M, Vera E, et al. Clinical effects of the extract of the seeds of the Indian celery-Apium Graveolens-in horses affected by chronic osteoarthritis. Animals (Basel) 2019;9(8):585.
87. Taintor JS, Wright J, Caldwell F, et al. Efficacy of an extract of Blue-Green Algae in amelioration of lameness caused by degenerative joint disease in the horse. J Equine Vet Sci 2014;34(10):1197–200.
88. Brien S, Lewith GT, McGregor G. Devil's Claw (Harpagophytum procumbens) as a treatment for osteoarthritis: a review of efficacy and safety. J Altern Complement Med 2006;12(10):981–93.
89. Tippler B, Syrovets T, Loew D, et al. Harpagophytum procumbens: Wirkung von Extrakten auf die Eicosanoidbiosynthese in Ionophor A23187-stimuliertem menschlichem Vollblut. In: Loew D, Rietbrock N, editors. Phytopharmaka II, vol. 231. Heidelberg: Steinkopff; 1996. p. 95–100.
90. Axmann S, Hummel K, Nöbauer K, et al. Pharmacokinetics of harpagoside in horses after intragastric administration of a Devil's claw (Harpagophytum procumbens) extract. J Vet Pharmacol Ther 2019;42(1):37–44.

Staying on the Right Side of the Regulatory Authorities

Ruth Bishop[a],*, David A. Dzanis, DVM, PhD[b]

KEYWORDS

- Equine nutrition • Regulatory • Feed safety • Prohibited substances

KEY POINTS

- Regulatory governance of equine nutrition exists to protect the animal, the purchaser, and the companies involved; it also provides for fair competition in the marketplace and in equestrian sport.
- In addition to the feed safety, accurate labeling, and claims regulations that apply to all animal feeds, horse feeds are also regulated by some sectors for controls in relation to prohibited substances in sport.
- Although there may be international agreements on regulatory approach, legislation can be enacted at federal, state or national level; considerable differences can therefore occur in different geographies.

INTRODUCTION

Discussions on nutrition between horse owner and their advisors (eg, veterinarian, trainer, nutritionist, or commercial supplier) on the feeding program for the horses in their care may lead to review, changes, or amendments to the various nutritional inputs in the horse's diet (eg, forage [turnout or conserved forages], prepared feeds, single-ingredient feeds, supplements, or even treats).

At such times, the regulatory compliance of the components of the feeding program is often assumed or assured with a verbal or simple statement and infrequently considered in detail. However, the regulatory responsibilities surrounding the supply of feedstuffs are numerous and complex and vary by country in which the products are being sold. Furthermore, should the horse be destined to compete, additional regulatory requirements apply, beyond those related to placing a product on the market.

In any industry, the role of regulation is to protect individuals, provide for acceptable business practices, and permit fair sporting competition. Each of these principles underpins the regulations impacting on equine nutrition.

[a] Premier Nutrition Ltd, The Levels, Rugeley WS15 1RD, UK; [b] Regulatory Discretion, Inc, 16256 Ravenglen Road, Santa Clarita, CA 91387, USA
* Corresponding author.
E-mail address: ruth.bishop@premiernutrition.co.uk

Vet Clin Equine 37 (2021) 223–244
https://doi.org/10.1016/j.cveq.2020.12.006
0749-0739/21/© 2021 Elsevier Inc. All rights reserved.
vetequine.theclinics.com

This review outlines the principal regulatory frameworks governing the supply of feed products, focusing on the United States and Europe.

The content of this article is applicable to all parties either advising on nutrition or placing products on the market, whether veterinarians, feed and supplement companies, or independent nutritionists, and whether manufacture is in house or contracted to a third party.

Finally, as regulations are continually evolving, some information in this article may become dated; however, principles covered remain "timeless."

Key regulatory perspectives are summarized in **Table 1**.

GOVERNANCE

Companies and individuals operating within equine nutrition operate within the 3 following distinct regulatory frameworks:

- Feed law: designed to ensure that feedstuffs manufactured are safe and fit for purpose
- Laws concerning medicinal products: in respect of the use of ingredients or the presentation of the product such that it may be classed as a medicine or drug rather than a feed
- Sporting integrity: regulations pertaining to antidoping and prohibited substances

Table 2 summarizes some of the different regulatory bodies impacting equine nutrition and sport.

STATUTORY REGULATION OF FEEDS AND SUPPLEMENTS

The classification of a feedstuff varies per geography. Differences are marked between the European Union and the United States.

Feed Regulatory framework in the United States

Overview
In the United States, animal feeds are regulated at 2 levels. At the federal level, "food" is defined within the Federal Food, Drug, and Cosmetic Act (FFDCA) in part as "articles used for food or drink for man or other animals (and)... articles used for components of any such article." As "food" then, the law applies to all animal feeds and feed ingredients in interstate commerce, including products imported into the United States, which are subject to regulation by the Food and Drug Administration (FDA) in the Department of Health and Human Services. The arm within the FDA with principal oversight of animal products (including animal feeds) is the Center for Veterinary Medicine (CVM).

In addition, most individual states have the authority to regulate animal feeds in distribution within their respective jurisdictions and have published their own laws and regulations to enforce provisions to ensure feed safety and proper labeling. The governmental body that regulates animal feeds within a given state varies, but most often it lies within that state's department of agriculture.

Role of Association of American Feed Control Officials
It would be exceedingly difficult for producers of animal feeds to distribute product on a nationwide scale if each state adhered to a wholly different set of rules. Fortunately, many of these state laws are based on the Model Bill as published by the Association of American Feed Control Officials (AAFCO).[1] Although AAFCO is a private

Table 1
Key stakeholders and their responsibilities in relation to regulatory conformance

Stakeholder	Regulatory Governance	Principal Responsibilities
Practicing veterinarian or nutritionist	Feed	• Provision of a safe diet • Use of permitted or otherwise safe and suitable ingredients • Recommended diet supplies nutrients consistent with sound nutritional principles and within regulatory minimum and maximum permitted limits • Recommended diet does not supply ingredients/substances above known safe limits
	Sport	• Products recommended do not cause violation of rules of competition or racing
Brand holder: equine nutrition products (also includes veterinarians marketing their own feeds/supplements)	Feed	• Manufacture and sale of safe feeds for the purpose intended • Product design does not exceed any known safe limits or maximum permitted levels for nutrients/ingredients • Use of permitted or otherwise acceptable ingredients only (as it applies for use in the target geography) • Permitted truthful and non-misleading claims • Complete and accurate labeling in accordance with geographically applicable laws and regulations • Use of assured supply chains
	Sport	• Avoidance of use or contamination with prohibited substances

Person responsible for feeding horses	Sport	• Products fed are fit for the purpose of feeding to horses
		• If competing or racing:
		  ○ Products used are assessed for risk of prohibited substances
		  ○ Stable management practices are designed to minimize the risk of prohibited substances entering a horse

Competitors, trainers, and those responsible for the direct feeding and care of competition and racehorses	Sport	• Considered the "Responsible Person" in the eyes of the sporting regulators • Responsible for ensuring no prohibited substances are present in the horse at the time of competition
Nutrition research scientist	Feed	• Conducts reviews and trials, considers ingredient regulation (eg, authorization status of ingredients, feed safety, research outcome)

Table 2
Overview of regulatory governance impacting equine nutrition and sport

Geographic Scope	Regulatory Area			
	Feedstuffs	Medicines	Competition[a]	Thoroughbred Racing[b]
International	Codex Alimentarius	World Organisation for Animal Health (OIE)	Federation Equestre Internationale	International Federation of Horseracing Authorities
United States	Food and Drug Administration/ state feed control officials	FDA	US Equestrian Federation	Association of Racing Commissioners International (ARCI); State Horse Racing Commissions[c]
United Kingdom	Food Standards Agency Department of Food, Environment, and Rural Affairs (DEFRA)	DEFRA via the Veterinary Medicines Directorate Agency	British Equestrian	British Horse Racing Authority
European Union	European Feed Standards Agency, then per member state food and feed agencies	European Medicines Agency working via national competent authorities	Examples include Ireland: Horse Sport Ireland France: Fédération Française D'equitation Germany: Deutsche Reiterliche Vereinigung	For example, Ireland: Turf Club; France: France Galop Germany: German Racing and Breeding Authority (Direktorium für Vollblutzucht und Rennen)

[a] Refers to Olympic discipline of dressage, show jumping, and 3-day eventing.

[b] Refers specifically to thoroughbred racing; other racing formats may follow similar principles within their own regulatory frameworks.

[c] Regulation of US Horseracing is fragmented with different rules and regulations in different states. However, similarly to the role of AAFCO in relation to feed controls, the ARCI provides Model Rules for racing in the United States as a standard for the independent and impartial regulation of horseracing. In some states, the Model Rules have the force of law as they have been adopted by statutory reference or through regulatory rule making. In other states, they form the basis upon which rules are written. ARCI is not a member of the IFHA, although there are US-based IFHA members, such as the Jockey Club and Breeders Cup International. Federal control is forthcoming however with the signing of the Horseracing Integrity and Safety Act into law in late 2020. With entry into force no later than July 2022, the intent is to bring regulatory uniformity across all US racing jurisdictions, with a particular focus on eliminating the use of performance-enhancing drugs.

organization, its membership is restricted to representatives of state and other governmental agencies whose duty is to regulate animal feed. The mission of AAFCO is to reach a consensus of regulators as to how feeds should be regulated and to provide guidance to the states to help achieve uniform interpretation and enforcement. Thus, the AAFCO Model Bill is not enforceable in and of itself, but when adopted and applied as appropriate by a state's legislature, the result has the power of law in that state.

Status of Supplements in the United States

Equine supplements are "food" under the FFDCA. The Dietary Supplement Health and Education Act (DSHEA, 1994) makes provision for human dietary supplements to allow for ingredients and claims that normally would not be acceptable for foods in conventional form. However, the FDA has determined that DSHEA was not intended by Congress to apply, nor does it apply to animal foods, including supplements. Thus, there is no formal "dietary supplement" regulatory classification for animal substances and products. Rather, under strict interpretation of the law, supplements for animals must wholly conform to the requirements set for feeds at both the federal and the state levels, without exception. Thus, nutritional supplements containing vitamins, minerals, fatty acids, and other recognized nutrients must contain ingredients and bear claims in full accordance with regulations set forth for animal feeds.

A cursory review of equine supplements on the market in the United States today reveals that many do not meet the above burden. Those supplements whose formulations include unapproved feed ingredients are subject to enforcement action as "adulterated foods." Furthermore, those whose labeling bears "drug" claims, including any explicit or implicit indication for use for the treatment, prevention, or other effect on a disease or condition, or an effect on the structure or function of the body beyond accepted nutritional precepts (including performance claims), would be objectionable to regulators as well.

Under the FFDCA, what makes a product a "drug" is determined by intended use (as established by the labeling or elsewhere), not the material composition per se. Therefore, products whose ingredients might suggest it would normally be a "feed," but whose labeling includes drug claims, would be considered a "drug." Furthermore, it could additionally be considered an "adulterated" or "misbranded" drug if that ingredient/intended use has not been expressly approved by FDA as a drug. The regulatory status of a product is determined by CVM on a case-by-case basis, using criteria provided in Guide 1240.3605–Regulating Animal Foods with Drug Claims.[2]

The apparent contradiction between what is on the market and what is permitted by applicable law is a matter of "enforcement discretion." Many of the supplement products that contain unapproved ingredients and/or bear drug claims are labeled to conform to guidance by the National Animal Supplement Council (NASC), a trade organization. The NASC has coined its own category of "dosage-form animal health products." Under its framework, products are formulated and labeled in a manner that roughly mimics that for human dietary supplements under DSHEA, which allows for inclusion of ingredients that normally are not acceptable for use in horse feed (eg, herbs, metabolites) as well as for drug claims that fall into the "structure/function" realm, such as "supports XXXX health" (by nonnutritional means). Claims to treat or prevent disease would not be acceptable under the NASC guidance.

Importantly, there is no formal regulatory construct to allow for the NASC format of labeling. However, notwithstanding this discrepancy, regulators may choose to exercise enforcement discretion, that is, to elect not to take action even though the product does not wholly abide by the law. Membership of NASC requires the company (manufacturer or distributor) to be subject to audits and inspections by the Council and to participate in a mandatory adverse event reporting system. Under those conditions, the CVM is reasonably assured as to the suitability of the product on the market and typically opts to regulate the product as an "unapproved drug of low regulatory priority." Because the product is not labeled as a feed, it often escapes scrutiny by state feed control officials. However, the product still falls under FDA scrutiny, and the CVM can act against any supplement product on the market that it deems to pose a safety issue or whose labeling bears treatment/prevention drug claims or false, misleading, or otherwise unsubstantiated claims. Also, companies and products under the NASC guidance must conform to any requirements set forth by the few states that enforce "animal remedy" laws. Briefly, these state laws require review and registration of animal drug products as a condition of distribution in that state, including those that are not formally approved as a drug by the CVM.

Labeling

At the federal level, animal feed labeling is subject to the regulations set forth in Title 21 of the Code of Federal Regulations Part 501 (21 CFR 501).[3] These regulations establish basic labeling requirements, including the need for a statement of identity (ie, "what it is" in common terms), a net content statement, a complete and accurate ingredient declaration, and the manufacturer's or distributor's name and address. FDA assists in enforcement of the US Customs and Border Protection regulations with respect to country-of-origin declarations, when applicable. The FDA regulations do not address many other aspects of the labeling, such as nutrient content declarations. Also, the FDA does not have expressed regulations covering claims. However, any "drug claim" or unsubstantiated food claim can be subject to enforcement through general "false and misleading" principles as set forth in the FFDCA.

In addition to the AAFCO Model Bill, most states have also adopted the "Model Regulations under the Model Bill" as published by AAFCO. These regulations are intended to complement as well as expand upon the federal regulations. Components of the Model Regulations include the following:

- Product name and brand name, if any
- Purpose statement: Identification of intended species and classes (although not required on the label, a manufacturer must also be prepared to substantiate nutritional suitability for that purpose)
- Guaranteed analysis: Declaration of nutritional content (varies depending on intended species, class, and type of product), declared in a prescribed format
- Ingredient declaration: A complete and accurate list, in descending order of predominance by weight, using the "common or usual names" of the ingredients as defined by AAFCO (or otherwise established through common use when an AAFCO definition does not exist). Under specified circumstances (AAFCO and FDA), "collective terms" (eg, "Grain Products") are permitted to replace the actual ingredient names to allow the manufacturer some flexibility in formulation, provided all substituted ingredients are included in the list for that collective term (wheat, rye, barley, and so forth)
- Directions for use/precautionary statements: As applicable and appropriate depending on the type of product and its ingredients to ensure safe use
- Manufacturer's or distributor's name and address: Regulatory officials must be able to visit the principal place of business unannounced in case of an emergency
- Net content statement: Generally in terms of weight, but can also be in volume for liquid products or count in the case of capsules, tablets, and so forth

An example of an appropriately labeled horse feed label can be found in **Box 1**.

As mentioned, equine "supplements" must conform to both FDA and AAFCO labeling requirements if they are to be subject to regulation as feed. Except for minor provisions (for example, the units used in the guaranteed analysis), the labeling needs to appear just like any other feed. However, those labeled as per NASC guidance have a decidedly different presentation. An example of a label as per NASC guidance appears in **Box 2**.

Safety-related regulations

Under the Food Safety Modernization Act (FSMA), all feeds and feed ingredients must conform to 21 CFR 507, which dictates responsibilities of all animal feed manufacturers and handlers to follow current Good Manufacturing Practices, conduct a hazard analysis (eg, Hazard Analysis and Critical Control Point [HACCP]), and implement risk-based preventive controls. Facilities are subject to inspection by federal and state agencies to confirm compliance with these requirements. Furthermore, under the

---

Box 1
Example of an acceptable equine feed label under the Association of American Feed Control Officials Model Regulations

Your 12% Textured Horse Feed

For maintenance of mature horses
  Guaranteed analysis

Crude protein (min)	12.0%
Crude fat (min)	3.0%
Crude fiber (max)	12.0%
Acid detergent fiber (max)	23%
Neutral detergent fiber (max)	18%
Calcium (min)	1.0%
Calcium (max)	1.5%
Phosphorus (min)	1.0%
Copper (min)	20 ppm
Selenium (min)	0.20 ppm
Zinc (min)	40 ppm
Vitamin A (min)	2000 TU/lb

  Ingredient statement
    Grain products, plant protein products, processed grain by-products, molasses products, roughage products, vitamin A supplement, vitamin D3 supplement, vitamin E supplement, vitamin B12 supplement, riboflavin supplement, folic acid, biotin, thiamine mononitrate, calcium carbonate, salt, dicalcium phosphate, manganous oxide, ferrous sulfate, copper sulfate, magnesium oxide, zinc oxide, ethylenediamine dihydroiodide, cobalt carbonate, potassium chloride, sodium selenite.
  Feeding directions:
    Feed ½ to 1 lb of feed per 100 lb of body weight for the maintenance of mature horses. Feed good-quality hay at the rate of 1 to 2 lb per 100 lb of body weight daily. Provide fresh, clean water at all times.
    Important: Feed hay along with this ration, as per directions.
      Manufactured by:
      YOUR NAME FEEDS
      City, State, Zip
      Net Wt.: 50 lb (22.67 kg)

From AAFCO (2020). Official Publication. Association of American Feed Control Officials, Inc., Champaign, IL; with permission.

Box 2
Example of a "dosage-form animal health product" for horses labeled as per National Animal Supplement Council guidance (courtesy of [4]).

Melanie's Happy Hoof Co.

Healthy Joint Support for Horses
  Product Facts

    Active ingredients per ounce:

Glucosamine HCl (shellfish)	1500 mg
Chondroitin Sulfate (poultry)	800 mg
Proprietary Herbal Blend (Ginger Root, Boswellia, Turmeric)	250 mg
Ascorbic Acid (Vitamin C)	100 mg
Manganese (manganese amino acid complex)	15 mg

  Inactive ingredients:
    Artificial apple flavor, beet molasses, British Horseracing Authority (BHA) and BHT (preservatives), dehydrated alfalfa meal, oat hulls, propionic acid (preservative), and silicon dioxide

  Cautions:
    Safe use in pregnant animals or animals intended for breeding has not been proven.
    If lameness worsens, discontinue use and contact your veterinarian.
    Administer during or after the animal has eaten to reduce incidence of gastrointestinal upset.

  For use in horses only.
  Recommended to support healthy joint function.
  Directions for use:
    Enclosed scoop holds 1 ounce.
    Give 2 scoops morning and night for initial loading dose (3–4 weeks).
    For maintenance, give 1 scoop daily (based on a 1000-lb adult horse).

  Warnings:
    For animal use only.
    Keep out of the reach of children and animals. In case of accidental overdose, contact a health professional immediately.
    This product should not be given to animals intended for human consumption.

  Questions?
    Distributed by: Melanie's Happy Hoof Co, San Angeles, CA 90298
  Call us at 1-800-555-4959 or visit www.melanieshappyhoof.com

Lot #:   *Best before:*

From Dzanis DA (2018). Veterinary Products. In: Pacifici E, Bain S. An Overview of FDA Regulated Products. Academic Press, Cambridge, MA; with permission.

Bioterrorism Act, all facilities that produce or handle feed must be registered with the FDA. Also, under FSMA, importers must give prior notice of any animal feed or feed ingredient before it arrives at the port of entry.

Prohibited Ingredients and Residues

By US law, it is prohibited for an equine feed to contain a poisonous or deleterious substance that may render it injurious to horse or public health. This poisonous or deleterious substance may include chemical, physical, or microbiological hazards. In the case of a substance that may be directly added to a feed (eg, food additive, color additive, or animal drug that has not been approved by FDA for that use), it is deemed "unsafe" by default, and hence, the product containing it is considered to be "adulterated" and subject to enforcement action. Tolerances for residues in the meat, milk, and eggs of animals treated with approved drugs are established in the FDA regulations (21 CFR 556), but this is probably less an issue with horse feeds compared with those intended for carnivorous species. Tolerances for pesticide and herbicide residues in agricultural commodities and processed feeds are set by the Environmental Protection Agency and appear in 40 CFR 180. There may also be action levels set by the FDA in guidance or policy for naturally occurring substances in feed, such as mycotoxins, heavy metals, and PCBs, as well as for microbiological contaminants such as *Salmonella*.

Approval of Ingredients

Under the FFDCA, all ingredients in feed/feed ingredients/supplements must be approved by the FDA as a food additive unless it is generally recognized as safe (GRAS) for its intended use. Products containing a food additive that is not expressly approved and/or whose conditions of use (eg, level, species, purpose) are not consistent with the food additive regulation are adulterated foods under the law and subject to enforcement action, at either the state or the federal level.

The requirements for a food additive and the Food Additive Petition process are laid out by FDA regulation (21 CFR 570 and 571). Briefly, petitioners must provide data on composition, manufacturing processes, and a full assessment of safety and functionality for its intended purpose in feed. The petitioner is usually expected to submit proprietary data, including animal safety trials, for review. The subject of a successful petition is codified in the FDA regulations (21 CFR 573), which includes the name of the substance, any specifications it must meet, and any restrictions on use (eg, species, amounts, type of feed).

The determination of a substance as GRAS, on the other hand, must be based on publicly available information, which is sufficient in the view of qualified experts to be safe when used as intended. GRAS status can be established either through scientific procedures (eg, data in the published literature) or through experience based on common use in food before 1958 (the year the Food Additives Amendment was passed). FDA regulations (21 CFR 582 and 584) provide lists of substances that have been previously determined by the agency to be GRAS for use in animal feed or were subsequently affirmed as GRAS after review of materials submitted by an outside petitioner. These substances include many flavorings, nutrient sources, and technical additives (eg, preservatives, anticaking agents, stabilizers).

In 2010, the CVM moved away from the GRAS affirmation process to allow for GRAS Notifications, wherein a petitioner reaches a conclusion of GRAS for a substance based on its review by qualified experts and informs the agency of its findings. In those cases, the CVM does not directly affirm the substance's status as GRAS, but if the supportive data are found to be adequate, then the CVM provides the submitter with a "no questions" letter. Substances for which there are "no questions" are not codified in FDA regulations, but their status is made publicly known through FDA's Web site and by AAFCO. Legally, a company is not obligated to file a GRAS Notification with the FDA to meet federal requirements, but some states will not accept an independent conclusion of GRAS without this tacit acceptance by FDA.

The FDA recognizes that it is infeasible for the agency to exhaustively list all GRAS substances. By example, the FDA notes that ingredients, such as salt, sugar, and vinegar, are GRAS, although there is no specific regulations codifying them as such. By extension, many equine feedstuffs may be implicitly GRAS, such as hay, oats, apples, and other feeds that have long, safe histories of common use in the United States. In other words, no one had to prove to a government agency that apples are safe for consumption by horses before including it in a commercial feed. Importantly, though, that does not mean that apples are necessarily safe in all circumstances, but rather their inclusion in feed must be in accordance with good manufacturing and feeding practice. Also, the manufacturer must practice due diligence to ensure that the substance is not contaminated with a deleterious substance or otherwise adulterated under the law.

Many equine feed ingredients are also deemed acceptable for use through the AAFCO Feed Ingredient Definition process. This process was originally developed to help ensure consistency in terminology between states. Notwithstanding the requirements as per FFDCA, not all defined ingredients are expressly GRAS or approved food additives, although these substances are generally included in the listing of acceptable ingredients in the AAFCO Official Publication. Rather, establishment of a new or amended AAFCO definition is considered an informal determination of safety and suitability. In an agreement with AAFCO, the CVM reviews data sufficient to support safety and utility before acceptance of the definition by AAFCO. Furthermore, the CVM assists AAFCO in establishing the name, specifications, and any limitations in use of the defined substance. In this way, although not formally approved as a food additive or necessarily GRAS for use in feed, the CVM and states are satisfied as to the ingredient's safety. Thus, they practice enforcement discretion and are not inclined to seek action against products based solely on inclusion of AAFCO-defined ingredients.

Enforcement: United States

There is a great deal of cooperative effort between the CVM and state feed control officials, individually and with AAFCO. For example, in contemplation of an enforcement action, the CVM may provide scientific and regulatory expertise to the state feed control official to facilitate its efforts. On the other hand, the states may have the ability to move faster or more effectively against a violative product compared with the FDA. Many states also have agreements with the FDA to conduct facility inspections and/ or product sampling and analysis on the FDA's behalf as part of a routine surveillance program. As previously stated, the AAFCO is a nongovernmental body, although all members must be regulators. In addition to representatives from each US state and territory, as well as those from countries such as Canada and Costa Rica, the FDA is also a member of the AAFCO. In that capacity, FDA representatives participate and assist in many AAFCO functions.

Most often, regulatory bodies will strive for voluntary compliance as the first step. When a violative product is found by the FDA (either in terms of safety or labeling), it often sends an "untitled letter" informing the company of its findings and asking for a timely remedy. If that request goes unanswered or the response does not sufficiently address the violation, that may be followed by a "warning letter." Letters so titled are indications that the FDA is sufficiently prepared for legal action.

The FDA does not require premarket submission of labels for review and registration of products before interstate distribution. Thus, unlike most states, it lacks the ability to deny product registration as an enforcement tool. Also, the FDA lacks the authority to fine companies for violations of the FFDCA. However, there are other options at its disposal to help ensure compliance. For one, it can initiate a "seizure" against the violative product. A seizure involves the physical detainment of the product and filing of a legal suit against the product rather than the manufacturer or distributor per se (eg, "United States vs 5000 bags of horse feed"). Unless the manufacturer or other owner of the detained product can satisfy the FDA's demands for remedy (eg, relabeling or reconditioning), the product is typically destroyed. Of course, this can have a severe economic impact on the owner. In more egregious cases or when violations continue or recur, the FDA may also seek an injunction against the company, legally barring it from certain practices. Other options include suspension of the manufacturers' food facility registration, refusal of entry for imported goods, and in some cases, criminal prosecution of the principals of the company.

Unlike the FDA, most state feed control officials do have the authority to impose product registration and/or company licensure requirements before distribution in that state. In either case, premarket submission of labels for review is usually required. As such, a quick and effective means of addressing labeling violations includes denial of registration and/or licensing by the state. With that action, unless and until the product is brought into compliance, it may not be entered into distribution. Technically, that action only restricts movement in that state, and the company could still be free to distribute product into other states. However, because states frequently interact between themselves and the CVM on these types of matters, one initial complaint can quickly grow to dozens. Also, on a practical basis, it is usually unfeasible for companies to have different labels for different jurisdictions, or for distributors to effectively prevent product from moving into some but not all states. Thus, if products are intended for nationwide distribution, companies must generally conform to the requirements of the most demanding state.

Product that is denied registration but is found in distribution anyway may be subject to a "stop sale." This state action is essentially the same as a "seizure" action by the FDA. Depending on the state, it may also have authority to file an injunction, impose criminal penalties, or issue fines for noncompliance.

Regulatory Frameworks in the European Union

Overview
In the European Union, feeds are defined as "[a]ny substance or product, including additives, whether processed, partially processed or unprocessed, intended to be used for oral feeding to animals."[5]

Relevant to horses are forages, compound feeds, and straights (eg, grains, single ingredients with or without simple processing). In EU law, compound feeds are classed as either "complete" (capable of supplying the entire ration), or "complementary"/"complementary mineral" feedstuffs (for use in combination with other feeds). Most equine feeds fall into the latter 2 categories. Also, in EU law, there is no specific provision for supplements; these are also classed as complementary or complementary mineral feeds, such that in EU regulatory parlance, the same terms can be used for products offered to horses at feed rates from 10 g per day to more than 10 kg, whereby the horse also receives some forage as a base to the diet.

Under EU law, there is considerable governance on the placing of feed products, including supplements, on the market. These regulations are designed to ensure quality and feed safety in animals that may enter the human food chain. The horse is classed as a food-producing animal under EU law, and so comes under these regulations. The principal EU regulations impacting equine feeds are described in **Table 3**.

It should also be noted that the United Kingdom withdrew from the European Union on February 1, 2020. During a defined transition period that ended on December 31, 2020, EU law in its entirety applied to and in the United Kingdom. After this date, the United Kingdom will develop its own regulatory frameworks, including those for feed, although it is expected that in the short to medium term thereafter, EU frameworks for feed will continue to be applied.

Supplements: European Union
In the European Union, as in the United States, the term "supplement" is not universally recognized as a distinct category of animal feedstuff. In the absence of a regulatory

Table 3	
Principal European Union regulations impacting equine feedstuffs	
Regulation	**Scope**
EU Regulation (European Community [EC]) No. 178/2002, laying down the general principles of food law	Governs food and feed (feed safety in particular) at EU and member state level
Regulation (EC) No. 183/2005 on feed hygiene	Feed hygiene, traceability of feed, registration, and approval of feed establishments. Applies to the whole feed chain
Regulation (EC) 767/2009 on the marketing and use of feed as amended by regulation EU 2017/2279	Rules for placing products on the market in the EU, including labeling and claims
Regulation (EC) 1831/2003 on feed additives for use in animal nutrition	For the authorization and labeling of feed additives (vitamins, preservatives, binders and gelling agents, colorants, antioxidants, stabilizers, trace elements, and enzymes and microorganisms)
Directive 2002/32 on undesirable substances and products	Sets out undesirable substances and limits for their presence in animal feeds
Regulation (EC) 1829/2003 on genetically modified food and feed	Traceability and monitoring of the impact of products consisting of or containing genetically modified organisms (GMOs), and food and feed produced from GMOs
Regulation (EC) 999/2001 concerning transmissible spongiform encephalopathies (TSEs)	Lays down rules for the prevention, control, and eradication of certain TSEs

EU Regulations are applied over all EU member states and are applicable to feed business operators therein and those importing products into the region. A similar overarching regulatory framework is not emulated in the United States, as the regulatory governance models have evolved over 2 centuries and are distributed across many authorities/states.

definition, a reasonable description has been put forward by some nutritionists[6] to mean a feed product that does not form more than 5% of the total ration by weight and tend to be fed in gram per day (and are not items such as carrots, apples, and mints).

Therefore, within the European Union, supplements are considered complementary feedstuffs, alongside other equine nutrition products fed at higher rates, typically kilogram per day.

Specific regulatory obligations: European Union

Feed business operators (FBO) are those who place feeds on the market in the European Union, whether they veterinarian, feed, or supplement manufacturer or brand holder. The principal regulations requiring specific action from the FBO, the person placing a product on the market, are as follows.

European Union Regulation (European Community) 183/2005 on feed hygiene (as amended). This regulation requires FBOs to register or seek approval of their establishments as feed businesses with the local authority Trading Standards department. FBOs are expected to comply with obligations relating to hygiene and traceability and manage feed safety risks based on HACCP principles via a system of written procedures.

European Union Regulation (European Community) 767/2009 on the placing on the market and use of feed (as amended). This regulation lays down rules on the placement on the market and use of feed, for both food-producing animals and non-food-producing animals. It also lays down labeling, packaging, and presentation requirements. The scope covers products intended for sale in store, over the Internet, and through veterinary practices.

Key requirements are as follows:

- Traceability: The traceability of feed is required to be guaranteed at all stages of production, processing, and distribution. FBOs must therefore be capable of identifying any person or organization that has provided them with feed or any substance intended or likely to be incorporated into feed. Feed must also be labeled or identified appropriately in order to facilitate its traceability.
- Accurate labeling and presentation: Labeling has a broad definition that covers more than the information provided on the bag or pot. EU regulation 767/2009 article 3 defines labeling as *"the attribution of any words, particulars, trademarks, brand names, pictorial matter or symbol to a feed on any medium referring to or accompanying such feed, such as packaging, container, notice, label, document, ring, collar, or the internet, including for advertising purposes."*

The regulation also states that labeling and presentation of feed must not mislead the user concerning the intended use or characteristics of the feed.

Mandatory labeling particulars should be clearly legible and indelible. The Regulation requires that the label be written in at least one of the official languages of the Member State or region in which the feed is marketed.

In addition, in the European Union, for distance selling, for example, Internet sales, the following mandatory labeling particulars should be available on the site where product selection and purchase takes place:

- Ingredients: Within EU labeling requirements, feed ingredients are classed as either feed materials or feed additives. The former are listed in the EU Catalogue of Feed Materials (EU Regulation 2017/1017), or for those not listed there, FBOs can voluntarily declare them on the EU Feed Materials Register.[7] Only feed additives listed in the EU Register of Feed Additives can be used in compound feedstuffs placed on the market in the European Union.
- Claims relating to feed must be justified; medicinal claims are not permitted. Medicinal claims are those suggesting a beneficial effect in relation to a disease process or clinical condition. Product claims can be judged medicinal in 2 ways: *"by presentation,"* where expressed indication, recommendation, or implication is given for treating or preventing a disease, or if it gives the averagely well-informed consumer the impression that the product treats or prevents disease; and also *"by function"* if it is endowed with properties for treating or preventing disease or for correcting, modifying, or restoring a function of the body, or if it contains an ingredient that has a significant pharmacologic effect.[8]

Labeling and claims regulations in the European Union are complex in themselves; for the horse, it is further complicated in that equine feed products are classed as for food-producing animals, whereby the principal typologies of claim are different, for example, in terms relevant to "more meat, more milk, more eggs," compared with the typology of equine claims, for example, supports digestive health, supports optimal muscle function, and so forth.

Article 25 EU767/2009 further provides for guidance on claims and labeling via Community Codes of Good Labelling Practice. For equine feeds and supplements, claims guidance is provided by the Fédération Européenne des Fabricants d'Aliments Composés (FEFAC) Comité des organisations professionnelles agricoles-Comité général de la coopération agricole de l'Union européenne / Committee of Professional Agricultural Organisations-General Confederation of Agricultural Co-operatives (COPA COGECA) Federation of European Compound Feed Manufacturers (EU) Code of Good Labelling Practice for Compound Feed for Food Producing Animals.[9] This code details the typology of claims, details labeling requirements, and gives guidance regarding acceptable claims justification. It should be noted that individual countries within the European Union may interpret this guidance differently. An example of a feed label for a complementary feed in the European Union is given in **Box 3**.

These represent the minimum label requirements; further voluntary additions are permitted. Also, if a claim is made for the presence of a particular feed material, then its inclusion in percent must be stated under composition.

Table 4 summarizes actions required by stakeholders to be compliant with the regulatory requirements for feed manufacture and marketing in the European Union and United Kingdom.

Demonstrating compliance

In the European Union, feed assurance schemes help to provide consumers and businesses with confidence that feeds have been produced to particular standards. Such schemes are independently run and externally audited and validated. Many retail customers make certification to an assurance scheme a specification requirement for their suppliers.

Examples of such schemes are GMP+ (www.gmpplus.org), UFAS (Universal Feed Assurance Scheme; www.agindustries.org.uk/sectors/trade-assurance-schemes/ufas-universal-feed-assurance-scheme.html), QS (Quality Scheme for Food; www.q-s.de), OVOCOM (https://www.ovocom.be), and FAMI-QS (www.fami-qs.org).

The primary focus of these schemes is quality and feed safety, based on HACCP principles, and regulatory conformance.

Box 3
Example label for a European Union complementary feed (with no voluntary labeling particulars)

Product Code and Name: *Horse and Pony Pellets*

Complementary feed for horses and ponies

Composition
Wheat feed, oat feed, barley, dried sugar beet pulp molasses, dehulled soya (bean) meal (produced from genetically modified soya), (sugar) cane molasses, calcium carbonate, soya oil (produced from genetically modified soya), sodium chloride, magnesium oxide

Additives (per kg)
Vitamins: vitamin A (3a672a): 10,000 IU; vitamin D3 (3a671): 1500 IU
Trace elements (source in brackets): iodine 5 mg (3b202/calcium iodate anhydrous); copper 30 mg (3b405/copper (II) sulphate pentahydrate 20 mg, and 3b406 copper (II) chelate of amino acids hydrate, 10 mg); manganese 50 mg (3b502/manganese (II) oxide 35 mg, and 3b504 manganese chelate of amino acids hydrate, 15 mg); zinc 100 mg (3b606/zinc oxide); selenium 0.5 mg (3b801/sodium selenite).

Analytical constituents
Crude protein 18%, crude fiber 7.5%, crude fats 5.5%, crude ash 8.0%, sodium 0.4%

Instructions for use
Feed 1kg per 100kg body weight.
Batch Number: XXX, Best before: MM/YY, Net weight: 20 kg
Establishment No.: α GB123456
Company name and address

Table 4
Summary of responsibilities and actions required to achieve European Union feed law compliance in equine nutrition

Regulatory Area and Key Persons Responsible	Examples of Non-compliance	Consequences	Actions Required
Feed safety Feed Business Operator and Brand Holders, for example, feed & supplement companies; veterinarians marketing own feed/supplement products	Not registered as a feed business operator Incorrect additions of ingredients	Potential for litigation Potential for harmful effect on the horse; product recall, reputational damage	Registration with relevant local authority. Documented Supplier QA Program based on HACCP; traceability procedures
Feed safety Feed business operator (manufacturers and brand holders); veterinarian; consulting nutritionist; research scientist	Use of unauthorized ingredients Use of ingredients at levels above safe limits (eg, garlic[10]) Inclusion of nutrients at level above known safe limits (eg, selenium) Ingredient contains undesirable substance at above maximum permitted limit (eg, heavy metals, mycotoxins)	Potential recall, reformulation, relabeling Potential for harmful effect on the horse; product recall, reputational damage; reformulation, relabeling	Knowledge of regulatory limits and safe upper limits; detailed understanding of ingredient provenance
Feed labeling Feed business operator (manufacturers and brand holders)	Misleading claims; illegal claims; ingredients and nutrients labeled incorrectly	Potential recall, relabeling; potential claims, and reputational damage	Knowledge of regulatory requirements for labeling nutrition products
Veterinary law Feed business operator (manufacturers and brand holders)	Medicinal claims made for feed or supplement	Product judged as unlawful medicine; product recall and relabeling	Knowledge of permitted claims for feed, and what constitutes a medicinal claim

REGULATIONS CONCERNING PROHIBITED SUBSTANCES
Introduction

The issue of doping is high profile in equine athletes. One notable example is the Queen's horse, Estimate, disqualified from the 2014 Gold Cup at Royal Ascot because of the presence of morphine in a commercially prepared feed. Another is the disqualification of Clifton Promise and rider, Jock Paget, from Burghley Horse Trials (United Kingdom) in 2013 as a result of reserpine consumed via a calming supplement.

The control of prohibited substances in equestrian sport and racing resides within their specific governing bodies and not at a state or federal level.

Racing

Some governance is achieved on technical aspects of substances and threshold setting via the International Federation of Horseracing Authorities (IFHA).[11] However, rules are enacted at the country or state level. Racing definitions of prohibited substances are broad, generally stating substances capable of acting on various physiologic systems.[11,12]

Equestrian sport

The Federation Equestre Internationale (FEI) provides governance over the Olympics and other sporting disciplines and addresses sporting integrity via its Clean Sport initiative[13] administered according to World Anti-Doping Agency (WADA) principles via the Equine Anti-Doping and Controlled Medicine Program.

The FEI publishes an Equine Prohibited Substances List (EPSL),[14] which is updated annually. This list includes a wide range of substances, including drugs (therapeutic or performance enhancing) and other substances, including those naturally occurring in feedstuffs. The presence or absence of a substance can be checked via a searchable database.

Table 5 provides definitions for the prohibited substances that appear on the FEI EPSL.

Regulatory considerations for feeds and supplements

Sporting regulators may consider feeds and supplements differently in respect to prohibited substances. For example, Article 10.5 of the FEI Equine Anti-Doping and

---

Table 5
Definitions of prohibited substances within the Federation Equestre Internationale Equine Prohibited Substances List

Category	FEI Definition
Banned substance	...no common legitimate use in the competition horse and/or have a high potential for abuse...
Controlled medication	...have therapeutic value and/or to be commonly used in equine medicine, ...have the potential to: (a) affect performance, and/or (b) present a welfare risk to the horse, ...generally prohibited in competition, but may be exceptionally permitted ...
Specified substance (relating to prohibited substances)	...substances that are more likely to have been ingested by horses for a purpose other than the enhancement of sport performance, for example, through a contaminated food substance (not ...considered less important or less dangerous than other prohibited substances)

A key difference between racing and sport definitions of prohibited substances is that in racing they tend to be described by category, whereas in equestrian sport, in following the WADA approach, substances are listed by name.

Controlled Medication Regulations (EADCMRs) differs for feeds and supplements: periods of ineligibility to compete after a doping offense can be eliminated whereby no fault or negligence can be proved by the responsible person with respect to feed but does not apply "where the presence of the Banned Substance/Controlled Medication Substance in a Sample came from a mislabelled or contaminated supplement."[15]

The division between feed and supplements is derived from human sport but is more problematic in the equine sphere, where feeds and supplements manufacture can be carried out in similar facilities, with multiple inputs often using common ingredients sourced from similar supply chains. This situation is further complicated by the nondistinction, in the European Union at least, between feeds and supplements, and the lack of a definition within the FEI on what constitutes as supplement. The resulting legal position therefore is complex.[16]

In racing, several jurisdictions have strict rules governing what can be administered to a horse on race day. In the context of nutrition, for example, the British Horseracing Authority (BHA) (United Kingdom) rules that on race day "[n]o substance may be administered to a horse other than normal feed and water." The use of supplements at that time, even if they are labeled as feedstuffs, has been considered outside of this rule.

Recognizing the need for more flexibility in relation to cases whereby contamination might have occurred, the FEI has amended the EADCMRs from January 2021 to expand the scope of Atypical Findings to include Specified Substances and 2 other contaminants, the beta-agonists ractopamine and zilpaterol via a new Atypical Findings Policy.

This allows for further investigation in the event of postcompetition blood or urine samples containing these substances. A defined process will now allow persons responsible to demonstrate how they consider the substance to have entered the horse beyond their control, the management steps they had taken to prevent such occurrences happening, and to demonstrate how to put forward other mitigating circumstances, such as multiple incidences of the contaminant at a competition. Upon presentation of the evidence, the FEI panel will then review the evidence and decide as to whether the occurrence was in fact an adverse analytical finding subject to tribunal, or whether the explanations are such that it remains classed as an atypical finding, in which case no further action is taken.

This change will likely reduce the number of contamination-related disqualifications in FEI competitions. However, the requirement remains for due diligence on the part of the rider and their support teams to ensure products used are safe and an antidoping risk assessment is conducted before use.

Incidences of Prohibited Substances Related to Equine Nutrition in Equestrian Sport
According to FEI Tribunal Decisions in the period 2016 to 2019, contamination associated with ingestion of feed accounted for 24% of cases. **Fig. 1** shows FEI Tribunal Decisions related to in-feed contamination in this period.

Of the 31 FEI Tribunal reports related to contaminants associated with ingestion in that period, manufactured feed was the largest source (11 cases), followed by forage (9), supplements (6), and other unidentified sources (4 cases).

These reports detected 10 different substances associated with feedstuffs. Most frequently reported across all classes of feedstuff were caffeine and theophylline (6 cases), followed by morphine and its derivative oripavine (6 cases). Scopolamine, theobromine, and harpagoside accounted for 3 cases each.

Seven of the substances were considered "specified substances" by which the FEI accepts that the levels found could have occurred naturally and outside of the rider's

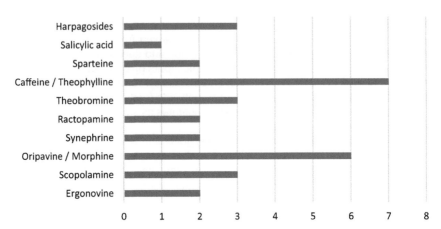

FEI Tribunal decisions 2016-2019 related to in-feed contaminants

Fig. 1. In-feed contaminants related to FEI tribunal decisions 2016 to 2019.

control in the diet of the horse. However, 3 substances (harpagoside, salicylic acid, and ractopamine) did not have this specific acknowledgment of source.

Responsible Persons

The regulations of both racing and competition state that an individual is held responsible for the presence of a prohibited substance in the postrace or competition urine sample. In racing, the trainer is considered the responsible person, whereas in equestrian sport, it is the rider, even if the rider is not directly involved in the daily management of the horse and the yard. Veterinarians, nutritionists, feed/supplement brands/manufacturers, and other advisors may be held liable by the responsible persons for any advice or products given that result in a positive dope test result.

The consequences of a positive test finding are disqualification and loss of prize money, furthermore, in the case of championship events, loss of individual and team medals. Even if the contamination is subsequently proven and the responsible person is cleared of intentional "doping," the consequences remain, although the finding will mitigate against any fines and suspensions incurred.

Sources of Prohibited Substances in Equine Diets

It is incumbent for responsible persons and their support teams to take an active understanding on how prohibited substances might be present in the horse at the time of competition.

The primary routes in are the following:

- Cross-contamination in stable management (either from other horse medication residues or from humans that care for the horses)
- Via the feed, either
  - The prohibited substance is inherent in the material itself (note "herbal" and "natural" ingredients provide no assurance that a product is free from such contamination)

○ Cross-contamination has occurred during processing of the feed ingredients, during storage and transport of feed ingredients, or during manufacture of the feed itself

Natural or Environmental Occurrence of Prohibited Substances

Racing and sport regulators recognize that there can be dietary or environmental sources of prohibited substances, which may occur out with the responsible person's direct control.

Certain prohibited substances, frequently termed naturally occurring prohibited substances (NOPS), are acknowledged to be naturally present within certain ingredients or occur as a result of inadvertent cross-contamination during processing before arriving at a feed manufacturing facility. These NOPS are not to be confused with nonnatural substances added by accident, for example, ractopamine via cross-

Table 6	
Principal naturally occurring prohibited substances in feed and examples of their primary sources	
Naturally Occurring Prohibited Substance	**Example of Primary Source**
Caffeine Theobromine Theophylline	Cacao, coffee, tea. Either naturally present in certain feed ingredients (eg, bakery waste, green tea) or through cross-contamination during processing
Morphine (and other derivatives from the source plant)	Opium poppy (*Papaver somniferum*): through cross-contamination in ingredient processing
Hyoscine/scopolamine Atropine/hyoscyamine	Deadly nightshade (*Atropa belladonna*) Jimson weed (*Datura* spp); usually present as a natural contamination of certain ingredients whereby the source species grow as weeds; can be present as weeds in field margins in certain geographies
Hordenine	Germinating barley
Cannabis: natural cannabinoids, synthetic cannabinoids, and other cannabimimetics	*Cannabis sativa* spp via cross-contamination in ingredient processing; potentially naturally present cannabinoids in hemp products
Lupanine/sparteine	Lupin (*Lupinus luteus*) Scotch (common) broom *Cytisus scoparius*
Bufotenine	Canary grass (*Phalaris* spp), toads, and toadstools
Cathinone/cathine	Khat (*Catha edulis*)
Digitoxin	Foxglove (*Digitalis* spp)
Ephedrine/pseudoephedrine	Ephedra spp
Reserpine	Indian snakeroot, Devils pepper (*Rauwolfia* spp)
Synephrine	Teff hay (*Eragrostis tef*), Orange (*Citrus* spp)
Harpagoside	Devil's claw
Salicylic acid[a]	Willow bark, meadowsweet
Valerenic acid	Valerian (*Valeriana officinalis*)
Yohimbine	Yohimbe tree (*Rauwolfia* spp)

[a] A threshold of 750 µg/mL in urine, or 6.5 µg/mL in plasma applies.

contamination, or furthermore, with substances well recognized as feed ingredients that are administered at high levels for a specific purpose, such as the use of sodium bicarbonate as an alkalizing agent.

Table 6 gives the principal contaminants that can be naturally occurring in feed and examples of their primary sources.

Certain substances on prohibited substances lists may also occur on various feed safety "undesirable substances" lists, but it should be noted that amounts provided for as safe within feed safety regulations do not automatically provide protection from prohibited substances rules since the critical limits, and regulatory enforcement priorities for each, are different.

Management Practices to Reduce the Risk of Prohibited Substances Entering the Horse

Given the varying sources of potential contamination, best practice for the responsible person is to ensure that they or their representatives adopt the following best practices:

- Ensure high standards of stable management to ensure no cross-contamination from other horses receiving medication in feed.
- Respect medication withdrawal times before competition.
- Ensure companies supplying feed are appropriately registered and insured.
- Only use product in proper packaging.
- Check the feed or supplement company has documented procedures for the control of prohibited substances in their products.
- Maintain a feed and supplements logbook to record products used and batch numbers, and if possible, retain a small sample of each batch of product used for a period of at least 3 or ideally 6 months.

Assurance Schemes

Products are sometimes held out by their suppliers to be safe for use in racing and competition; this can be via a statement on the pack or by some form of validation by laboratory analysis of the product for known feed contaminants. However, brand holders should consider both ingredients and their supply chains as risk factors for possible contamination in products destined for competition and racehorses. Robust quality assurance procedures based on risk assessment will help mitigate any identified risks; relying solely on batch testing has a high risk of false negatives without such supply chain scrutiny.

For feed and supplement companies, the BETA NOPS scheme[17] run by the British Equestrian Trade Association offers an externally validated certification to demonstrate they have procedures in place to control the potential incidence of prohibited substances in feeds and supplements. The scheme does not constitute a guarantee but aims to show best practice by companies working to reduce the risk of NOPS occurring in feed and supplements from raw material sourcing through to end-product packing.[17] It should also be noted that the regulators do not operate specific product antidoping approval schemes.

SUMMARY

The regulations relating to feed safety, manufacture, claims, labeling, and sporting rules regarding antidoping are many and complex. Above all, persons or companies manufacturing and/or marketing equine nutrition products or recommending their use have a duty or care to ensure that the products they recommend are safe and legal.

Practitioners operating in equine nutrition should be aware of the various regulatory requirements and how to comply with them; ignorance is no defense in the court of law. These rules and regulations apply to product brand holders, be they veterinarians, feed and supplement companies, or independent nutritionists with their own line of products, whether the manufacture is in house or contracted to a third party.

The subject is detailed and labyrinthine; however, those in doubt should seek expert advice to help maintain the accuracy and integrity of the products and services they offer.

DISCLOSURE

R. Bishop is employed by Premier Nutrition Ltd. Premier Nutrition Ltd manufactures premixes and complementary feeds / supplements for animal feed businesses. Regulatory Discretion, Inc (D.A. Dzanis) offers independent consulting services to the animal feed and related industries on matters relating to US regulation, labeling, and nutrition.

REFERENCES

1. AAFCO (2020). Official publication. Published by Association of American feed Control officials, Inc; 1800 South Oak Street, Champaign, IL. www.AAFCO.org.
2. FDA Guide 1240.3605 – Regulating animal foods with drug claims. Available at: https://www.fda.gov/media/69982/download. Accessed May 29, 2020.
3. US animal feed labelling regulations: electronic code of federal regulations title 21: ;501—animal food labeling. Available at: https://www.ecfr.gov/cgi-bin/text-idx?SID=1a63c813a688c831fcc9893f9e53c4ac&mc=true&node=pt21.6.501&rgn=div5. Accessed May 29, 2020.
4. Dzanis DA. Veterinary products. In: Pacifici E, Bain S, editors. An overview of FDA regulated products. Cambridge (MA): Academic Press; 2018.
5. Regulation(EC) No 178/2002 OF THE EUROPEAN PARLIAMENT AND OF THE COUNCIL of 28 January 2002 laying down the general principles and requirements of food law, establishing the European Food Safety Authority and laying down procedures in matters of food safety. Official Journal of the European Communities (2002) L31;45:1-24.
6. Harris P, Dunnett CE. Nutritional tips for veterinarians. Equine Vet Educ 2018; 30(9):48–496.
7. EU register of feed additives (July 2020). Available at: https://ec.europa.eu/food/sites/food/files/safety/docs/animal-feed-eu-reg-comm_register_feed_additives_1831-03.pdf. Accessed August 5, 2020.
8. UK Veterinary Medicines Directorate Guidance on marketing non-medicinal products.. Available at: https://assets.publishing.service.gov.uk/government/uploads/system/uploads/attachment_data/file/823727/medicinal_words_and_phrases.pdf. Accessed August 8, 2020.
9. FEFAC/COPACOGECA code of good labelling practice for compound feed for food producing animals (2018).. Available at: https://www.fefac.eu/files/86306.pdf. Accessed August 8, 2020.
10. National Research Council. Safety of dietary supplements for horses, dogs, and cats. Washington, DC: The National Academies Press; 2009. https://doi.org/10.17226/12461.
11. IFHA screening limits.. Available at: https://www.ifhaonline.org/Default.asp?section=IABRW&area=1. Accessed July 2, 2020.

12. British Horseracing Authority equine anti-doping rules (valid from 1 September 2020). Available at: http://media.britishhorseracing.com/bha/AntiDoping/rules.pdf. Accessed June 6, 2020.

13. FEI clean sport for horses webpage. Available at: https://inside.fei.org/fei/cleansport/horses. Accessed July 2, 2020.

14. FEI 2020 equine prohibited substances list effective 1 January 2020.. Available at: https://inside.fei.org/sites/default/files/2020%20Prohibited%20Substances%20List_0.pdf. Accessed June 6, 2020.

15. FEI Equine Anti-Doping and Controlled Medication Regulations, 2nd edition (2020).. Available at: https://inside.fei.org/sites/default/files/EADCMRs%20-%20effective%201%20January%202020%20-%20Final%20Version%20for%20Website%20-%20Clean_0.pdf. Accessed June 6, 2020.

16. Pheasant J. Feed, supplements and contamination risks under FEI rules: insight from the Guerdat and Bichsel decisions. Equine Vet J 2016;48(2):135–7.

17. BETA NOPS Code.. Available at: http://www.beta-uk.org/pages/feed-safety/beta-nops-scheme.php. Accessed June 6, 2020.

Printed and bound by CPI Group (UK) Ltd, Croydon, CR0 4YY

03/10/2024

01040484-0006